AF477151

MODERN DISPENSING PHARMACY

Second Edition

MODERN DISPENSING PHARMACY

Second Edition

Dr. N. K. Jain
M. Pharm., Ph.D., LL.M., FIC
Professor
Department of Pharmaceutical Sciences
Dr. H. S. Gour Vishawavidyalaya,
Sagar – 470 003 (MP)

Dr. G. D. Gupta
M. Pharm., Ph.D.
Professor and Director
ASBASJSM College of Pharmacy
BELA (Ropar) - 140 111 (Punjab)

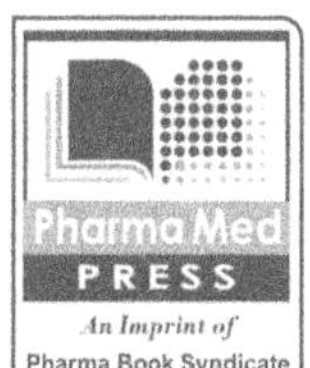

PharmaMed Press
An imprint of Pharma Book Syndicate

A unit of BSP Books Pvt., Ltd.

4-4-309/316, Giriraj Lane,
Sultan Bazar, Hyderabad - 500 095.

Published by

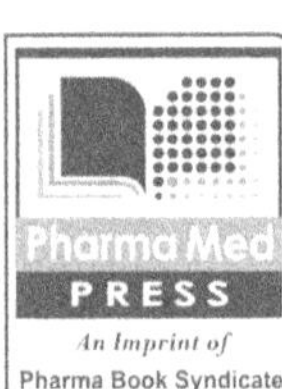

PharmaMed Press

An imprint of Pharma Book Syndicate

A unit of BSP Books Pvt., Ltd.

4-4-309/316, Giriraj Lane, Sultan Bazar, Hyderabad - 500 095.
Phone: 040-23445605, 23445688; Fax: 91+40-23445611
E-mail: info@pharmamedpress.com

ISBN : 978-93-52300-46-4 (HB)

Preface to Second Edition

The authors derive satifaction in presenting the second edition of the book, which has been widely accepted by professional and students as a textbook of various Universities and Institution in India.

The subject chapters has been updated and remove all types of errors. As per the AICTE syllabus, A new important chapter 'Community Pharamcy' has been added.

It is anticipated that this thoroughly revised edition would enjoy even greater popularity and the authors would be happy to receive any suggestion or criticism for further improvement of contents and quality of book.

- Authors

Preface to First Edition

The spectrum of pharmaceutical knowledge has undergone radical changes in the last half century. Newer concepts like bioavailability, pharmacokinetics and biopharmaceutics have emerged as therapeutically significant considerations. The traditional role of a pharmacist as compounder and dispenser of pharmaceutical dosage forms, based mostly on crude drugs, has witnessed a paradigm shift to that of a drug consultant and a member of health care team. Numbers of potent synthetic drugs and their formulations available in the market have largely replaced galenicals, traditional mixtures and similar preparations, which essentially required compounding. Over-the-counter medicines do not need compounding and are formulated with longer shelf-lives. However dispensing of medication remains an art and a most exacting science, which pharmacists are supposed to master. Obviously modern pharmacists have to cope with their changing role and this has been the focal theme in presenting this text on Modern Dispensing Pharmacy.

Precisely, an attempt has been made to inculcate the newer concepts and latest knowledge relevant to a pharmacist as dispenser of medicines that is greatly facilitated with the knowledge of computers and user friendly software. This leads to error free dispensing of complex, potent and toxic drugs, radiopharmaceuticals and biotechnology based drugs. A thorough grinding in forensic pharmacy, pharmaceutical calculations, pharmacology and toxicology etc. are essential for a dispensing pharmacist. To maintain a balance between the traditional and the modern practice of dispensing, this text covers briefly the basic techniques of compounding and introduces the modern concepts in adequate details. Appendices provide useful information relevant to the dispensing pharmacist.

Authors are open to suggestions for further improvement in the subject matter of this book and shall welcome criticism as well as feedback.

- Authors

Contents

Preface to Second Edition.. (v)

Preface to First Edition... (vii)

1. Introduction 1
- Pharmaceutical Profession and Ethics
- Career Scope for Pharmacy Professionals
- Classification of Dosage Forms
- Definitions of Some Dosage Forms
- New Drug Delivery Systems

2. Dispensing Procedure 14
- Prescription Processing
- Sources of Information
- Operational Aspects
- Principle of Size Reduction

3. Containers and Closures 29
- Aim of Packaging and Labelling
- Materials Used for Packaging
- Common Polymers and Their Typical Uses
- Safety Cover
- Closures

4. Pharmaceutical Calculation 39
- Weights & Measures
- Percentage Solution
- Proof Spirit
- Reducing and Enlarging Recipes
- Alligation
- Isotonic Solutions

5. Posology **72**

- Factors Affecting the Dose and Action of Drugs
- Calculation of Dose
- Young's Formula
- Dilling's Formula
- Cowling's Formula
- Fried's Formula
- Bastedo's Formula
- Clark's Formula
- Doses and Uses of Different Drugs

6. Prescription **101**

- Prescription
- Latin Terms Commonly Used in Prescription
- A Model Prescription
- Pricing, Filing and Delivery of the Prescription
- Medication Errors

7. Solid Dosage Forms **124**

- Powders
- General Compounding Methods
- Wrapping of Powders
- Classification of Powders
- Cachets
- Special Powders
- Pills
- Pastilles
- Lozenges

8. Tablets **144**

- Classification of Tablets
- Compounding
- Compressed Tablets
- Wet Granulation

- Dry Granulation
- Direct Compression
- Evaluation Parameters
- Tablet Defects
- Coating and Polishing
- Sugar Coating
- Film Defects
- Compression Coating
- Enteric Coating

9. Capsules 160

- Hard Gelatin Capsules
- Soft Gelatin Capsules

10. Liquid Dosage Forms 166

- Internal Liquid Preparations
- External Liquid Preparations
- Syrups
- Elixirs
- Solutions
- Linctuses
- Lotions
- Liniments
- Throat Paints
- Collodions
- Douches
- Enemas
- Nasal Drops
- Nasal Sprays
- Inhalations
- Gargles
- Mouthwashes

11. Suspension **195**

- Ideal Suspension
- Purpose of Suspension
- Classification of Suspensions
- Dispensing of Suspensions
- Common Suspending Agents in Dispensing Practice
- Marketed Products of Suspension

12. Emulsion **205**

- Emulsion Types
- Differences between *o/w* and *w/o* Emulsions
- Routes of Administration of Emulsions
- Emulsifying agents
- Methods of Preparation of Emulsion
- Evaluation of Emulsions
- Tests for Identification of Emulsion Type
- Instability of Emulsion
- Some Marketed Emulsion Products

13. Semisolid Dosage Forms **220**

- Semisolid Preparations
- Ointments
- Ideal Ointment Base
- Ointment Bases
- Properties of Ointment Bases
- Ophthalmic Ointments
- Rectal Ointments
- General Comments on Compounding Ointment Bases
- Creams
- Jellies
- Pastes
- Poultics
- Plasters

14.   Suppositories **240**

- Advantages of Suppository Medication
- Classification
- Suppository Bases
- Classification of Suppositories Bases
- Preparation of Suppositories
- Displacement Value of Medicaments
- Mould Lubricant

15.   Ophthalmic Preparations **252**

- Isotonic Solutions
- Common Preservatives for Ophthalmic Preparations
- Design of an Aseptic Laboratory
- Ophthalmic Products
- Eye Drops
- Eye Ointments
- Eye Lotions

16.   Parenteral Formulations **266**

- Routes of Administration
- Adjustment of Tonicity and Specific Gravity
- Sterilization
- Aseptic Technique
- Container Materials

17.   Incompatibility **282**

- Physical Incompatibility
- Liquefaction of Solid
- Chemical Incompatibility
- Therapeutic Incompatibility

18.   Community Pharmacy **292**

- Types of Drug Store and Design
- Site Selection
- Layout Design

- Legal Retirements for Establishment of Drug Stores
- Wholesaler of Drugs
- Retail Sale of Drugs
- Storage of Drugs
- Records of Sale of Drugs
- Patient Counseling
- Role of Pharmacist in Health Care and Education
- Important Terms

19. Dispensing of Proprietaries **317**

- Proprietary Medicine
- Bioavailability of Proprietary Preparations
- Nostrums

20. Drug Interaction **323**

- Classification of Drug Interaction
- Modification of intestinal absorption
- Effect on transport system
- Complex formation
- Displacement of drug from storage tissue components
- Modification of drug action at receptor site
- Interaction at adrenergic neuron
- Biotransformation
- Alteration of urinary excretion
- Direct effect on kidney
- Increase or decrease of synthetics

21. Future Trends in Dispensing **330**

Appendix A : 333

Appendix B : 339

Appendix C : 343

Appendix D : 347

Index 351

CHAPTER 1

Introduction

Pharmaceutical Profession and Ethics

Pharmacy is an integral part of the health profession. Occurrence of disease is inevitable and an evil that has to be accepted and fought against. Thus drugs will be used as long as human beings exist. A pharmacist therefore, as one having insight into drugs and their intricacies, will always enjoy a status in the society. Amongst the professions too, pharmacy as a career will be considered as one of the noblest. All occupations cannot be designated as professions. Usually such occupations that serve the more important functions in the society are classified as professions such as pharmaceutical, medical, nursing, teaching etc. A society leans heavily for its development and existence on the quality of its professionals.

A profession not only caters to the requirements of specialized services to the society but is also considered as an embodiment of integrity and ethics. One feels safer in confiding in a professional without any apprehension of humiliation or loss to his reputation. In brief, both the society and an individual regard him as a reliable and trustworthy person. The pharmacist has to reciprocate this faith by superior professional services and conduct. However, a professional too is as much a part of the society as anyone else and if a highly ethical standard of performance is expected of him, the society has to grant him an income that is sufficiently high to keep him free from monetary worries. High standards of services in a materialistic society cannot be based on ideals alone.

Society will have to recognize the necessity of higher income to a professional as compared to a non-professional. One of the motivating factors of a professional is to enjoy respect in society. This can be achieved by service, dedication and sincerity to the patrons. Pharmacists are known to have acquired a stature when the patient trusts their judgment more than anyone including his own.

A pharmacist performs his duties on the basis of his specialized knowledge and its application to his job. The knowledge comprises of his intellectual conception of the pharmaceutical sciences as well as laboratory skills. His recognition is not due to his skills e.g. attractive packaging and labeling but depends upon his intellectual caliber to apply his specialized knowledge. Merely undergoing a formal education and training does not make a professional. Professionalism is an attitude towards work. The income is a reward of his hard work and sense of service and not a calculated objective.

A professional man is characterized by certain values he cherishes in life. He functions ethically and by dint of his conduct wins not only the individuals but makes a mark in the society. A large number of ethically oriented persons in a profession create an impression and exercise an impact on the government. They win recognition not only for them- selves but also for the profession as a whole. Ethics practiced over generations becomes a tradition and a way of life for the new entrant to a profession. Moral involvement eventually generates higher ethical standards, which keep improving and in course of time raise the social acceptability of a profession. Welfare government normally provides legal measures for safe guarding the health of a nation against antisocial and unethical practices. Thus both professional ethics and the law try to regulate and encourage a clean code of conduct, the former voluntarily and the latter by legal provisions. To what extent can law control human behavior is a question difficult to answer but one thing is certain that a code of conduct evolved by the profession has much deeper roots and compliance. Ultimately, in a specific situation, it is the man who applies the law and draws the line of balance as to what extent could a law be stretched. It is the judgment of the individual that finally, keeping in view that all human activities should be governed by the motto-**good to others**.

The relationship between a pharmacist and a patient is not that of a seller and buyer. Its basis is trust and not suspicion. It is difficult to prescribe and standardize the extent of professional services as they are based on personal traits and attitudes of an individual. The desirable qualities even if reduced to writing vary considerably in practice from one pharmacist to another. Such qualities cannot be purchased but inculcated. The patient is an ignorant person and is in a vulnerable position. He should be treated with understanding and sympathy and given all possible advice and assistance even without demanding. A pharmacist is not born with these qualities and acquires them with experience for which there is no short cut. Education followed by a long period of work experience alone enables him to develop professional conscience and ultimately a respectable status.

In countries where the profession of pharmacy is highly developed, professional societies and associations have evolved a code of ethics, which governs pharmacist's behavior to the patient, public, physician, nurse and the fellow pharmacists. The Pharmacy Council of India has also drafted a code of Ethics for pharmacists in India (For details the readers may refer 'A textbook of Forensic Pharmacy' by N.K. Jain, Vallabh Prakashan, New Delhi).

The code of ethics in short, is a framework within which a professional is expected to function and operate for the benefit of the suffering society, respect and abide by law and place service before self. It is expected of him that the society is served with utmost initiative and superior performance both in fields of specialized knowledge as well as human consideration. A pharmacist ought to constantly endeavor to idealize in perfection and hold the safety of the patient paramount.

The spectrum of the scope of activities of a pharmacist is broad and comprehensive. It may range from trade to hospital, dispensing to manufacturing and accountancy to management. The nature of duties and challenges may differ from situation to situation. In the realm of trade whether wholesale or retail, the job may consist of procurement, storage, maintenance of records and accounts, stocking, distribution, window display, sale of drugs over the counter, and compounding and dispensing of medication. These functions may involve knowledge and experience in areas other than those covered during his formal education. Besides, dealing with a large variety of clientele demands understanding of human behavior, attitudes and response in situations, which are not always pleasant. Neither the prestige of one's knowledge and the power of salesmanship nor the extent of his learning and the precision of planning can be substitutes for the originality of approach, keenness of observation and sincerity of purpose. In a nutshell, a successful career in pharmacy warranty the qualities of both head and heart and capability of applying them wherever necessary. These may include scientific knowledge, precision and accuracy, alertness and aesthetic leanings. Salesmanship is a skill and window display an art. The functions of a pharmacist working in a hospital may be considerably different than those who practice trade. It may be dispensing of medication in the out-patient department or compounding in bulk behind the counter. If a manufacturing unit is attached to the hospital, the pharmacist is required to supply both parenteral as well as non-parenteral preparations and exercise control over their quality. Most hospitals maintain their own stores for the supply of drugs and allied materials and it is the job of the pharmacist to indent stores and maintain stocks for proper supply. He may have to create proper storage conditions and sort out and prevent issue of date expired drugs. In larger hospitals, he may have to discharge managerial functions and duties for proper regulation of medicinal agents, drug information centre, as well as sterile supplies.

As a consultant he may have to carry out clinical duties along with the physicians and accompany him during visit to indoor patient wards. He may have to participate in meetings of the policy-making bodies of the hospital. In better-developed hospitals he may have to do patient counselling and maintain their record. The role of a pharmacist in the present and future context has become considerably intricate. The complexity increases each day as the number of drugs and their formulations continue flowing in. The scientific investigations are becoming more and more intensive revealing the hazards of drug safety and drug interaction. Thus from one expected to fill prescriptions, a pharmacist is now recognized as an expert member of the health team.

What does the professional pharmacy cater for? A simple answer would be the 'patient'. Thus, for a well managed system of health services, the entire attitude has to be patient-care oriented, particularly so in hospitals and nursing homes where the total environment and the performance of all professional personnel – the physician, the nurse and the pharmacist has to be directed to the convenience, comfort and care of the sick. Lately, the public is becoming increasingly conscious of restoration of normal health and suffering to minimal extent. 'Why to suffer' and 'how to keep fit' have acquired universal appeal.

The present status of the nature and complexity of drug formulation and anxiety of the sick and his relatives for a speedy recovery and best possible treatment and medication have put very specific demands not only on the knowledge and its application by the pharmacist but also on his mannerism and performance in the presence of those concerned. Today a prescription is the result of a long series of clinical tests and is a very valuable document to the patient and he does not expect it to be handled in a casual, careless and non-challant manner. On the first reading of the prescription, a pharmacist has to say nothing or do anything such as making a remark, pulling a face or shaking his head, which may be indicative of his disapproval of the prescribed drug(s). Such a reaction is likely to create doubt about the competence of the physician and, for all that matters, it may lead to the avoidance of taking the medicine by the patient. In such situations, it is best to refer to the 'drug profile' and ascertain by diplomatic questions the condition to be treated by the prescription *vis a vis* the intention of the prescriber. The drug profile must list chronic diseases e.g. diabetes, hypertension, cardiac irregularities etc., if any. Privacy must be ensured while consulting the patient on such personal matters. A finished prescription must be presented, as far as possible, to the patient himself by the pharmacist in order to avoid any confusion with regard to administration of medication. 'Take as directed' is an ambiguous statement, which may require a lot of elaboration and explanation and hence must not be employed in prescription writing. 'One capsule four times a day ' leaves much to imagination - every six hours, between meals, bed time etc. As a compensation for pharmaceutical services, it is necessary that the public appreciate the importance of service besides the drug being supplied at cost. Inefficient use of drugs has two aspects, lose of drug due to improper use and the imminent danger to the patient. Clinical pharmacy, due to closer involvement of the pharmacist has brought about improved efficiency, safety and reduction in drug cost. Drug interaction is another area in which the advice of the pharmacist has considerably reduced the dangers due to simultaneous administration of several drugs. Patients must be advised by the pharmacists to use medication calendar that helps patient compliance and most effective and safe treatment.

For a satisfactory regulation of professional services the government makes legal provisions, which are amended, as and when necessary. These laws cover essential requirements to be met, in absence of which the services are not expected to be adequately reliable. The prescribed requirements are to be fulfilled by the organization or the individual service provider. Several laws are in force in India at present, which has provision for direct or indirect controls over the pharmaceutical profession; the most important are the Pharmacy Act, 1948 and the Drugs and Cosmetics Act 1940 and the Rules there under. The Pharmacy Act embodies all aspects pertaining to the minimum qualification necessary for practicing the profession and prescribes educational standards and training requirements for a pharmacist. Besides, it incorporates the authorities that will have a statutory control over the profession. The Drugs and Cosmetics Act, in the main, is directed to regulating the import, manufacture, sale and distribution of drugs and cosmetics in India. Under Schedule N, it lays down the requirements for the efficient running of a Pharmacy. The minimum requirements include specifications for the entrance, premises, furniture and apparatus and other general provisions. Schedule X deals exclusively with the drugs designated as prescription drugs. A thorough understanding of all laws pertaining to Pharmacy is essential and those who wish to practice the profession must satisfy all legal aspects. The Narcotic Drugs and Psychotropic Substances Act and Rule 1985 is another important legislation for a pharmacist which has repealed the Opium Act 1857: the Opium Act 1878; the Dangerous Drugs Act, 1930; the Central Opium Rules, 1934; the Dangerous Drugs Rules 1957; and the Central Manufactured Drugs Rules, 1962. The Consumer Protection Act, 1986 is public welfare legislation equally important for pharmacists because the term 'services' under the Act includes 'health services' and hence, by interpretation, pharmaceutical services in a hospital. For detail the readers may refer to 'A Textbook of Forensic Pharmacy' by N.K. Jain, Vallabh Prakashan, New Delhi.

Career Scope for Pharmacy Professionals

From ancient times Pharmacy is known as a branch of healthcare services. Today, the discipline of Pharmacy has made enormous progress in production and research. It has attained independent status as pharmaceutical sciences encompassing all the stages in product development of a drug, from its discovery, identification, purity, development, action, safety, formulation, application, quality control, packaging, storage, marketing, stability studies etc. Thus, today's pharmaceutical professional is a drug expert in a true sense.

In India Pharmacy education is two-tier system after higher secondary passed with PCM or PCB both types of students are eligible for any of the two courses, D. Pharm. (Diploma in Pharmacy) and B. Pharm. (Degree in Pharmacy). All Institutes conducting courses in Pharmacy are regulated by two bodies namely, the All India Council for Technical Education (AICTE) and the Pharmacy Council of India (PCI).

Scope for Diploma Students

- Community Pharmacy (retail shop)
- Wholesale pharmacy
- Pharmacist in Hospital
- Lab Technician in degree teaching institutes
- Higher Education- direct admission to B.Pharm. II yr (Lateral Entry)
- Marketing (Medical representative)
- Production assistant

Scope for Pharmacy Graduates

Graduate pharmacists have opportunities in the field of production, marketing, regulatory affairs as well as academia. Government and Private sectors are open with excellent job opportunities and pay packages.

- **Hospital Pharmacy**

  A Registered Pharmacist can work in hospitals or drug stores. Retail Pharmacy in U.S.A. and Canada is a highly demanded opportunity. This facility is set in many hospitals in the country. This is a key position and the pharmacist plays an important role in dispensing /compounding the prescription, maintaining patient's medical history and all patient profile.

- **Community Pharmacy**

  Pharmacist is a link between production, patient and physician.

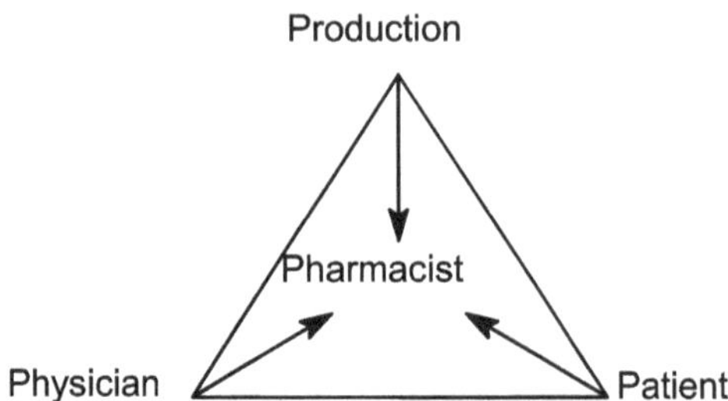

Other responsibilities of Pharmacists :

- Patient counselling regarding the use of the drugs and dosage forms, storage condition, etc.

- Providing detailed drug and product, storage and handling information.

- Detail history of patient and genetic problems

- Maintaining patient records

- Providing self-diagnostic kits for highly sensitive patient for disorders like diabetes, hypertension etc.

- **Academics**

  After 5th pay scale and AICTE rules and regulation, most of Post Graduate candidates are choosing academic field as profession because of job satisfaction, facility for higher education and research, social status and comfort. Promotion scheme in academia is well defined by the regulatory bodies with a definite service length i.e., Lecturer, Sr. Lecturer, Reader, Associate Professor, Professor, Principal/ Director.

- **Higher Education**

  There are many opportunities in higher education M.Pharm in various branches are sanctioned by AICTE in those institutes, which have prescribed facilities for the same. Branches of Master in Pharmacy – Pharmaceutics, Pharmaceutical Chemistry, Pharmacognosy, Pharmacology, Quality Assurance, Regulatory Affairs, Biotechnology etc.

- **Drug Inspector**

  The Central and State Governments are empowered to appoint Drugs Inspectors and to assign them definite areas. Drug Inspectors are deemed to be public servants and are officially sub-ordinate to Licensing Authority. Drug inspectors are important component of drug regulatory activity.

- **Production**

  A pharmacy graduate can work as a production person, chemist, Production Manager, officer, executive, manager, Director, President, Vice-president etc. involved in the production of dosage form and policies, research in different areas. Pharmacy professionals also have opportunities in production of ayurvedic preparations and veterinary products as well as bulk drugs and cosmetics.

- **Research**

  After Graduation a student can opt for M Pharm and PhD courses. Personnel with adequate experience in research are in great demand in the various areas of Pharmacy; Novel Drug delivery system, Quality control, New Drug Discovery Research, Designing of Dosage Form, Process Development (P & D), Contract Research etc.

  Formulation and Development, Biological Products, Clinical Trials and Bioequivalence.

- **Analysis and Testing**

  Excellent quality and purity of drugs /dosage forms are required for human use. Identification and characterization of these are required in production, storage and during the handling of finished product. Quality control and quality assurance have assumed enormous importance in view of current GMP regulations.

- **Marketing**

  Marketing is one of the challenging jobs in the field of Pharmacy because it is different as compared to other business. The Pharmaceutical Sales and Marketing is a highly technical field and offers excellent opportunities for the pharmacy graduates. MBA degree after B. Pharm. enhances job opportunities.

- **Regulatory Affairs**

  Drug Control Administration is the main regulatory body governing and implementing the rules and regulations for the pharmaceutical industry. The job opportunities for Pharmacy graduates are excellent but challenging in this field. In the current scenario pharmacy graduates and postgraduates are in high demand for patent filing and global expansion of drug manufacturing activities.

Journalism

Pharmaceutical journalism has great potential. This requires specialist technical personnel to cover various aspects related to the field of Pharmacy.

- **Consultancy**

  Most of experienced pharmacy professionals are providing consultancy to Industry and also earning a handsome amount in hand and popularity. Consultancy services in Pharmacy are offered in various fields i.e. regulatory affairs, manufacturing, analytical services, documentation, approvals, research, marketing policies, etc.

- **Scope Abroad**

  In the field of Pharmacy, India is one the countries producing many Pharmacy Graduates. Many countries have demand for qualified Pharmacy professionals including U.S.A., Canada, European Countries like U.K., France, Germany, African Countries like S.

Africa, Nigeria, Yemen, Gulf Countries like Saudi Arabia, Kuwait, South East Asian Countries like Singapore, Korea, Japan, etc. and the Australian continent including New Zealand. A registered pharmacist commands very high salary and repute in developed countries including USA and UK.

Pharmacy Graduates have are placement opportunities in Higher Education, Druggist and Chemist, Councilor, Retailer, Pharmacist, Manufacturing and Clinical Pharmacy

Classification of Dosage form

A pharmacist is required to dispense a wide range of preparations. Some of them may require compounding and others dispensed in manufacturer's package or packed by the pharmacist according to the quantity required. However it is desirable that a pharmacist is familiar with all varieties of preparations that he handles. A classification of preparations along with a brief description is given. Preparations that may require compounding are underlined.

Table 1.1 Classification of Dosage forms.

Dosage Form					
Solid	**Semisolid**	**Liquid**	**Sterile Products**	**Gas**	**Miscellaneous**
Internal	**Internal**	**Internal**	Injection	Aerosols	Novel Drug
• Powders	• Gels	• Solution	Infusion	Inhalations	Delivery System
• Tablets	• Jellies	• Suspension	Ophthalmic	Insufflations	
• Capsules	**External**	• Emulsion	Drops	Sprays	
• Cachets	• Ointments	• Elixirs			
• Tablet	• Creams	• Syrups			
triturate	• Pastes	• Collodions			
• Pills	• Gels	• Spirits			
• Lozenges	• Jellies	• Mixtures			
• Pastilles	• Suppositories	• Draughts			
External	• Pessaries	**External**			
• Dusting	• Applications	• Irrigations			
Powders	• Poultices	• Lotions			
	• Paints	• Liniments			
		• Mouth washes			
		• Nasal drops			
		• Ear drops			
		• Enemas			
		• Inhalations			
		• Irrigations			
		• Paints			
		• Sprays			
		• Applications			

Definitions of Some dosage Forms

Aerosols : Aerosols are suspensions of fine, solid or liquid particles in a gas. This preparation is also known as pressurized preparation. These are dosage forms for spraying in a solution, suspension or emulsion form with an atomizer device or nebulisers. Aerosols are packed in pressurized containers with suitable propellants that provide a steady stream of the liquid. They are most popular in the treatment of asthma or respiratory tract infection and skin conditions.

Applications : These are fluid or semi-fluid preparations intended for application to the skin. These formulations are generally in the form of emulsion and suspension. Some official examples are used as antiparasites and also in other skin diseases.

Cachets : Cachets are disc or cylinder shaped devices made from rice paper and consist of a lower and upper part, the latter having a slightly broader flange. Medication of disagreeable taste is enclosed between the two halves and sealed.

Capsules : These are similar to cylindrical cachets and are available in different sizes. The material is however gelatin, hard or flexible (hard or soft gelatin capsules).

Collodians : Fluid preparations for external use in the form of collodians contain susbstances dissolved in a volatile solvent which, after evaporation, leaves a thin film of the material on the surface.

Creams : Highly viscous oil-in-water or water-in-oil emulsions meant for external application are considered as creams. Medicament may also be incorporated in them.

Draughts : Liquid oral preparations packed as a single dose in separate containers and in large volumes are known as draught.

Dusting Powders : This form of medication comprises of extremely fine particles to be dusted on the affected part.

Elixirs : These are sweetened, clear and coloured, aromatic, hydroalcoholic liquids.

Emulsions : Emulsions are mixtures of two immiscible liquids in which one phase is dispersed into the other in the form of minute globules. An emulsifying agent is employed to bring about emulsfication. Usually unpalatable oils may be conveniently administered as emulsions dispersed in water.

Ear drops : Solutions of drugs meant for dropping in the ears are classified as ear drops.

Enemas : Drugs in solution or in dispersed form meant for rectal administration are called enemas.

Gargles : Aqueous solutions employed for local action in the throat are called gargles. They may be diluted with luke-warm water before use.

Gels : Insoluble substances presented as suspension of their colloidal state in a hydrated form are known as gels.

Granules : These are free flowing, dry conglomerates of particles ranging from 1 to 5 mm in diameter. The medicament and the excipients are rendered to a cohesive mass with a suitable moistening agent and the mass is pressed through a sieve of required granule size and dried.

Inhalations : Inhalations are the preparations meant for relieving congestion of the throat. These preparations are either volatile and inhaled directly, or contain volatile substances which can be inhaled by adding the preparation to hot water.

Insufflations : Insufflations, commonly known as snuffs also, provide a medicament intimately mixed with a dusting powder to be deeply inhaled or blown into body cavities by an insufflator.

Irrigations : These preparations are used as antiseptics for washing the urinary bladder or vagina, the solution being introduced through a soft tube.

Jellies : Jellies are non-greasy semi-solid preparations containing a high proportion of gelatin, gum or starch.

Lozenges : The medicament, sugar and gum are made into a solid form for local action and slow release of the drug meant for the mouth and the throat.

Liniments : Emulsions, viscous, oily or free flowing solutions of drug in alcohol meant for application to the skin usually by rubbing are called liniments.

Lotions : These are preparations in solution or suspension form to be applied to the affected part without friction. The lotions may be applied as such or with the support of a dressing material.

Mixtures : Solutions and suspensions meant for oral use are classified as mixtures. The vehicle is usually water and their stability is limited from a few days upto a few weeks.

Mouth washes : Mouth washes are liquid preparations for treating mouth infections or providing a freshening feeling. They are usually diluted before use.

Nasal Drops : Solution of drugs meant for instilling in the nasal cavity with the aid of a dropper are considered as nasal drop.

Ointments : These are semi-solids meant for external use. The medicament is incorporated in the base usually comprising of greasy substances.

Pastilles : The drug along with gelatin and glycerin is converted into a solid form for slow dissolution in the mouth.

Pills : Pills are spherical dosage forms containing the drug and excipients. Pills have now been almost completely replaced by capsules and tablets. As dosage form pills are very popular in Ayurvedic medicine and are known as *vati.*

Powders : The medicament with or without excipient in fine state of subdivision is supplied in either bulk or individually wrapped in a paper.

Pessaries : The medicament is either compressed in a suitable shape or moulded with the help of a base so that it is released when inserted into vagina by solution or melting.

Pastes : Pastes contain a very high proportion of the solid medicament in relatively small proportion of the base, meant for external application.

Poultices : These are thick and pasty preparations. Due to good heat retention property, they may be applied on a dressing while hot and bandaged on to the affected part to relieve inflammation.

Paints : Solutions in viscous vehicles or suspensions that are meant to be applied to the skin or mucus with a soft device such as brush or cotton are called paints.

Solution Tablets : These are tablets designed to dissolve quickly in water. After dissolution, the solution can be applied to the skin or mucous.

Syrups : These are concentrated solutions of sucrose or any other sugars. Syrups are less commonly prescribed as such except cough syrups but are very often prescribed as sweetening and flavouring vehicles.

Sprays : Drugs dissolved in alcoholic or glycerin media and sprayed in the form of fine droplets to the mucous with the help of a spraying device are called sprays.

Suppositories : These are semi-solid to solid moulded preparations meant for insertion into the rectum. They resemble pessaries which are meant for vagina. The medication is incorporated in a suitable base that liquefies at the body temperature and releases the medicament. Some of the bases may dissolve in the rectum and release the medicament.

Tablets : These are solid dosage forms in which the medicament is compressed in different shapes and sizes. They may be plain or coated. Tablets remain the most popular dosage form.

New Drug Delivery Systems

The current approach is on the improvement of therapeutic effectiveness of known drugs and exploring their lesser-known pharmacological actions. Simultaneously the formulation pharmacists all over the world are also engaged in research leading to the discovery of newer drug delivery systems. Sustained action dosage forms are just one of the examples. In conventional drug delivery systems only a fraction of the administered dose reaches the blood circulation and hence most of the dose is wasted and causes undesirable side effects and toxicity. Even when the drug reaches blood circulation, the action may be desired in only a specific organ or at a specific site. Newer drug delivery systems are aimed at maximizing the drug effectiveness and reduce the side effects. Newer drug delivery systems are now available which would deliver the drug for selective action only on cancer cells leaving other cells and organs unaffected. As these drug delivery systems affect only the target organ, site or receptor, they are also called targeted drug delivery systems or 'magic bullet'. Although a number of new drug delivery systems have been introduced in the market, the following discussion is restricted to the most popular types:

Liposomes

Liposomes are artificial microscopic bilayer vesicles or sacs made of phospholipids and enclosing an aqueous compartment. They resemble cell membranes in structure and composition. Drugs incorporated in liposomes and administered into the body can be delivered at the desired site, in desired concentrations, without being toxic. Several products are available in the market including doxorubicin; amphotericin B, gentamycin and daunorubicin.

Microspheres

These are small, solid particulate carriers containing dispersed drug particles either in solution or crystalline form. Microcapsules are made from natural and synthetic polymers and administered by injection or nasal route. Magnetic microspheres have great potential in the localized tumour treatment. Drugs that can be enclosed in microcapsules include mitomyein C, 5-flurouracil, adriamycin, cisplation, enzymes and proteins.

Resealed Erythrocytes

These are the erythrocytes in which the pores (200-500 Å diameter) are created within the cell membrane, drug is allowed to enter the cell through these pores and finally pores are closed causing the erythrocytes to 'reseal';. This system can be used to attain targeted delivery of drugs to the liver or spleen mainly in the treatment of lysosomal storage diseases and metal toxicity.

Nanoparticles

Nanoparticles are colloidal particulate systems in the submicron size range acting as carriers of drug molecules. Their size varies from 10 to 1000 nanometers. These carriers are solid spheres and their surface is amorphous and lipophilic with a negative charge. Magnetic nanoparticles can be used to enhance site specificity. As a drug delivery system they enhance the therapeutic efficacy of the drug and minimize adverse effects and toxic reactions. Major applications include treatment of infections of the reticuloendothelial system (RES), enzyme replacement therapy in the liver, treatment of cancer, and vaccination.

Monoclonal Antibodies

Monoclonal antibodies are artificially produced proteins, which exhibit specificity for one single antigen. The inherent specificity of the monoclonal antibodies provides the rationale for their use in drug targeting for therapeutic applications. The major therapeutic applications of monoclonal antibodies as drug delivery systems would be in cancer treatment.

Microcapsules

Microencapsulation is the process of applying relatively thin, reproducible coatings to small particles of solids or droplets of liquids and dispersions. The process can be adapted to a wide variety of dosage forms and product applications. It provides a means for converting liquids to solids, altering colloidal and surface characteristics, or providing environmental protection, and of controlling the release characteristics of coated materials. Commercial products based on microcapsules include leuprolide acetate for prostrate cancer, doxycycline and aspirin. Microcapsules are most popular in the development of sustained release dosage forms.

Osmotic pumps

Osmotic pumps exploit the tendency of a fluid to equalize the concentration of substances on both sides of a semi-permeable membrane. The system can be designed to deliver different drugs at different rates. Marketed products include Acuteim and Acusystem C to release phenylpropanolamine and vitamin C, respectively.

Ion exchange resin systems

This system involves preparation of drug charged resin and its drying to form beads. In the GI tract the drug molecule is exchanged for an appropriately charged ion and hence the drug is released at controlled rates. The major ion exchange system commercialized todate is the Pennkinetic System, which has been used to deliver a variety of antitussive agents.

Transdermal drug delivery systems

These are laminated patches which adhere to the skin and permit absorption of drugs from the skin surface through its layers into the general blood circulation, at controlled rates, resulting in sustained blood levels. Important products in the market include Transderm-Scop, Nitro-Dur, Nitrodisc for delivery of nitroglycerin; and Catapress-TTS for delivery of clonidine.

Implants

Implants are sterile polymeric devices of varied shapes containing one or more medicaments for introduction into body tissues. They release the drug in a controlled manner for prolonged time extending to several months. They must be surgically implanted, subcutaneously or intramuscularly. The major areas of application of implants include contraception, diabetes, cancer, cardiovascular diseases and brain diseases. Marketed systems include Progestasert, Norplant, Today™, Vaginal Ring and Dual Release Ring for contraception, the Lacrisert for artificial tear therapy, the Alzet Osmotic Pumps for various drugs, and the Occusert for glaucoma.

Nasal drug delivery systems

Conventional nasal formulations in the form of spray and drops have used delivery systems like the rhinyle catheters, single dose pipettes, metered dose spray pumps (non-pressurized) and metered aerosol valve devices. Out of these the spray pumps and the aerosol valve orifices lend themselves to controlled delivery of nasal formulations. Both systems are simple to use and provide multiple dosing facility. They also provide ease of administration, rapid absorption and onset of action, and bypass of presynaptic clearance. Marketed products include calcitonin for metabolic bone diseases and desmopressin acetate for primary noctural enuresis.

Intrauterine devices

Intrauterine device (IUD) is the device inserted in the uterus and is a popular method of contraception. The Tatum-T (T-shaped, commonly known as Copper T) and the Cu-7 (7 shaped) are examples of devices containing contraceptive metal, made of polypropylene with copper wire wrapped around the vertical limb. Copper acts as the contraceptive agent and a single IUD is effective for up to 40 months. The Progestasert is a commercially available hormone-releasing device. In this device progesterone (contraceptive hormone) is dispersed with barium sulphate in silicone oil within an ethylene/vinyl acetate copolymer membrane. The device releases progesterone at a constant rate of 65 µg per day for a year. Tatum-T is marketed by Searle and Progestasert by Alza Corporation.

CHAPTER 2

Dispensing Procedures

In India only registered pharmacists are authorized to dispense, sell, or compound a drug or supervise the part of a Pharmacy where drugs are kept. Dispensing includes the selection, preparation, and transfer of one or more doses of a drug to a patient. The process of dispensing mainly comprises of the following components.

1. Technical Component
   - receiving and reading the prescription,
   - adjusting an order according to approved policy,
   - entry of order,
   - selecting the drug or determining the product to dispense,
   - checking the expiry date,
   - reconstituting a product as per the requirement,
   - labeling a product,
   - final physical check for accuracy of finished product,
   - maintaining but not interpreting medication profiles, and
   - maintaining, preparing and operating equipment.

2. Cognitive Component
   - assessing the therapeutic appropriateness of a prescription,
   - making a recommendation to a prescriber, and
   - developing the formula for a drug that needs to be specifically prepared by a pharmacist;

Following activities do not constitute dispensing: (a) administration of medications, (b) repackaging of medications, (c) supplying medications.

Prescription Processing

Following precautions are essential during the processing of a prescription

    (a) Collect important information relating to the patient.

    (b) Carefully scrutinize the prescription for quantity and dose, therapeutic use and incompatibilities of ingredients.

    (c) Dispensed prescriptions should be compared with their originals for accuracy.

    (d) Check label of large quantity container.

    (e) Properly affix labels on container having necessary information.

    (f) Another pharmacist should finally check filled prescriptions.

    (g) Following information should be clearly recorded on all new prescriptions:
- Name of patient
- Age of patient
- Weight of patient
- Type of disease
- Any allergic reaction
- Identification of agent acting on behalf of patient.
- Contact person on delivered prescriptions

Prescription records of Schedule X drugs and Narcotic Drugs and Psychotropic Substances must be maintained.

Important Instruction while working in the dispensing laboratory

    (a) Laboratory should be neat and clean.

    (b) All chemicals and other articles should be in proper place.

    (c) Electric points, washing and weighing area and working table should be arranged properly to reduce the risk of mistakes, errors and contamination.

    (d) Protect the clothes and reduce contamination of dispensed product using neat and clean white overcoat (apron), gloves, napkin etc.

    (e) Before dispensing, read the prescription carefully. In case of any doubt in understanding clarify the confusion with the prescriber.

    (f) For formula and quantity consult Pharmacopoeia or other reference book (do not apply any trial and error method or approximate quantity).

    (g) Following things are also checked – dose, number of doses prescribed, incompatibility.

    (h) Check the calculation of different ingredients used in prescription.

(i)   Selection of containers for dispensing.

(j)   Weighing, mixing, and other steps performed as per the process.

(k)   Label should have all information regarding product, instruction for use and storage.

(l)   Paste the label on the container properly.

(m) Wrap the container according to suitability of transportation.

(n)   Check the finished product before delivery to the patient or consumer.

(o)   Ensure that the patient or his representative has followed the instructions regarding mode of administration and storage of the prescription.

(p)   Maintain the record of the prescription having all basic requirements.

Sources of Information

The pharmacist should rely on following sources of information.

1. Official books

- Indian Pharmacopoeia [IP]
- United States Pharmacopoeia [USP]
- Extra Pharmacopoeia [Martindale]
- British Pharmacopoeia [BP]
- British Pharmaceutical Codex [BPC]
- European Pharmacopoeia [EP]
- International Pharmacopoeia

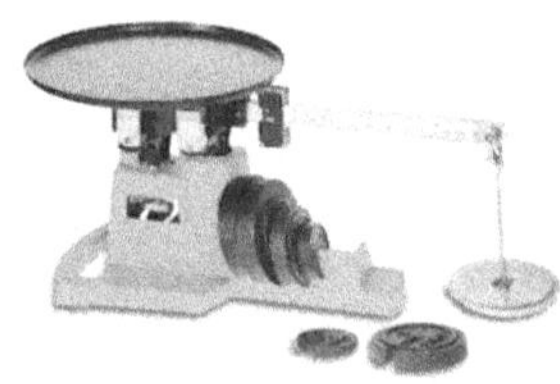

Mechanical Beam Balance

2. Reference books

- Remington's Pharmaceutical Sciences
- Pharmaceutical Handbooks
- National Formulary of India
- Drug Today
- Monthly Index of Medical Specialties [MIMS]
- Current Index of Medical Specialties [CIMS]
- Physician Desk Reference [PDR]
- Indian Drug Review [IDR]
- Indian Pharmaceutical Guide [IGP]

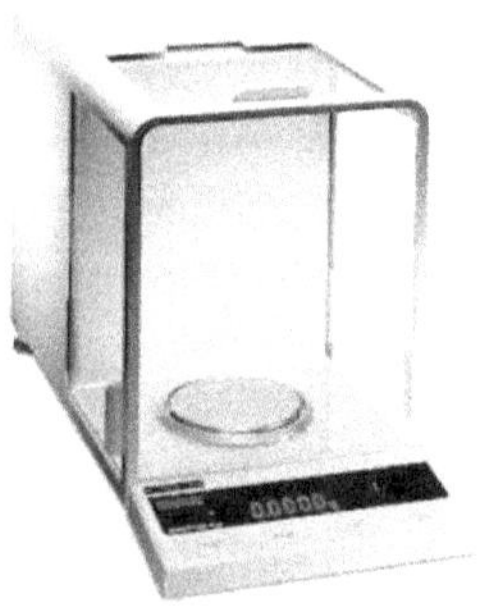

Analytical Balance

3. JOURNALS

Name of Journal	Frequency of publication	Address
Bhartiya Vegyanic Avam Audhyogik Anusandhan Patrika	Half Yearly	The Sales and Distribution officer, NISCAIR, CSIR, Dr. K. S. Krishna Marg, New Delhi – 12
CSIR News	Bimonthly	The Sales and Distribution officer, NISCAIR, CSIR, Dr. K. S. Krishna Marg, New Delhi – 12
Current Literature of Science	Bimonthly	The Sales and Distribution officer, NISCAIR, CSIR, Dr. K. S. Krishna Marg, New Delhi – 12
Drugs and Pharmaceutical Industry Highlight	Weekly	Scientist-in-Incharge, Central Drug Research Institute, Chattar Manzil Palace, Lucknow-226 001
IDMA, Bulletin	Weekly	Indian Drug Manufacturer's Association 102-B, A-Wing, Poonam Chambers Dr. A.B.Road, Worli, Mumbai-400 018
Indian Drugs	Monthly	The Editor, Indian Drugs Indian Drug Manufacturers Association, 102-B, Poonam Chambers, Dr. A.B.Road, Worli, Mumbai – 400 018 publications@idmaindia.com
Indian Journal of Chemical Technology	Bimonthly	The Sales and Distribution officer, NISCAIR, CSIR, Dr. K. S. Krishna Marg, New Delhi – 12
Indian Journal of Biotechnology	Quarterly	The Sales and Distribution officer, NISCAIR, CSIR, Dr. K. S. Krishna Marg, New Delhi – 12
Indian Journal of Chemistry Section B	Monthly	The Sales and Distribution officer, NISCAIR, CSIR, Dr. K. S. Krishna Marg, New Delhi – 12
Indian Journal of Pharmaceutical Education & Research	Quarterly	The Editor, Indian Journal of Pharmaceutical Education & Research, J.S.S. College of Phramcy, S.S.Nagar, Mysore – 570 015 (Karnataka) ijpeindia@lycos.com www.ijpe.org
Indian Journal of Pharmaceutical Sciences	Bimonthly	The Editor, Indian Journal of Pharmaceutical Sciences Kalina, Sanatacruz, (E), Mumbai – 400 098 ijps 2002@rediffmail.com www.Indianpharma.org
Indian Journal of Pharmacology	Monthly	Publishers (Medknow Publications 12 Manisha Plaza, MN ROAD, Kurla (W) Mumbai- 400 070 [ijp@jipmer.edu, subscription@medknow.com]

Contd….

Name of Journal	Frequency of publication	Address
Indian Journal of Physiology and Pharmacology	Monthly	The Editor, Department of Physiology, All India Institute of Medical Sciences,Ansari Nagar, **New Delhi**-110 029
Indian Journal of Traditional Knowledge	Quarterly	The Sales and Distribution officer, NISCAIR, CSIR, Dr. K. S. Krishna Marg, New Delhi – 12
Journal of Scientific and Industrial Research	Monthly	The Sales and Distribution officer, NISCAIR, CSIR, Dr. K. S. Krishna Marg, New Delhi –12
Indian Journal of Natural Products	Quarterly	The Editor, Deptt. of Pharamcy, Dr. H. S. Gaur University, Sagar- 470 003 (MP)
Pharma Pulse	Weekly	The Editor, Indian Express Newspapers (Bombay), Ltd. First Floor, Express Towers, Nariman Point Mumbai – 021 Bpdsubscriptions@expressindia.com
Pharmabiz	Weekly	The Editor, iPharma India Pvt. Ltd. Rajmahal, 4th Floor, 84, Veer – Nariman Road, Church Gate, Mumbai – 400 020 (Mah)
Pharma Times	Monthly	The Editor, Pharma Times Indian Pharmaceutical Association, Kalina, Santacruz (E) Mumbai – 400 089
Probe	Quarterly	The Editor, Dr. S.K.Mitra, Probe, The Himalaya Drug Company, Makali, Banglore – 562 123
The Indian Journal of Hospital Pharmacy	Bimonthly	The Editor, The Indian Journal of Hospital Pharamcy, R-566, New Rajinder Nagar, New Delhi – 110 060
The Indian Pharmacist	Monthly	The Circulation Manager The Indian Pharmacist, Bazaz Publications 507, Ashok Bhawan, 93, Nehru Place, New Delhi – 110 019 subscription@indianpharmacist.com
The Pharma Review	Bimonthly	The Editor, The Pharma Review, Kongposh Publications Pvt. Ltd. C-19 Commercial Complex, SDA, New Delhi fpc@vsnl.com website: www.kbpub.com
Drug One	Monthly	The Editor SCO-252, Basement, Sector-44-C, Chandigrah-160047 (India)

4. Internet

In 21st centaury, Internet is one of the easiest and quickest method for collection of the literature and latest information; news, discoveries and other scientific development in the field of pharmaceutical sciences. Some important Pharma-websites are listed below.

Website	Information
www.apti.org	Association of Pharmaceutical Teachers of India
www.aicte.ernet.in	All India council for Technical Education, New Delhi
www.pharmweb.net	Pharmacy Information
www.who.ch	World Health Organization
www.aaps.org	American association of Pharmaceutical Sciences
www.nih.gov	National Institute of Health, Bethesda
www.nlm.nih.gov	National Library of medicine
www.acs.org	American Chemical Society
www.pharminfo.com	Pharm. Infonet
www.chemport.org	Chemical Abstracts and Chemistry Journals
www.biomednet.com	Bio-medical Journals
www.ideallibrary.com	International digital electronic access library
www.pharmweb.net/pharmweb/fip.html	International Pharmaceutical Federation (FIP)
www.isinet.com	Current contents
www.elsevier.com	Elsevier Publishing company
www.pharmweb.net/pharmweb/pharmwebyp.html	List of Pharmaceutical Companies on the internet
www.pharmweb.net/pharmweb/pharmpress.html	Pharmaceutical press
www.pci.ac.in	Pharmacy Council of India, New Delhi

Operational Aspects

The following operations are commonly required in pharmaceutical dispensing:

1. Weighing
2. Measuring
3. Dissolution
4. Solubilization
5. Size reduction
6. Size separation
7. Mixing
8. Filtration

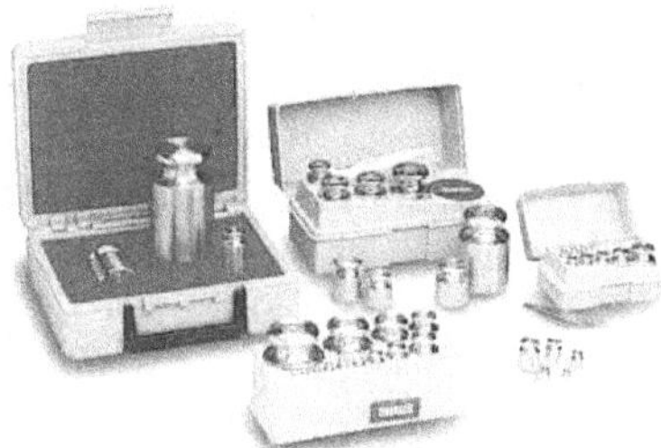

Weights

Weighing

Several varieties of dispensing scales and weight boxes are available. Three to four varieties of balances capable of weighing different quantities and of desired accuracies should be available in a pharmacy and a pharmacist exercises his choice for use while dispensing a prescription depending on the quantity to be weighed and accuracy desired. The balances should be installed on a heavy, stable platform in a corner free from drift of air or fumes. The balance meant for daily use may be installed at a suitable place on the working table. The balance should be adjusted in level with the help of a spirit level and checked for the null point and oscillations of the beam before use. While commissioning a new balance, the pharmacist should carefully read the literature supplied by the manufacturer and understand its operation and accuracy. Quantities lesser than 50 mg of ingredients and lesser than 100 mg of potent medicaments should be weighed on an analytical balance. After testing a balance, pieces of white paper should be placed under each pan. The weights should be handled and picked with the help of forceps and kept in the left pan of the balance. Solid is slowly added to the right pan or removed there from using a spatula of suitable size. Greasy and sticky substances are weighed by placing them on a greaseproof (butter or waxed) paper and then weighing using a counterpoise. After the weighing operation, the weights are rechecked while returning them to the weight box. The solid is then removed from the right pan, which is usually made of glass or stainless steel. Corrosive and oxidizing agents should not be put directly in a stainless steel pan but weighed in a watch glass providing a suitable counterpoise in the left pan. It may be borne in mind that weighing operation, if executed without care, may lead to serious errors.

Measuring

The devices used for this operation are measures and pipettes. The measures may be cylindrical or conical and between the two varieties, the former are easier to read and more accurate and reliable. The latter are however, easier to clean, rinse and handle. Nature of meniscus and its reading influence the degree of measuring accuracy considerably. It is desirable that one acquires practice and experience in taking meniscus readings with different measures and liquids of different colours. A measure should rest on a flat surface perpendicular to the surface while taking readings and should be straight before the eyes to avoid parallax errors. Errors are also possible in removing the liquid from the measure. Viscous liquids may stick to the measure and deliver lesser volumes, the error sometimes being as high as 20%. In practice, one should use a clean, dry measure closest in volume to the quantity to be measured. The liquid from the bottle may be poured carefully in the measure upto the proper graduation from the side opposite to the label holding the bottle in the right hand The stopper of the liquid bottle should either be held in between two fingers of the right hand or placed on the table with the surface that touches the liquid pointing upwards so as to avoid the contamination by the wet surface coming in contact with the surface of the table top. After the requisite volume has been filled in the measure the container should be removed from the hand and stopper put back in position. The liquid may then be poured in the container or mortar as the case may be and rinsed if the liquid is viscous, adding the rinsing to the original lot. Small volumes can be accurately delivered with the help of graduated pipettes calibrated from 0.01 to 0.1 ml. Pipette should be of a proper size, clean and dry. A rubber teat should be attached to the upper end of the pipette. The air may be expelled by pressing the teat with right hand thumb and the lower end of the pipette immersed in the liquid to be sucked in. If excess liquid is sucked in, it can be removed by pressing the teat till the meniscus reads the required volume. The liquid inside the pipette can now be delivered to the container or mortar as the case may be. One can also remove the teat after sucking the pipette and can control delivery of the volume with the help of the thumb or the forefinger. Use of measuring pipettes based on vacuum (Vaccupet etc.) should be encouraged for reasons of accuracy and avoiding hazard while sucking the liquids through mouth.

Solubilization

It is the process of dissolving poorly soluble solute molecules in water in the presence of surfactants. Mc Bain introduced this term in 1937. The exact mechanism of solubilization is not clear yet. When surfactants with proper HLB values are added to a liquid in very low concentrations, the solution behaves as an ideal one. Surfactant molecules in the solution tend to orient themselves at the liquid-air interface. Addition of surfactant may be continued until all available space is saturated and beyond which the surfactant is forced back into the bulk of the liquid. At still higher concentrations, the surfactant molecules or ions tend to aggregate to form micelles. Thus micelles are the aggregates of 100 to 150 surfactant molecules. Solubilization concept has been profitably employed in pharmaceutical practice. Water insoluble substances are solubilized using various techniques of solubilization. Generally low toxicity soaps are used to provide micelles. Cholesterol can also be solubilized to an appreciable extent by soaps. Proprietary disinfectants such as Lysol, chloroxyxylenol solution and hexachlorophene liquid soaps are formulated on the basis of solubilization phenomenon. Lyophilic surfactants with HLB values higher than 15 are considered to be the best solubilizing agents.

Dissolution

It is presumed that a student is familiar with the theoretical aspects of solution. When a soluble solid is incorporated in a liquid, its physical form is changed. Essentially it is a phenomenon of mass transfer. After due scrutiny of the prescription, one should be able to envisage and assess whether the prescription would yield a clear product. Lack of comprehension may result into filtering out and rejecting the therapeutically active precipitate in an over enthusiastic attempt to supply a clear product. Such instances are not rare and it is vital that a pharmacist fully understands the likely reactions that may occur and act suitably. Once it is established that a solution will result he may take steps to affect it rapidly. Drugs in fine state of subdivision have a greater specific surface and dissolve faster than larger particles or crystals. Secondly, stirring the particles in the vehicle expedites dissolution as highly concentrated solution around the particle is replaced by dilute solution till the equilibrium is established. Raising the temperature usually accelerates the rate of solution. However, heating may not be advisable to if the drug is thermo-labile. Rise in temperature increases the diffusion coefficient and reduces the viscosity, two important factors that favor solution. As a rule, the pharmacist should not rely on his memory regarding the solubility of ingredients. It is advisable that he makes use of tables and texts for ascertaining solubility of the substances in given vehicle under the overall conditions of the prescription. When two substances are present to the optimum amount of their solubility, it is likely that the resultant product may not be clear. Further, the pharmacist should thoroughly examine the possibility of a chemical reaction resulting into precipitate formation. The drug is first powdered and the requisite quantity weighed. Stirring or shaking with a liquid may be done preferably in a conical flask large enough to prevent spilling during shaking. Another method for affecting solution of relatively less solute substances is to transfer the solid and a portion of the vehicle in a mortar and mixing with the help of pestle. Wherever volatile substances are prescribed, heating should be avoided as a precautionary measure and shaking done in a closed container with a suitable closure to prevent loss of volatile medicament. Whenever heating has been employed, the solution should be first cooled to room temperature, if need be, under running tap water. Filtration, dilution, making up the volume and transference to the container should be done thereafter.

Size reduction

In dispensing practice drugs and excipients are used in the preparation of dosage forms in specified size for effective result or action. Size reduction is necessary to some extent. 'Grinding', 'comminution' and 'milling' are the terms commonly used to signify size reduction of solids.   Size reduction of a drug may include one or more of the operations e.g. cutting, slicing, chopping, rasping or grating, contusion, grinding, pulverizing, milling, micronizing etc. Selection of the processes and equipment depends on type of material, desired degree of size reduction, moisture content etc. in the material, mechanism of size reduction, stability of final product and economic and fast method of size reduction.

Some manual processes employed in the size reduction of substance used in the dispensing of prescription are explained below.

Trituration

The term trituration refers to the process of size reduction of substances to a fine powder but it is also applied for the process whereby a mixture of fine powders is intimately mixed in a mortar. The circular mixing motion causes blending and also breaks up soft aggregates of powders. Crushing or grinding can also be effected by means of application of force on the pestle.

Pulverization by intervention

This is the process of powdering a substance with the help of another substance, which can be removed easily after the pulverization has been completed. Substances such as camphor, which are gummy and tend to re-agglomerate or which resist grinding, can be powdered by this method. Camphor cannot be pulverized by trituration because the particles tend to cohere as quickly as they are powdered. This difficulty is overcome by addition of a small amount of alcohol or other volatile solvent during trituration. The solvent can be removed after pulverization process is complete, by spraying the powdered camphor in a thin layer. Spermaceti wax may also be powdered in this manner. Iodine crystals may be pulverized with the help of a small quantity of ether. Picric acid is often mixed with 10 to 20% of water for safety in transportation. The water content serves a dual purpose. When picric acid is to be powdered for use in ointments, it prevents dangerous explosion during comminution, and aids in the grinding process by intervention.

Levigation

A pharmacist often uses this process to incorporate solids into dermatological and ophthalmic ointments and suspensions. The term refers to the reduction of a substance to an extremely fine state of subdivision by rubbing it, in a glass mortar or on a slab with the aid of an insoluble liquid called the levigating agent. The process is one of wet grinding. Levigating agent should be selected on the basis of its ability to form a paste with the substance to be levigated, and its compatibility with other ingredients in the product. For instance, water cannot be used as levigating agent with zinc oxide, intended to be incorporated into an oleaginous ointment base. Liquid paraffin is the levigating agent of choice in this case.

Principle of Size Reduction

Size reduction involves four different mechanisms.

1. *Cutting :* This implies cutting of materials by means of sharp blade(s).
2. *Compression :* This is accomplished by application of force by a suitable device.
3. *Impact :* Impact implies hitting of a more or less stationary material by an object moving at high speed or striking the moving particles at a stationary surface. In either case, the material is shattered to small pieces.
4. *Attrition :* Attrition occurs when the material is subjected to pressure as in compression but the surfaces are mobile in relation to each other, resulting in shear forces, which break the particles. The mechanisms of impact and attrition may be combined as in ball mill and fluid energy mill.

Equipment in Small Scale : Mortars and pestles (China and Glass), Household mixer, Grinder, Hand mill and Laboratory mill.

Large Scale Equipment

Following mill are commonly used in industry for size reduction. Selection of a mill is based on types of material, size required, cleaning, and mechanism of milling.

- Cutter mill
- Hammer mill
- Ball mill
- Rod mill
- Fluid-energy mill
- Roller mill
- Colloid mill
- Disc mill
- Edge runner mill
- Vibration ball mill

Size Separation

Control of particle size and size range is of great importance in dispensing pharmacy. Size reduction affected by the use of various types of equipments does not necessarily ensure the desired size distribution and therefore at times it is necessary to classify or grade the powdered materials. The process of fractionation of particles on the basis of size range is known as 'grading' or 'sifting'. Sieving has been used conventionally for the close control of particle size after size reduction. The wire sieves, used in sifting powdered drugs, are distinguished by numbers, which indicate the number of meshes (openings) included in a length of 2.54 cm, in each transverse direction parallel to the wires. It should be noted that it is the number of meshes that is specified and not 'the number of wires. Thus, a No. 20 sieve has 20 meshes per 2.54 cm in each transverse direction, but if there were 20 wires there would be 19 meshes only. According to I.P. 1996, "sieves for pharmacopoeial testing are of wire cloth woven from brass, bronze, stainless steel or other suitable material and not coated or plated. The wires are of uniform circular cross-section."

Mixing

Mixing is probably the most widely used operation in dispensing of medicine. Mixing may be defined as an operation, which tends to result in a state in which each particle of one material lies as nearly adjacent as possible to a particle of the other material.   Mixing tends to minimize non- uniformity or gradients in composition, properties, or temperature of material in bulk. The desired degree of mixing depends on the purpose of the product and the objective of mixing depends on types of dosage form being dispensed.

Types of Mixtures

Mixtures are mainly three types -

1. *Positive mixtures :* This type of product results when there is an irreversible mixing of materials such as gases or miscible liquids.

2. *Negative mixtures :* These are more difficult to obtain and a higher degree of mixing efficiency is essential. Negative mixtures require work for their formation and the components of such mixtures separate out unless work is continually expended on them e.g. suspension.

3. *Neutral mixtures :* These mixtures are static in their behavior and the components neither have tendency to mix spontaneously, nor do they segregate after mixing. Examples are pharmaceutical mixtures e.g. pastes, ointments and mixed powders.

Common Mixers used in Pharmaceutical Laboratories : Propeller mixers, Turbine mixers, Sigma-blade mixer, Triple-roller mill, Planetary mixer and Colloid mill.

Homogenization

Homogenization is the process, which renders a material to uniform quality, consistency or structure. The process is used in the preparation of fine suspensions, emulsions etc. Usually, in a homogenizer, the mixed phases of dispersion are passed through a finely ground valve and seat under high pressure, which causes atomization. This is further enhanced by the impact received by the atomized mixture as it strikes the valve seat.

(a) **Hand homogenizer :** It is suitable for homogenizing small amounts of materials. This type of homogenizer is specially meant for laboratories and is moderately priced. It is probably the most efficient homogenizer apparently available to the prescription pharmacist.

(b) **Silverson mixer-homogenizer :** Processes of mixing and homogenizing may be combined in some machines e.g. Silverson mixer-homogenizer. It consists essentially of an emulsifier head in which a set of rotor blades is surrounded by a fine-meshed stainless sieve. The materials are sucked through the mesh by the rotor blades and are reduced to a homogeneous dispersion before being expelled. The blades are adjusted so as to give a powerful shearing action. Two stage homogenizers are so constructed that the dispersion, after treatment in the first valve system, is passed on directly to a second one; wherein it receives a second treatment.

Filtration

Filtration is a unit operation by which solid particles are removed from a fluid by passing the mixture through a porous, fibrous or glandular medium. The object of simple filtration is to obtain sparkling and optically transparent liquids, free from insoluble liquid drops whereas sterile filtration is aimed at the removal of microorganisms in addition to other foreign matter. When the solids are present in small proportions (not exceeding 0.15%), the process is usually spoken of as *clarification*. Filter media are the porous devices, which retain solids by mechanical separation and allow liquid to pass through. The accumulated layer of solids deposited on the filter medium during the filtration of a slurry or feed is known as *filter cake*. *Slurry* is a suspension of solids in a liquid to be filtered. It may also be referred to as feed. *Filtrate* is the clear liquid passing through the filter.

The mechanism of filtration basically involves a two-step operation -

(i) the flow of solid materials is resisted by the filter medium while the liquid is allowed to pass through; and

(ii) the solid material retained on the filter medium during the course of operation gradually builds up a filter cake which acts as a secondary, and sometimes as a more efficient filter medium.

Filtering Media

1. **Filter paper :** Filter papers are most commonly used for the retention of very fine solids and for the clarification of liquids containing only a small amount of solids. Rapid filtration rate is achieved because the pores on the paper are small and in a large number. As filtering medium may be a possible source of contamination in the finished product, a high quality of filter paper should always be used in pharmaceutical operations.

2. ***Membrane filters :*** These are employed for micro-filtration e.g. in the preparation of sterile solutions. These are made of pure cellulose or cellulose derivatives mainly cellulose esters or from nylon, teflon, polyvinyl chloride, or silver. Absence of fibers or particles in the integral structure is a particular advantage in the filtration of ophthalmic solutions. The thickness of the membrane filters ranges from 50 to 200 μm with millions of pores per square meter of filtering surface. The pores are extremely uniform in size ranging from 0.05 to 14μm and may occupy up to 90 percent of filter volume. To avoid rapid clogging of membrane filler, because of surface screening characteristics, pre-filtration is often required. Thermo-labile materials can be economically and rapidly filtered/sterilized in one cycle by the membrane filtration process.

3. ***Cotton filters :*** Large particles of extraneous matter from a clear liquid may be removed by loosely inserting a small pledget of absorbent cotton wool in the neck of the funnel. However, as fine cotton fibers may be frequently imparted to the filtrate, it is sometimes necessary to recycle the filtrate a number of times to attain transparency.

4. ***Glass wool :*** Filter paper, cotton-wool etc., are not suitable when solutions of highly reactive or corrosive substances as strong acids, alkalis and oxidizing agents are to be filtered. In such cases glass wool may be used as it is resistant to ordinary chemical action. Although it provides very effective filtration, glass wool may contaminate the filtrate with glass-fibers.

5. ***Asbestos :*** Asbestos pads are also used for the reasons stated above and placed under glass wool. They are prepared by compressing shredded asbestos lightly under pressure and are available in various size ranges. However, asbestos pads are of limited application because they impart an alkaline reaction to the filtrate. Calcium and magnesium ions released from the pads may cause incompatibility etc.

6. ***Sintered glass filters :*** These are made from borosilicate glass and the filtering medium is a flat or convex plate consisting of particles of Jena glass powdered and sifted to produce uniform solid granules, which are moulded or sintered together at a very high temperature. Depending upon the powder size used during sintering, these filters are available in different pore sizes.

Filtration Equipment

The selection of filtering equipment depends on the nature of the material, the volume to be filtered and the object of the operation. The one that satisfies all the requirements at the minimum overall cost is considered to be the most suitable process of filtration. Various types of filtering equipment may be conveniently discussed under the following three main headings:

A. *Small Scale Filtration :*   Filter Funnels, Porcelain Funnel, Hot filtration and Sintered glass filter

B. *Large Scale Filtration :*   Gravity filter, Pressure filter, Vacuum filter, Filter press, Leaf filter, Cartridge filter, Edge filter and Continuous rotary drum filter

C. *Sterile Filtration :*   Candle filter, Seitz filter, Edge Filter, Sintered glass filter and Membrane filter

Clarification

Clarification is the process of removal of relatively small amount of suspended solid present, without the use of filters. The term applies when the solids do not exceed 0.15%. The filtrate clarity is seldom absolute even when brilliance is called for. The process is employed in the preparation of aromatic waters, fruit juices, syrups and honey. The selection of specific procedures and equipment for clarification depends on a number of factors.

(i)   the particle size of the suspended matter,

(ii)   the physical state of the suspended matter,

(iii)   the quantity of the suspended matter,

(iv)   the characteristics of the fluid medium, and

(v)   the speed of the operation.

Clarification methods

1. ***Sedimentation and decantation :*** Gravity sedimentation is the simplest method of clarification although it may not always be feasible. The method consists of allowing the suspension or slurry to stand in a suitable container until the suspended matter either settles down or rises to the top of the liquid, depending on the density of the suspended matter. Thus, if the suspended matter is colloidal or if its density is approximately equal to that of the liquid phase, the method cannot be used fruitfully. The insoluble matter can be separated from the clear liquid phase by siphoning, decantation or straining. Process of settling down can be accelerated by centrifugation. Simple batch sedimentation can be demonstrated in a laboratory by using graduated cylinders whereas for continuous sedimentation operations, thickeners and large sedimentation tanks are employed. Gravitational sedimentation is usually employed for clarification of fixed oils.

2. ***Colation (straining) :*** In Latin colare means 'to strain'. Colation or straining is crude filtration. Like a filter, the strainer also acts by simple sieving action i.e. impeding the passage of suspended particles with diameters greater than that of the pores, while allowing the liquid to pass. The process consists of separating large, visible particles of a solid from liquid by pouring the mixture through a coarse cloth or a porous substance. Glass wool or asbestos is used for corrosive liquids such as potassium permanganate solutions, acids etc. The straining cloth may be freed from sizing materials e.g. starch glue, gelatin, albumin etc., by soaking it for a few hours in cold distilled water, rinsing thoroughly, and covering with distilled water or boiling for a few minutes. Final rinsing with distilled water will remove the last traces of sizing material.

3. ***Siphoning :*** It is an efficient method of removal of clarified supernatant liquid and students are expected to be familiar with basic principle underlying siphoning.

4. ***Absorption and adsorption*** *:* In addition to 'sieving' action of filter media, absorption and adsorption processes also help in efficient clarification. 'Soaking up' or trapping of the foreign particles within the media is called adsorption whereas adherence of foreign particles to the surface of the media is referred to as absorption. The absorption and adsorption properties may also be enhanced by addition of the filter aids. Albumen, gelatin and some synthetic coagulants are used as clarifying agents. These agents convert the solids to be removed into a conveniently filterable size either by precipitation or coagulation followed by physical adsorption.

5. ***Temperature*** *:* If the suspended solids are free filtering, their characteristics may be improved by varying the temperature or pH of the medium. Increase in the temperature of a viscid liquid reduces its viscosity and specific gravity and hence the particles suspended into it separate readily. This process was formerly *"official"* for the clarification of honey.

CHAPTER 3

Containers and Closures

A container-closure system is the sum of packaging components that together contain and protect the dosage form. A packaging component is defined as a single part of a container closure system.

Packaging components are mainly of two types-

Primary packaging component : A packaging component that is or may be in direct contact with the dosage form e.g. ampoule, vial, bottle, etc.

Secondary packaging component : It means a packaging component that is not and will not be in direct contact with the dosage form. It is intended to provide additional protection to the drug product. A **packaging system** is equivalent to a container closure system e.g. carton, box, lamination etc.

Typical components are –

- Containers- ampoules, vials, bottles
- Container liners – tube liners
- Closures – screw caps, stoppers
- Closure liners
- Stopper over seals
- Container inner seals
- Administration ports - Large volume parenterals (LVPs)
- Over wraps
- Administration accessories
- Container labels

A package refers to the container-closure system and labeling, associated components such as measuring devices (e.g., dosing cups, droppers, spoons), and external packaging (e.g., cartons or shrink wrap). Cost of container-closure is included with the final product. Container-closure is helpful to maintain the quality of finished product and also protect from physical, chemical, microbiological, biological, and other types of contamination and enhance the stability of drug product. Many containers are also suitable for identification of quality product.

Current Good Manufacturing Practice (cGMP) requirements for the control of drug product containers and closures include quality, purity and protection from the environment and contamination of the finished product.

The United States Pharmacopoeia/National Formulary (USP/NF) has established requirements for containers, which are described in many of the drug product monographs.

For capsule, tablets, liquid dosage forms : Tight, well-closed or light-resistant containers

For parenteral products : Preserve in single-dose or in multiple-dose containers, preferably of Type I glass, protected from light

The container is the device that holds the product. The immediate container is that which is in direct contact with the article at all times. The closure is a part of the container. The container is designed so that the contents may be taken out for the intended purpose in a convenient manner. It provides the required degree of protection to the contents from environment hazards.

The container should not interact physically or chemically with the product placed in it so as to alter the strength, quality or purity of the article beyond the official requirements. Special precautions and cleaning procedures may be necessary to ensure that each container is clean and that extraneous matter is not introduced into or onto the article.

Terminology

(a) ***Well-closed container :*** A well-closed container protects the contents from extraneous solids and liquids and from loss of the product under normal conditions of handling, shipment, storage and distribution.

(b) ***Light-resistant container :*** A light-resistant container protects the contents from the effects of light by virtue of the specific properties of the material of which it is made. The container should bear a statement "store in dark place" until the contents have been used up.

(c) ***Tightly-closed container :*** A tightly-closed container protects the contents from contamination by extraneous liquids, solids or vapors and from loss or deterioration of the product from effervescence, deliquescence or evaporation under normal conditions of handling, shipment, storage and distribution.

(d) ***Hermetically sealed container :*** A hermetically sealed container is impervious to air or any other gas under normal conditions of handling. It may be closed by fusion of the material of the container as in ampoules.

(e) ***Single unit container :*** A single unit container is one that is designed to hold a quantity of the drug product intended for administration as a single dose or a single finished device intended for use promptly after the container is opened.

(f) *Single dose container :* A single dose container is intended for product for parenteral administration and is designed to hold a quantity of the drug equivalent to a single dose.

(g) *Unit dose container :* A unit dose container is a container for articles intended for administration by other than parenteral route as a single dose, direct from the container – drought, application, etc.

(h) *Multiple unit container :* A multiple unit container is a container that permits withdrawal of successive portions of the contents without changing the strength, quality or purity of the remaining portion.

(i) *Multiple dose Container :* A multiple dose container is a multiple unit container for articles intended for parenteral administration only.

(j) *Tamper-evident container :* A tamper-evident container is fitted with a device or mechanism that reveals irreversibly whether the container has been opened.

Cold : Any temperature not exceeding 8 °C and usually between 2 °C and 8 °C. A refrigerator is a cold place in which the temperature is maintained thermostatically between 2 °C and 8 °C.

Cool : Any temperature between 8 °C and 25 °C.

Room temperature : The temperature prevailing in a working area.

Warm : Any temperature between 30 °C and 40 °C.

Excessive heat : Any temperature above 40 °C.

Protection from heat : Where, in addition to the risk of breaking of the container, freezing results in loss of strength or potency.

Storage under non-specific conditions : Where no specific storage directions or limitations are given. It is to be understood that storage conditions include protection from moisture, freezing and excessive heat.

Table 3.1 Suitability of Containers and Considerations

Dosage Form	Protection
Aerosols, Oral solutions, Oral suspensions, Topical delivery Systems, Topical aerosols, Topical solutions Topical suspensions	Light, Solvent loss and Microbial contamination
Capsules, Oral powders, Powders for injection Sterile powders, Tablets inhalation Powders	Light, microbial contamination and water vapor
Aerosols, Inhalation, Injections, Injectable suspensions Nasal sprays, Ophthalmic solutions, Ophthalmic suspensions	Light, solvent loss, microbial contamination, water vapor and reactive gases

Packaging is used to enclose the object physically, typically a product that will be offered for sale. Labelling refers to any written information of the finished product or graphic communications on the packaging or on a separate label.

Aim of Packaging and Labelling

Physical protection : The main aim of packaging is to protect the finished product during handling and in transportaiton by pressure, heat, sunlight, physical force, rain, cold, airborne contamination, etc.

Protection from duplicacy : Laymen can identify the quality and originality of a product by the packaging and labeling system of the substance or finished product. Proper packaging system is helpful in reducing duplicay of the product and also protect it from hazards of transportation.

Marketing : Proper packaging and labelling can enhance the marketability of the product like its elegance, storage properties, usefulness of the container and packaging.

Handling of product : Suitable containers and packaging system is helpful in the handling of product during administration and also for storage.

Shape and Size : Suitable shape and size of packaging render the product ease of transportation at low cost and may reduce the storage space.

Information transmission : Important information for user is available on the label or package i.e. how to open, how to use, how to store, indications and contraindications, if any; expiry, transport, or disposal of the remaining product etc. Some times special information is also available on the label prescribed by the governments or authorized official body i.e. FDA, for example 'under Employees' State Insurance Scheme (ESIS)'.

Factors Affecting Selection of Packaing Materials

Different types of materials are commonly employed in the packaging depending on –

- Type of product (solid, liquid, gases etc.)
- Sensitivity of product
- Chemical composition of finished product
- Toxicity and contamination
- Types of damage depends on container during transportation
- Product prize
- Application and utility of product
- Product size
- Product weight
- Duration of storage
- Method of transportation and distance

Materials used for Packaging

Following materials are commonly used in packaging of pharmaceutical products i.e., Corrugated cardboard, Wood; wool, Jute, Paper, Plastic, Wood and Bubble wrap.

Packaging types

Pharamaceutical products are packed into different types of packages and containers such as Boxes, Pallets, Bags, Bottles, Cans, Cartons, Aseptic packages, Wrappers and Blister packs

Packaging machines are of the following main types:

- Vertical Form, Fill, Seal (FFS) machines
- Horizontal FFS machines
- Bottling machines
- Cartoning machines
- Case packing machines
- Palletizing machines

Paper

Paper is a thin, flat material produced by the compression of fibres. The fibres used are usually natural and based upon cellulose. The most common material is wood pulp from pulpwood (largely softwood) tree such as spruces, but other vegetable fibre materials including cotton, linen, and hemp may be used. The edges of paper sheets can act as very thin, fine-toothed saws, leading to paper cuts. The material to be used for making paper is first converted into pulp, a concentrated mixture of fibres suspended in liquid. These fibres are mainly obtained from natural sources. Fibres extraction from natural source requires many stages of separation and washing. Once the fibres have been extracted, they may also be bleached or dyed to alter the appearance of the final product.

Plastic /Polymer

Plastic is a term that covers a range of synthetic or semisynthetic polymerization products. They are composed of organic condensation or addition polymers and may contain other substances to improve performance or economics. There are few natural polymers generally considered to be "plastics". Plastics can be formed into objects or films or fibres. Their name is derived from the fact that many are malleable, having the property of plasticity. Plastics are designed with immense variation in properties such as heat tolerance, hardness, resiliency etc. Combined with this adaptability, the general uniformity of composition and light weight of plastics ensure their use in almost all industrial segments.

Plastic may also refer to any material characterized by deformation or failure under shears stress, plasticity and ductility.

Plastics can be classified in many ways

(a) On the basis of polymer backbone - Polyvinyl chloride, Polyethylene, Acrylic, Silicone, and Urethane

(b) On the basis of synthesis – Addition and Condensation

(c) On the basis of properties – Thermoplastic, Thermoset, Elastomer and Engineering plastic

(d) On the basis of nature – Crystalline and Amorphous

Polymers are high molecular weight compounds whose structures are made up of a large number of simple repeating units. The repeating units are usually obtained from low molecular weight simple compounds referred to as **monomers**. The reaction by which monomers are converted into polymers is known as **polymerization**. Polymers are giant molecules (also called macromolecules) that are essential to our existence. They are important chemicals in our bodies [proteins, poly (nucleic acids)], in plants (starch, cellulose), and in our everyday lives (fibers, plastics, elastomers). Although the chemical properties of polymers are similar to those of analogous small molecules, their physical properties are quite different. Every polymer has its own characteristics, but most polymers have the following general properties.

1. Polymers can be very resistant to chemicals.

2. Polymers can be both thermal and electrical insulators.

3. Generally, polymers are light in weight with varying degrees of strength.

4. Polymers can be processed in various ways to produce thin fibers or intricate parts.

Polymer characterization

A variety of techniques are used to determine the properties of polymers: Determination of crystalline structure, Determination of number average molecular weight, Glass transition technique, Melting point etc.

1. Hompolymers

Polymers which are synthesized from only one kind of monomers.

Polypropylene
(Monomer-propylene)

Polyethylene
(Monomer -ethylene)

Polyvinyl chloride
(Monomer-vinyl chloride)

Orlon
(Monomer - Vinyl chloride

Teflon
(Monomer -Teterafluoroethylene)

Polystrene
(Monomer - Styrene)

2. Copolymers

Polymers which are prepared from more/different than one kind of monomers.

$$-\!\!+\!CH_2\!-\!CH_2\!-\!OOC\!-\!\!\left\langle\!\bigcirc\!\right\rangle\!-\!COO\!+_{n}$$

Terylene (Dacron)

Rubber

Rubber is an elastic hydrocarbon polymer, which occurs as a milky emulsion (latex) in the sap of a number of plants but can also be produced synthetically. The latex from various trees are collected into flat pan containers and this is mixed with formic acid act as a coagulating agent. After a few hours, the very wet sheets of rubber are pressed and then sent to factories for vulcanization and further processing to remove impurities. Sulfur is mixed to improve resilience and elasticity of rubber. The process of vulcanization greatly improves the durability and utility of rubber. Carbon Black is commonly used as an additive to rubber to improve its strength. Natural rubber is essentially a polymer of isoprene units, a hydrocarbon diene monomer. Synthetic rubber can be made as a polymer of isoprene or various other monomers. Using various types and ratio of elastomers can modify properties of rubber.

Table 3.2 Common polymers and their typical uses

Polymer	Pharmaceutical Uses
polyethylene (PE)	wide range of uses, very economical
polypropylene (PP)	food containers, appliances
polystyrene (PS)	packaging foam, food containers, disposable cups, plates and cutlery
polyethylene terephthalate (PETE)	beverage containers
Polyamide (PA) (Nylon)	toothbrush bristles, fishing line
polyvinyl chloride (PVC)	plumbing pipes, flooring, erotic clothing, water bottle, liquid detergent containers
polycarbonate	compact discs, eye glasses
acrylonitrile butadiene styrene	electronic equipment cases (e.g., computer monitors, printers, keyboards)
polyvinylidene chloride (PVDC)	food packaging
Teflon	heat resistant, low-friction coatings, used in things like frying pans and water slides
Polyurethane	insulation foam, upholstery foam
Bakelite	electrical fixtures
Polyethylene Terephthalate (PETE)	soft drink bottles, cooking oil bottles, peanut butter jars.
High Density Polyethylene (HDPE)	detergent bottles, milk jugs

Bubble wrap Regularly spaced, protruding air-filled hemispheres (bubbles) which provide the cushioning for fragile or sensitive objects are generally available in different sizes, depending on the size of the object being packed, as well as the level of cushioning protection that is needed. They can be as small as 1/4 inch in diameter to as large as an inch or more, to provide added levels of shock absorption during transit.

Metals

(a) Aluminium

Aluminium is a soft and light weight metal with a dull silvery appearance, due to a thin layer of oxidation that forms quickly when it is exposed to air. Aluminium is nontoxic (as the metal) non-magnetic and non-sparking. Pure aluminium has a tensile strength of about 49 megapascals (MPa) and 700 MPa if it is formed into an alloy. Aluminium is about one-third as dense as steel or copper; is malleable, ductile, and easily machined and cast; and has excellent corrosion resistance and durability due to the protective oxide layer. It is also non-magnetic and non-sparking and is the second most malleable metal (after gold) and the sixth most ductile.

Pure aluminium has a low tensile strength, but readily forms alloys with many elements such as copper, zinc, magnesium, manganese and silicon. When combined with thermo-mechanical processing these aluminium alloys display a marked improvement in mechanical properties.

Pharmaceutical Applications : Aluminium collapsible tube, ophthalmic containers, aluminum foil, aluminium packing, etc.

General Applications :

- In transportation – automobiles, airplanes, trucks, railroad cars, marine vessels, etc.
- In packaging – cans, foil, etc.
- Water treatment
- Construction – windows, doors, siding, building wire, etc.
- Consumer durable goods- appliances, cooking utensils, etc.

Closures

Closures are the essential device by which containers of finished product can be opened and closed. It is important that cap size fits the bottle neck finish in order to obtain proper sealing. The first digit corresponds to the cap diameter (in mm.) The second digit stands for the height and thread design of the neck or cap finish.

Closure is the most important part of container because –

- It protects the product from environmental contamination.
- It prevents loss of material during transportation and storage.
- It enhances stability of product.
- It prevents microbial attack.

Closures are mainly following types –

1. ***Liner caps :*** Liner type consideration is an important part of the cap selection process. Some liners tend to withstand chemicals better than others, while other liner material types are better used for moisture barriers.

2. ***Thread caps :*** It is an uninterrupted spiral design threaded closure. The main purpose of a threaded closure is to match with corresponding bottle threads to provide sealing and resealing of containers. Threaded caps are available in a variety of styles including smooth, ribbed and dome cap.

3. ***Snap Caps :*** A closure held in place by a bead (a depressed or raised circle or ring around a container or closure) rather then a thread.

4. ***Lug Caps :*** A closure with raised internal impressions that inter-mesh with identical threads on the finish of the container.

5. ***Disc Top Caps :*** Disc top caps typical screw on to a bottle similar to a screw cap, though there is no need to unscrew and remove the cap in order to dispense. Disc top caps are made with a slight indent in the plastic top, which is designed to have a light amount of pressure applied to in order to expose the orifice where the product can be dispensed. Simply applying light pressure to the open end of the cap will easily close the cap.

6. ***Twist Top Caps :*** Twist top caps allow for greater control of the flow of product. Twist top caps are applied to the packaging the same way screw top caps are, though in order to dispense the product there is no need to unscrew the entire cap. Instead the top part of the cap is twisted to allow for the product to be dispensed through the top of the closure.

7. ***Snap Top Caps :*** The closure is screwed on to the packaging. To dispense the product the hinged cap is flipped up, product dispensed and then resealed by simply pressing the cap back on to the beaded finish.

8. ***Flip-Top Spout Caps :*** A closure designed to have the dispensing spout retract into the closure when not being used. The flip top is opened to dispense the product.

9. ***Glass Droppers :*** A closure that includes an attached dropper and rubber bulb.

10. ***Spout Caps :*** A closure designed to aid in the dispensing of the container contents through a hole at the end of the cone shaped cap.

11. ***Sifter Caps :*** A closure that allows for the shaking out of dry products.

12. ***Pump Type :*** Pumps allow for high viscosity products to be easily dispensed. Pumps can be used with glass, plastic or metal containers. Pumps allow for an equal amount of product to be dispensed each time.

13. ***Sprayer Type :*** Sprayers allow low viscosity products to be misted out of the container.

14. ***Orifice Reducer :*** Orifice reducer allow a great deal of control over the amount of product being dispensed. There are two types of orifice reducers, one that can be inserted into the bottle by the customer and the other that comes in the tamper-evident closure.

Safety Cover

Shrink bands : PVC sleeves, which slide over either the packaging, closure or in some cases the whole package. Shrink bands make products tamper evident increasing the safety of product.

Induction sealing : A specialized laminate containing an aluminum foil and a plastic heat sealable film which hermetically seals a container through the use of a cap sealing machine.

Child-resistant caps (CR caps) : A closure requiring dissimilar motions making removal by a child difficult. Child Resistant closures are subject to current Government Regulations.

Material for construction of closures

Cork : It is obtained from the bark of a certain variety of oak growing in Mediterranean countries. It is used in the manufacturing of stoppers for glass bottles. Cork is almost inert and does not impart any undesirable odour to product.

Glass : As compared to cork, glass stoppers are more elegant but unless properly ground, they may allow leakage. The use of glass closures is mainly restricted to laboratory glassware in pharmaceutical field.

Metals : In modern dispensing, metal closures are very common. They are made from aluminium and tin plate.

Plastics : Cork, glass and metal closures have been mostly replaced by plastic and metal closures with liners of cork or other resilient materials. They can be easily molded to various shapes and sizes easily. Plastics selected for stoppers should particularly be tested for any extractive matter present in them and for their reaction with contents of the containers.

Rubber : Natural rubber imparts a characteristic odor to product. Synthetic rubbers like silicone, neoprene, nitrile or butyl are expensive. Rubber closures are commonly used for vials of antibiotics and multidose injectable.

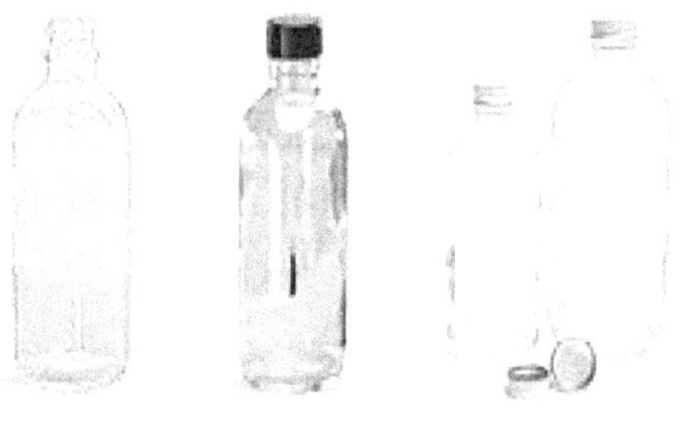
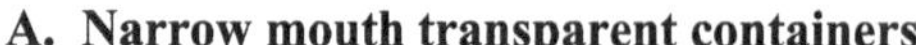
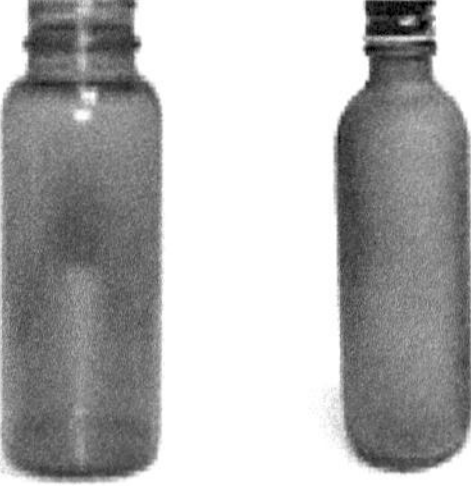

A. Narrow mouth transparent containers   **B. Narrow mouth colored containers**

CHAPTER 4

Pharmaceutical Calculation

Weights and Measures

In our day-to-day life as well as in the practice of pharmaceutical profession, it is always necessary to have some unit to measure a quantity. The science, which deals with weights and measures, is called **Metrology**. As each and every pharmaceutical operation implies the fundamental knowledge of metrology, it appears appropriate to acquaint us with various aspects of metrology.

The need for a system of weights and measures might have been felt as a basis for comparison in day-to-day dealings and therefore mechanical devices like balances or scales were devised. Historically, the ancient standards referred to various parts of human body e.g., fathom, cubit, span, foot and nail etc. Later, the objects around human beings like grains or wheat were preferred for comparison. As the facilities for trade and transport widened and the geographical barriers crossed, a need was realized to bring about uniformity in the system of weights and measures which might have started initially on a regional basis and developed through provincial to a national and international basis. Such an attempt to adopt an uniform, scientific and methodical system naturally culminated in most of the civilized countries of the world having adopted the metric system of weights and measures which is certainly the simplest and the best. However most of the elder physicians still don't follow the metric system in prescription writing and hence it is desirable that a pharmacist should be acquainted with other systems of weights and measures normally encountered in prescription writing. The Indian system of weights and measures having the units *tola, masha* and *ratti* etc., is no more official since April 1,1956 when the Government of India recognized the metric system as the only official one. In India the Standards of Weights and Measures Act controls the weights and measures and the Pharmacopoeia of India has also recognized the metric system.

Mass is a constant based on inertia while weight changes with altitude, latitude, temperature and pressure. The measure of the gravitational force acting on a body is directly proportional to its mass and is known as *weight*. The unit of weight is Gram, which is equal to 1/1000 of the mass of the International Prototype Kilogram. The extent of volume of a body is called *measure*. The units commonly employed are litre and metre for capacity and length, respectively.

The Standards of Weights and Measures Act, 1976 provides for the reference standard, secondary standard and working standard for calibration of weights and measures. The Act also provides for the preparation of national prototypes of the kilogram and metre by the Central Government. The Standards of Weights and Measures Act, 1976 provides the calibration standard of weights and measures. Under the Act, 'International Bureau of Weights and Measures' means the Bureau International des Poids at Sevres in France. 'International prototype of the kilogram' is defined as the prototype sanctioned by the First General Conference on weights and measures held in Paris in 1889, and deposited at the International Bureau of Weights and Measures. Kilogram is recognized as the base unit of mass and is equal to the mass of the International prototype of kilogram. **Metre** is recognized as the base unit of length and is equal to 1650763.73 wavelengths in vacuum of the radiation corresponding to the transition between the levels $2p_{10}$ and $5d_5$ of the krypton-86 atom.

The Act also provides for the preparation of national prototypes of the kilogram and metre by the Central Government.

English System : The earlier units were based on the weight of 32 grains of wheat, which equaled a silver penny (Sterling), 20 penny weights (Pence) made an ounce, twelve ounces a pound and eight pounds made a gallon of wine, etc. The word 'haberdupois' was used first in English laws in 1303. The 'troy' weight has still earlier origin. Troyes is a French city in which great fairs were held during 8th and 9th centuries. However these systems caused great inconvenience to buyers and sellers of medicines. In 1790 Washington recommended the establishment of uniformity in currency, weights and measures; and in 1836 the troy pound (5760 grains), the avoirdupois pound (7000 grains) along with yard were introduced.

Metric System : In 1783, James Watt first proposed the use of decimal system and the commensurability of weight, length and volume. Metric weights were officially recognized in Great Britain in 1864, in United States in 1866 and in India in 1956. The principal attributes of this system are its simplicity, brevity and adaptability to everyday needs. It is the system of decimal progression meaning thereby that every unit is multiplied or divided by the same number (i.e. 10) to obtain various denominations. Latin prefixes like *milli, centi, deci,* etc., are used to indicate subdivisions while Greek prefixes like *deca, hecto, myria,* are used to denote multiples of the principal units.

A brief account of different systems of weights and measures and relationships relevant to a pharmacist are given below.

(a) Measures of Mass

   The difference between weight and mass is that the weight changes with the altitude, as it is dependent on the gravitational force, whereas mass remains unchanged.

The unit of weight is the Gram, which is defined as 1/1000 of the mass of the International Prototype Kilogram. e.g.,

1 Tonne (T)	1,000 kilograms (Kg or kg or kilo)
1 Quintal	1000 kilograms
1 kilogram	1000 grams (g, G or Gm or gm)
1 Hectagram (Hg)	100 grams
1 Dekagram (Dg)	10 grams
1 Decigram 9dg)	1/10 gram
1 Centigram (cg)	1/100 gram
1 Milligram (mg)	1/1000 gram
1 Microgram (mcg), μg	1/1000 mg or 10^{-6} g
1 Nanogram	1/1000 μg = 10^{-9} g
1 Picogram	1/1000 of a nanogram = 10^{-12} g

(b) Measures of Length

The unit of length is the Meter (M), which is defined as the length of the International Prototype Meter bar

1 Kilometer (Km)	1000 meters (m.)
1 Centimeter (cm)	1/100 meter [0.01]
1 Millimeter (mm)	1/1000 meter
1 Micron (μ)	10^{-6} mm
1 Millimicron (mμ)	10^{-9} mm
1 Micromicron ($\mu\mu$)	15^{12} mm

(c) Measures of Capacity

The unit of capacity is the litre or liter (l. or L.) that is defined as the volume of 1 kg of water at 4°C. There is difference between millilitre and cc. 1 ml is the volume occupied by 1 g of water at 4°C, whereas 1 cc is the volume of a cube each side of which is 1 cm length. 1 cc = 0.99984 ml or 1 litre = 1000.028 cc.

However, for all practical purposes ml and cc are taken as the same.

1 Hectolitre	100 litres
1 Millilitre	1/1000 litre
1 litre	1000.028 cc = 1000 ml
1 Microlitre (μl)	0.001 ml = 10^{-6} litre
1000 litres	1 cubic meter

(d) Imperial System

Imperial system of weights and measures, commonly known as Avoirdupois system was recognized in the British Pharmacopoeia, though at present UK also has switched over to the metric system.

(i) Avoirdupois Weights and measures

Measures of mass

437.5 grains (gr.)	1 ounce (oz)
16 ounces	1 pound (lb)
14 pounds	1 stone
112 pounds	1 hundredweights (cwt)
20 hundredweights	1 ton

Measures of Capacity (Volume)

60 minims (min)	1 fluid drachm (dram) (fl.dr.)
8 fluid drachms	1 fluid ounce (fl.oz)
20 fluid ounces	1 pint (pt)
2 pints	1 quart
4 quarts or 8 pints	1 gallon

Relationship of capacity to mass

- 1 Gallon = the volume of 10 pounds or 70,000 grains of distilled water at 62°F
- 1 Fluid ounce or 480 minims = the volume at 62°F of 1 oz. or 437.5 grains of distilled water
- 109.71 minims (taken as 110 minims) = the volume at 62°F of 100 grains of distilled water.

(ii) Apothecaries' Weights and Measures

Measures of Mass

Grain is the same in both Avoidupois and Apothecaries systems.

20 grains	1 Scruple
3 Scruples	1 drachm (dram)
8 Drachms	1 ounce
12 Ounces	1 pound

The measures of volume are the same in both the systems. In Avoirdupois system the abbreviations are fl.dr and fl.oz while in Apothecarees system they are and for dram and ounce, respectively.

United States of America : Weights and Measures

1 Fluid ounce (480 minims) = 454.6 grains at 25°C (USA standard) = 437.5 grains at 16.7°C (Imperial Standard)

1 pint =16 fl.oz. (USA) = 20 fl oz. (Imperial)

1 Gallon = 128 fl. Oz. (USA) = 3.7853 liters

1 Gallon = 160 fl.oz. (Imperial) = 4.5436 litres

1 hundredweight = 100 pounds (USA) = 112 pounds (Imperial)

1 ton = 2000 pounds (USA) = 240 pounds (Imperial)

Household Measures

The accepted approximate dose equivalents for the household measures are given below-

Household measure	Apothecaries measure	Metric measure
1 Drop	1 minim	0.04 ml
1 Teaspoonful	1 fl.dr.	5 ml
1 Dessertspoonful	2 fl.dr.	8 ml
1 Tablespoonful	4 fl.dr.	15 ml
1 Wineglassful	2 fl.oz.	60 ml
1 Teacupful	4 fl.oz.	120 ml
1 Tumblerful	8 fl.oz.	240 ml

The drops of various liquids vary in size and it is therefore necessary to calibrate the dropper to get the correct dose of a potent liquid preparation.

Use of Equivalents

A pharmacist is sometimes required to convert a formula from one system to the other or to dispense prepared dosage forms like mixtures, lotions, ointments etc., in a suitable equivalent dose.

Imperial system	Approximate metric system	Exact metric equivalent
15 minims	1 ml	0.924 ml
16.23 minims	1 ml	1.0 ml
60 minims (1 fl.dr.)	4 ml	3.697 ml
480 minims (1 fl.oz.)	30 ml	29.573 ml
33.8148 or 33.815 fl.oz.	1 litre	1 litre
1 gallon (177.27 cubic inches)	4.5 L	4.5436 L
1/60 grains	1 mg	1.1 mg

Contd….

Imperial system	Approximate metric system	Exact metric equivalent
1 pound (lb)	454 g	453.59 g
1 grain	60 mg	64.7989 mg or 64.8 mg
7.5 grains	0.5 g	0.4864 g
10 grains	0.6 g	0.6480 g
15 grains	1 g	0.972 g
15.432 grains	1 g	1.0 g
60 grains = 1 dram	4 g	3.888 g
437.5 grains = 1 oz.	28 g	28.3495 or 28.35 g
480 grains = 1 ounce	30 g	31.1035 g
32.151 Apoth. ounces	1Kg	1 Kg
35.274 Av. Ounces (2.2046 lbs)	1 Kg	1 Kg
16 Av. Ounces (1 lbs.)	450 g	453.5924 g
1 Inch	2.5 cm	2.54 cm
1 Cubic Inches	16 cc	16.3872 cc
39.37 inches	1 meter	1 meter
1.196 sq. yards	1 sq. meter	1 sq. meter
1 mile	1.6 Km	1.6093 Km
0.6214 mile	1 Km	1 Km

Uncalibrated teaspoons may vary from 2.4 to 7 ml and tablespoons may vary from 13.4 to 27.2 ml. In pharmaceutical practice the teaspoonful and tablespoonful should be taken to be 4 ml and 15 ml, respectively. It is the duty of the pharmacist to educate the general public regarding the use of calibrated spoons for the measurement of medicinal preparations. As such the manufacturers usually supply calibrated spoons along with the packages and therefore the use of household spoons must be discouraged.

Following points must be borne in mind to avoid confusion and to facilitate memorizing:

1. The pharmacist uses avoirdupois system of weights (1 oz = 437.5grains) to buy and sell merchandise other than on prescription.

2. The pharmacist uses apothecary system of weights (1 oz = 480 grains) to dispense prescriptions and compound formulae.

3. The term 'ounce' or its abbreviation 'oz' means an Avoirdupois ounce. The avoirdupois ounce (abbreviated as oz) is 42.5 grains lighter than apothecary ounce.

4. The Apothecary or Troy pound is not used in pharmacy.

5. One pound avoirdupois (lb) (7000 grain) is heavier than one pound apothecary (lb apoth) (5760 grain) by 1240 grain.

6. The avoirdupois and apothecary grain are exactly equal (both abbreviated as gr).

7. The abbreviations for apothecary system are represented by the signs as mentioned in table.

8. Measures of volume in apothecary and avoirdupois systems are same and hence differ from US measures of volume.

9. The US fluid ounce or minim equals 1.04 imperial fluid ounce or minim, respectively.

10. The US gallon contains 128 fl oz whereas the imperial gallon contains 160 fl oz.

11. The US pint weighs 1.04 avoirdupois pound.

12. The apothecary fluid ounce weighs 453.6 grains while imperial fluid ounce weighs 437.5 grains at 25°C and 15.6°C, respectively.

13. The standard of capacity is the litre which is the volume of 1 kg of distilled water at its maximum density (approximately 4°C). A millilitre is the volume occupied by 1 g of water at 4°C whereas a cc is the volume occupied by a cubic each side of which is 1 cm in length. Actually 1 cc = 0.99984 ml.

14. The denomination scruple exists only in the Apothecaries system and there is no counterpart in the Avoirdupois system.

15. Drachm and dram should not be confused. Dram is 1/16 of the Avoirdupois ounce and is equivalent to 27.34375 grains whereas a drachm contains 60 grains.

16. The unit 'one' is often expresed by the letter. When two or more units are to be used, the first one is expressed as j, e.g. 3ij, 3iij, 3vj.

Practice Exercise

1. Convert the following
   - (a) 205 mg to grain
   - (b) 80 mg to grain
   - (c) 2.5 gram to grain
   - (d) 25 pounds to gram
   - (e) pounds to kg

2. Convert the following
   - (a) 2.5 scruple to grain
   - (b) 5 dram to scruple
   - (c) 32 dram to ounce
   - (d) 2.5 pound to ounce
   - (e) 60 grains to scruple

3. Fill in the blank –
   - (a) gr i = ______ mg
   - (b) 1 gal = ______ ml
   - (c) 1 oz = ______ g
   - (d) 1 kg = ______ lbs
   - (e) 1 pint (pt) = ______ ml
   - (f) fl oz I = ______ ml
   - (g) 1 lb = ______ g
   - (h) 1 qt = ______ ml
   - (i) 1 oz = ______ gr
   - (j) 1 g = ______ gr
   - (k) 1 (teaspoonful) tsp = ______ ml

4. Convert the following
   - (a) 1750 grains to ounce
   - (b) 2.5 kg to pound
   - (c) 26 gram to grain
   - (d) 155.5 gram to ounce
   - (e) 66 ounce to pound

5. Convert the following

    (a)   24 ml to fluid drachm   (b)   50 ml to minim

    (c)   352 fluid ounce to liter   (d)   2841 millilitre to fluid ounce

    (e)   185.9 millilitre to minim

6. Convert 1 gallon, 1 pint and 2 fluid ounce to ml.

7. A specific gravity bottle filled with water weighed 121.0 g, when 12.0 g of an insoluble powder was introduced and then filled with water the sp. gr. Bottle weighed 123.0 g. The weight of empty bottle is 21.0 g. Calculate the sp. gr. of the powder

8. What is the capacity in litres of a cylindrical percolator that is 3 feet high and 0.5 feet in diameter? (Capacity of a cylindrical percolator = $\pi\, r^2\, h$).

9. The dose of a liquid is 10 minims. How many doses are contained in 4 fl.oz. of the liquid?

10. 308 tablets each containing 1/2gr of a drug are to be prepared. How many gram of the drug will be required?

11. If a 3 feet deep, 6 feet long and 4 feet wide tank is filled with a liquid preparation, how many 2 oz. bottles can be filled out of it?

12. How many grains of a chemical are left in a bottle after 3ii are dispensed from it?

13. A pharmacist prepared 5000 tablets each containing 1/200 grain of a drug. How many grains of the chemical are left if the pharmacist started with 1/4 oz. of the drug?

14. A solution has been prepared by dissolving 32 grains of a drug in 1 fl oz. How many grains of the drug are contained in 200 mL of the solution?

15. A tank is 6 ft long, 4 ft wide and 2 ft deep and is filled with a cough syrup. How many 4 oz. bottles can be filled out of it?

16. Tetracycline suspension contains 250 mg of tetracycline per five cc's. How much of the suspension would be required to give a patient 125 mg of tetracycline? Give the answer in household equivalents.

17. Pyrantel pamoate is given as treatment for roundworms in a single dose of 1 ml for 10 pounds of body weight. What would be the dose in milliliters for a 44 lb child?

18. Meperidine hydrochloride injection contains 50 milligrams of meperidine HCl per milliliter of injection. How many milliliters must be administered to give a patient 75 milligrams of the drug?

19. Calculate the number of 1/2 grain phenobarbital capsules that can be made from 4 ounces of phenobarbital.

20. To lower a patient's elevated blood pressure, a physician has prescribed 500 mg of methyldopa to be taken each day. Tablets are supplied in 250-mg. How many tablets must be dispensed to give the patient a 30 day regimen?

21. How many 30-mg doses can be made from one ounce of a drug?

Answers

1. (a) 3.416 gr.   (b) 3.0 g   (c) 37.5 gr.   (d) 11339.75 g
   (e) 2.26795 kg
2. (a) 50 g   (b) 15 scruple   (c) 4 ounce   (d) 30 ounce
   (e) 3 scruple
3. (a) 65   (b) 3785   (c) 28.4   (d) 2.2
   (e) 473   (f) 30   (g) 454   (h) 946
   (i) 437.5   (j) 15.432   (k) 4 or 5
4. (a) 4   (b) 5.5   (c) 401.23   (d) 5.485
   (e) 5.5
5. (a) 6.76   (b) 845   (c) 10   (d) 100
   (e) 11
6. 5176.62 ml (1 one fl oz = 28.41 ml)
7. 1.2   **8.** 16.72 litres   **9.** 24 doses   **10.** 10.0 g
11. 8976 bottles   **12.** 317.5 grains   **13.** 84.4 grains   **14.** 14.2 grains
15. 11965 bottles   **16.** 1/2 teaspoonful   **17.** 4.4 ml   **18.** 1.5 ml
19. 3484   **20.** 60 tablets   **21.** 945 doses

Percentage Solution

Percentage rate per hundred is a convenient means of expression of the concentration of a solute in solution or amount of a potent drug in a dosage form or the quantity of an ingredient in a mixture. The common types of percent solutions or mixtures in Pharmacy are classified as follows-

1.   Percentage of solid in liquid usually expressed as % *w/v*
2.   Percentage of solid in solid usually expressed as   % *w/v*
3.   Percentage of liquid in solid usually expressed as % *v/w*
4.   Percentage of liquid in liquid usually expressed as % *v/w*
5.   Miscellaneous mixtures

Percentage of solid in liquid

The true percentage of solid in liquid is expressed as weight in weight e.g., 10% solution of sugar in water means 10 g of sugar dissolved in sufficient water to make up 100 g of solution or 10 grains of solution dissolved in sufficient water to make up 100 grains of solution.

In this type where the percentage strength is expressed as weight by weight (W/W) the solutions are to be done by weighing solids and liquids. It is not easy to weigh the liquids. It is also necessary to take into consideration the specific gravity of the solvent and the final solution when finding the amount of a substance in equal volume of two solutions of the same substance.

Useful Tips

1 fl oz of 1% *w/v* solution requires 4.375 grains of solute

1 pint of 1% *w/v* solution requires 87.5 grains of solute

1quart of 1% *w/v* solution requires 175 grains of solute

1 gallon of 1% *w/v* solution requires 700 grains of solute.

1 pound = 16 ounce

1 fl oz = 8 fl drachm

1 pint (568 ml)=20 fl oz

1 quart = 40 fl oz or 2 pint

1 gallon =160 fl oz or 8 pint or 4 quart

1 pound = 453.59 grams

Practice Exercise

1. How many grams of glucose will be required to prepare 10 litre of 2.5% *w/v* solution?
2. How many 5 grains tablet would be required to prepare 5 gallons of 2.5% *w/v* solution?
3. Calculate the amount of potassium permanganate to prepare 5 litres of 1 in 4000 solution.
4. How many grams of a drug are required to make 3 L of a 1 in 500 solution?
5. How many grains of glucose are required to make 6 fl oz of 0.4% w/v solution?
6. A mixture contains 2% boric acid and 1 in 2000 mercuric chloride. How many grains of each are contained in 4 fl oz?
7. How many grains of a substance should be dissolved to make 6 fl oz of a solution so that one fl dr. of it when diluted to a pint gives 1 in 4000 solution?
8. Calculate the weight of nux vomica seeds containing 1 % strychnine required to prepare 10 gallons liquid extract containing 1.5% strychnine.
9. How many g of a drug are required to make 8 L of a 1 in 500 solution?
10. How many grains of Pot. Permanganate are required to make 8 fl oz of a solution so that 2 fl dr when diluted to a quart makes a 1 in 500 solution?
11. How many ml of a 0.1% *w/v* solution of mercury bichloride can be prepared from 50 tablets each containing 0.47 g. of the drug
12. Fifty fl oz solutions have been prepared by dissolving 75 grains of scopolamine hydrochloride. What is the % *w/v* strength of this solution?
13. How many 5 grains tablets would be required to prepare 10 gallons of 5% *w/v* solution?
14. Calculate the % *w/v* strength of a solution prepared by dissolving 0.5 lb. of a salt in sufficient water to make one pint.
15. A sunsceen lotion contains 5% *v/v* of methyl salicylate. How many ml of methyl salicylate should be used to prepare 3 pints of the solution.

16. A pharmacist has in stock 200 grains of bichloride of mercury. How many ml of a 0.25% *w/v* solution of bichloride of mecury can the pharmacist prepare from his stock?

17. An inhalation aerosol contains 0.25% *w/v* of isoproterenol hydrochloride. If each actuation of the aerosol valve delivery 0.12 mg of the drug. How many doses are contained in a 28 ml aerosol package?

18. How many grains of a substance should be dissolved to make 8 fl oz. of a solution so that 1 fl dr. of it when diluted to a pint gives 1 in 2000 solution?

19. 850 g of sucrose are dissolved in sufficient water to make 1000 ml of syrup having sp. gr. of 1.313. Calculate the % *w/v* strength of the syrup.

20. An ophthalmic ointment contains 2 mg/10 g of mercury bichloride. Calculate the % w/v strength of mercury bichloride in the ointment.

21. Syrup is 85% *w/v* solution of sucrose in water and has specific gravity of 1.3131 g/ml. How many ml of water should be used to prepare 500 ml of syrup?

22. Ten pound of a cosmetic cream is to be preserved using a 0.04% mixture of methyl paraben (70 parts) and propyl paraben (30 parts). Calculate the quantities in grams of methyl and propyl parabens required.

23. How much 95 % alcohol is required to prepare 10 L of 70% alcohol?

24. How many grams of crystal violet should be used in preparing 5 gallons of a 0.025% *w/v* solution?

25. How many grains of gentian violet should be used in preparing of 8 fl oz of a 0.25% *w/v* solution

26. A pharmacist has to dispense 450 g of a 15 % *w/w* solution of zinc sulphate. How many grams of zinc sulphate should be used?

27. How many lit. of 2% solution can be made from 4 oz of a solid?

28. How many Lt. of 0.9% solution can be prepared from 500 g of sodium chloride?

29. How many grams of drug are needed to make 5 L of a 1 in 500 solution?

30. How much of a drug is required to make 2 quart of a 1 in 1200 solution?

31. How much solute is required to prepare 12 oz of a solution so that 3 teaspoonfuls to a quart will make 1/8% solution?

32. How much solute is required to prepare 8 oz. of a solution so that 1 tablespoon to half a gallon will make a 1 in 500 solution?

33. How much solute is required to make 4 oz. of solution so that 2 teaspoonfuls diluted to a pint will make a 1 in 1000 solution.

34. Rx

    Pot. permanganate : 3.0 g

    Distilled water 120.0 ml

    Sig. Dilute 2 teaspoonful to one quart calculate the % strength of the dilution

    How many grains of $KMnO_4$ are required?

Answers

1.	250 g	**2.**	1750 tablets	**3.**	1.25 g
4.	6.0 g	**5.**	10.5 gr	**6.**	35 gr and 0.88 gr
7.	105 gr	**8.**	150 lbs.	**9.**	16.0 g.
10.	1120 gr	**11.**	23500 ml	**12.**	33.33%
13.	7000	**14.**	48% w/v	**15.**	85.2 ml
16.	5184 ml	**17.**	583 doses	**18.**	280 gr
19.	64.7%	**20.**	0.02%	**21.**	231.5 ml
22.	Methyl para 12.5 g, Propyl Para 5.475 g.	**23.**	8.4211		
24.	5.67g	**25.**	8.7 gr	**26.**	67.5 g
27.	5.67 L	**28.**	5.5 L	**29.**	10 g
30.	1.59 g	**31.**	700 gr	**32.**	1120 gr
33.	140 gr	**34.**	700 gr		

Proof Spirit

Alcohol is an excellent solvent. It is used for many purposes in pharmaceutical practice and in formulation of cosmetic etc. In the United States Pharmacopoeia, all alcohol concentrations are expressed as volume-in-volume, based on the quantity of absolute alcohol present, as determined at 15.56 °C. Proof spirit was official in B.P. 1885. London Proof spirit mean that mixture of ethyl alcohol and water which weighs exactly $12/13^{th}$ part of an equal volume of distilled water at 51°F. Proof spirit has a sp. gr. of 091976 at 15.5 °C and contains 57.1% *V/V* of ethyl alcohol to 100 volume of proof spirit.

Proof spirit is therefore an aqueous solution containing 57.1% *v/v* of absolute alcohol. Any alcohol solution, which contains 57.1% v/v alcohol, is a proof spirit and it is said to be 100^0 Proof.

Over proof (°O/P) means strength of alcohol above the proof strength.

Under proof (°U/P) means strength of alcohol below proof strength.

Thus 25 (°U/P) mean that 100 volume of such alcohol are equivalent to 100-25 = 75 volume of proof sprit. 35 (°O/P) mean that 100 volume of such alcohol are equivalent to $100 + 35 = 135$ volume of proof spirit.

In India the rates of excise duty are prescribed in terms of rupees per litre of proof alcohol.

Example : Convert 90% V/V alcohol into proof spirit.

As 57.1 volume of ethyl alcohol = 100 volume of proof spirit

1 volume of ethyl alcohol = 100/57.1 = 1.7513 volume of proof spirit

90 volume of ethyl alcohol = 90 X 1.7513 volume of proof spirit

Hence Proof strength of 90% *v/v* alcohol = (90 X 1.7513) – 100 = 57.6°O/P

Similarly Proof strength of 30% v/v alcohol can be calculated as follows.

Proof strength of 30% V/V alcohol = (30 X 1.7513) – 100 = -47.5 or 47.5°U/P

Thus 70 °O/P = 100 + 70 / 1.7513 = 97% *v/v* of ethyl alcohol, and

70 °U/P = 100 - 70 / 1.7513 = 17.13% *v/v* of ethyl alcohol.

Practice Exercises

1. Convert the following degrees of Proof into percentage strength of ethyl alcohol by volume?

    (a)   12.1(°U/P)   (b)   17.1 (°U/P)   (c)   21.5 (°U/P)

    (d)   54.8 (°U/P)   (e)   75.0 (°U/P)

2. Convert the following degrees of Proof into percentage strength of ethyl alcohol by volume?

    (a)   44.6 (°O/P)   (b)   44.0 (°O/P)   (c)   35.3 (°O/P)

    (d)   24.0 (°O/P)   (e)   18.4 (°O/P)

3. How many proof gallons are contained in 5 gallons of 70% of ethyl alcohol?

4. How many gallons of 20 % *v/v* of ethyl alcohol would be equivalent to 20 proof gallons?

5. On the first of Dec. 1997 a hospital pharmacist had on hand a drum containing 54 gallons of 95 % alcohol. During the month he used the following amount

    (a)   10 gallons in the manufacture of bathing solution

    (b)   b. 15 gallons in the manufacture of soap solution

    (c)   8 gallons in the manufacture of medicated alcohol and at the end of month.

    (d)   How many proof gallons of alcohol did he have on hand?

6. On the first day of the month a hospital pharmacist had two drums (108 gallons) of 95 % alcohol and 10 pints of absolute alcohol (100%) on hand. During the month he prepared 25 gallons of 70% *v/v* of ethyl alcohol and .25 gallons of 50% *v/v* alcohol. He also dispensed two pints of absolute alcohol. How many proof gallons of alcohol did he have on hand at the end of the month?

7. How many proof gallons are represented by 50 wine gallons of 90% *v/v* alcohol?

8. 20 gallons of 70% *v/v* alcohol and 30 gallons of 50 % *v/v* alcohols were mixed. Calculate the proof strength in the mixture.

9. Five gallon proof spirit was diluted with two gallons of water. Calculate the alcoholic strength of the mixture

10. An alcoholic inventory shows 30 gallons of 95% and 7.5 pints of absolute (100%) alcohol. How many proof gallons of alcohol are represented in the inventory?

11. In what proportion should 95% and 25% alcohol be mixed to prepare 70 litre of 40 (°U/P) alcohol?

12. If the excise duty payable on spirit is Rs. 3.85 per LP gallon, calculate the duty to be paid on 25 gallons of rectified spirit containing 90% *v/v* alcohols

13. On a purchase of 10 gallons of rectified spirit containing 94% alcohol, hjgh a manufacturer paid Rs. 288 as excise duty. Calculate the rate of excise duty per Proof Litre

Answers

1. (a)   50.14%   (b)   47.29%   (c)   44.78%   (d)   25.78%
   (e)   14.26%

2. (a)   82.49%   (b)   82.14 %   (c)   77.18%   (d)   70.73 %
   (e)   67.54%

3.   6.13 gallons   4.   57.1 gallons   5.   34.39

6.   128.9 proof gallons   7.   28.8 Pg   8.   50.78 %

9.   40.78 %   10.   51.5 proof gallons

11.   95% -9.22 lt., 25% alcohol-60.78 lt   12.   Rs.727.65   13.   Rs. 3.85

Reducing and Enlarging Recipes

It is common practice to reduce a recipe for dispensing or enlarge the recipe as required for the purpose of patient. This is required when a manufacturing formula is to be taken from the laboratory scale to a manufacturing floor and a formula for the large scale manufacturing is to be adopted for prescribing to a patient. Such calculations may also involve conversions from one system of weights and measures to another.

The following rules are generally useful in such system

Rule 1. To convert a recipe in imperial system to metric system

"Write grams in place of grains, divide the minims by 1.1 and write the result as milliliters. For large batch, read avoirdupois ounce as grams and fluid ounces as milliliters"

Rule 2. To convert a recipe in metric system to imperial system

"For a small batch write grains in place of grams and multiply the milliliters by 1.1 and write the result as minims. For large batch, write ounce in place of grams and fluid ounce in place of minims"

Example 4.1

Rx

Sodium hypophosphite	gr. xx
Sulphuric acid	fl dr. I
Cinnamon water q.s. ad	fl.oz. ii
Dispense	50 ml

Calculation : Convert to metric system

Sodium hypophosphite 20 g. = 20 × 50/872.7 = 1.15 g

Sulphuric acid 60/1.1 = 55.5 ml = 55.45 × 50 / 872.7 = 3.2 ml

Cinnamon water q.s. ad 2 × 480/1.1 = 872.5 ml = 50 ml

Dispense 50 ml

However, the simpler solution of the problem would be to retain the original recipe and prepare 2 fl. oz. of the mixture, which corresponds to about 60 ml. Out of 2fl.oz, 60 ml, could be dispensed and the rest rejected.

Example 4.2

Rx

Pt. Nitrate	
Sod. Chloride	
Camphor of each	3 g
Tincture opium	15 ml
Alcohol to make	200 ml
Dispense	4 fl.oz.

Solution

4 fl oz of the prescription is to be dispensed hence quantities can be converted to Imperial system.

R

Pt. Nitrate	
Sod. Chloride	
Camphor each 3 grains	

Tincture opium = 15 × 1.1 = 16.5 minims

Alcohol = 200 × 1.1 = 220 minims

4 × 480 = 1920 minims

Quantity of Pt. Nitrate, Sod. Chloride and Camphor = 3 × 1920/220 =26.2 grains

So to avoid this we can prepare 9 times the formula1980 minims and dispense 4 fl.oz and reject 60 minims

Example 4.3

Calculate the amounts of ingredients required to make 50 ml of calamine lotion.

Rx

Calamine	150 g
Zinc oxide	50 g
Bentonite	30 g
Sodium Citrate	5 g
Liquefied Phenol	5 ml
Purified water, q.s.	1000 ml

Dispense 50 ml.

Solution

Formula is to be reduced by $50/1000 = 1/20$, hence each quantity is to be multiplied by $1/20$

Thus the calculated quantities of the ingredients will be –

Ingredient	Quantity for 50 ml
Calamine	150 g × 1/20 = 12.5 g
Zinc oxide	50 g × 1/20 = 2.5 g
Bentonite	30 g × 1/20 = 1.5 g
Sodium Citrate	5 g × 1/20 = 0.25 g
Liquefied Phenol	5 ml × 1/20 = 0.25 ml
Purified water, q.s. 1000 ml	1000 ml 1/20 = 20 ml

Practice Exercises

1. Calculate the quantity for making 50 ml of the given formula.

    Rx

Opium tincture	50 ml
Benzoic acid	5 g
Camphor	3 g
Anise Oil	3 ml
Alcohol (60%) q.s.	100 ml

2. How many grams of each ingredient are required to make 100 ml of lotion?

    Rx

Calamine	150 g
Zinc oxide	50 g

Bentonite	30 g
Sodium citrate	5 g
Liquefied phenol	5 ml
Purified water q.s.	1000 ml

3. Calculate the quantity of each ingredient required to prepare 1 ounce of the ointment.

   Rx

Benzoic acid	6 parts
Salicylic acid	3 parts
PEG ointment	91 parts

4. An antihistamine tablet contains the following ingredients. How many grains of each ingredient are required to prepare a batch of 2.5 million tablets?

   Rx

Reserpine	100 mcg
Hydralazine hydrochloride	25 mcg
Hydrochlorthiazide	15 mg

   A mixture contains 7.5 g of a drug per 100 ml. How many pounds of the drug will be required to make 5 gallons of the mixture?

5. From the following formula, calculate the quantity of each ingredient required to make 8 litres of the lotion

   Rx

Witch Hazel	4 parts
Glycerine	1 parts
Boric acid solution	15 parts

6. Calculate the quantities of each ingredient needed to make 2 lb of the mixture from the following formula:

   Rx

Potassium citrate	30.0 g
Hyoscyamine tincture	30.0 ml
Tween 20	0.4 ml
Distilled water q.s.	

7. A formula for 1000 capsules contains 5.0 g of amphetamine, 325 g of thyroid, 1 g of thiamine hydrochloride, 40 g of Phenobarbital, and enough lactose to make 500g. How much of each ingredient should be used in preparing 76 capsules?

8. Prepare 2 pints of the mixture

    Rx

Zinc oxide	2 g
Talc	2 g
Milk of Magnesia	3 ml
Bentonite magma	5 ml
Lime water qs ad	16 ml

9. What quantities will be required for 8 fl oz of the following recipe?

    Rx

Glycerine	25%
Zinc oxide	25%
Lanolin	50%

10. From the following formula, calculate the quantity of each ingredient that should be used in preparing 10 lb of the ointment base.

    Rx

Stearic acid	14 g
Triethanolamine	1 g
Cetyl alcohol	4 g
Glycerine	8 g
Water	63 g

11. From the following quantities to make 6 fl oz. Of an infusion of digitalis form the following preparation.

    Rx

Powdered digitalis	15 g
Alcohol	100 ml
Cinnamon water	150 ml
Boiling water	7000 ml
Cold water, to make	1000 ml

12. From the following formula, calculate the quantity of each ingredient required to make 10 lb of the powder.

    Rx

Bismuth subcarbonate	8 parts
Kaolin	15 parts
Magnesium oxide	2 parts

13. Calculate the quantity of each ingredient to make 500 ml.

    Rx

Boric acid	3.5
Sodium chloride	5.0
Glycerin	3.0
Camphor water	13.0
Purified water	75.5

14. Calculate the quantity of each ingredient required to make 25 ml of the following recipe.

    Rx

Ammonium bicarbonate	25.0 g
Strong ammonia solution	67.5 ml
Lemon oil	0.5 ml
Nutmeg oil	0.3 ml
Alcohol (90%)	37.5 ml
Purified water q.s.	1000.0 ml

Answers

1. Opium tincture – 25 ml, Benzoic acid – 2.5 g, Camphor- 1.5 g Anise Oil –1.5 ml Alcohol (60%) q.s. 50 ml.

2. Calamine -15 g, Zinc oxide- 5 g, Bentonite-3.0 g, Sodium citrate- 2.5 g. Liquefied phenol-2.5 ml, Purified water q.s. 100 ml.

3. Benzoic acid-300 g, Salicylic acid-150 g, PEG ointment –4550 g.

4. Reserpine-225 g, Hydralazine hydrochloride –62.5 g, Hydrochlorthiazide –37.5 kg. 0.75 lbs.

5. Witch Hazel-1.6 pint, Glycerine – 1 parts, Boric acid solution- 6 pint.

6. Potassium citrate- 9.6 oz, Hyoscyamine tincture-9.6 oz, Tween –1 fl oz, Distilled water to make 2 lb.

7. Amphetamine-0.38 g, thyroid-24.5 g, thiamine hydrochloride-0.76 g, Phenobarbital- 3.04 g, lactose-38 g.

8. Zinc oxide – 118.28 g, Talc – 118.2 g , Milk of Magnesia-177.42 ml, Bentonite magma-295.70 ml, Lime water – 2 pint.

9. Glycerine- 2 fl oz, Zinc oxide- 2 oz, Lanolin-4 oz.

10. Stearic acid-706 g, Triethanolamine-50 g, Cetyl alcohol-202 g, Glycerine-404 g Water-3178 g.

11. Powdered digitalis-39.5 gr, Alcohol- 4fl dr 48minims, Cinnamon water-7 fl dr 12 minims, Boiling water -4 fl oz 1 fl dr 36 minims, Cold water-6 fl oz.

12. Bismuth subcarbonate-1.4528 kg, Kaolin-2.724 kg, Magnesium oxide-363.2 g.

13. Boric acid-17.5, Sodium chloride-25.0, Glycerin-15.0, Camphor water-65.0 Purified water –377.5.

14. Ammonium bicarbonate-0.625 g, Strong ammonia solution-1.6875 ml, Lemon oil-0.0125 ml, Nutmeg oil-0.0075 ml, Alcohol (90%)-0.9375 ml, Purified water q.s.25 ml

Alligation

Alligation is a rapid arithmetic method used to solve problems that involve mixing two products of different strengths to form a product having a desired intermediate strength. The term alligation has its origin in Latin, *alligatio* which means the art of attaching and therefore refers to lines drawn during calculation to bind quantities together.

Alligation medial is used in calculating the strength of the mixture of two or more components of different strengths. It gives the weighed average percentage strength of a mixture resulting from components of known quantities and concentration.

Alligation method is used to calculate:

(a) The amount of diluent that must be added to a given amount of higher strength preparation to make a desired lower strength.

(a) The amounts of active ingredient that must be added to a given amount of lower strength preparation to make a higher strength.

(a) The amount of higher and lower strength preparations that must be combined to make a desired amount of an intermediate strength.

It is often more practical to dilute a known strength preparation than it would be to compound an entire preparation. Sometimes, a simple calculation using alligation allows us to calculate the amount of diluent to be added to an already prepared higher strength preparation to form the strength desired.

Sometimes, it is necessary to increase the strength of a preparation by adding an active ingredient for example if 1% coal tar ointment is available and required strength is 2 %, it can be accomplished by adding an unknown amount of coal tar (100 percent).The unknown amount may be found by using alligation method.

Procedure of Calculation

(a) Draw a problem matrix

(a) Insert quantities as shown

(a) Subtract along the diagonals

(a) Read along the horizontals

The desired strength always goes in the center square of the matrix. The desired strength is the strength of the preparation that one wishes to make.

Example : In what proportions should a preparation containing 15% of drug be mixed with one containing 30% of drug to prepare a mixture of 20% strength.

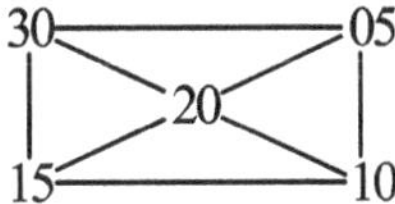

Thus 5 parts of 30% and 10 parts of 15% drug mixed together will give a mixture of 20% drug strength.

Proof of Alligation Method

Suppose a product of X percentage strength is to be prepared by mixing constituents of percentage Y (Higher) and Z (lower).

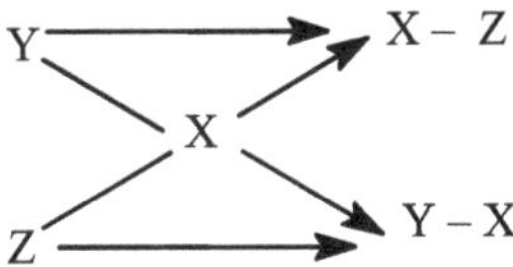

Hence desired percentage strength of X can be obtained by mixing together (X- Z) parts of Y and (Y-X) parts of Z

$$(X–Z) \times Y + (Y–X) \times Z = [(X–Z) + (Y–X)] \times X$$

Solving the equation

$$X Y – Z Y + Y Z – X Z = [X–Z + Y–X] \times X$$

$$X Y – X Z = [Y – Z] \times X = X Y – X Z$$

This equation proves the line diagram method of alligation is correct and most suitable in such calculation

Example 1

What is the % of alcohol in a mixture obtained by mixing 5 L of 25%, 1L of 50% and 2 L of 95% alcohol?

Solution

$$(1 \text{ Litre} = 1000 \text{ ml})$$

$$5000 \text{ ml} \times 25\% = 1250$$

$$1000 \text{ ml} \times 50\% = 500$$

$$2000 \text{ ml} \times 95\% = 1900$$

8000 ml	3650

$$3650 \ : \ 8000 : : X \ \times 100$$

$$X = \frac{3650}{8000} \times 100 = 45.6\%$$

Final mixture concentration = 45.6%

Example 2

What is the strength of zinc oxide in an ointment prepared by mixing 400 g of 10%, 100 g of 20% and 50 g of 5% ointment?

$$400 \text{ g} \times 10\% = \ 40$$

$$100 \text{ g} \times 20\% = \ 20$$

$$\underline{50 \text{ g} \times 5\% = 2.5}$$

$$\underline{550 \text{ ml}} \qquad \underline{62.50}$$

$$62.50 \ : \ 550 : : X \ \times 100$$

$$X = \frac{62.50}{550} \times 100 = 11.36\%$$

Final mixture concentration = 45.6%

Example 3

How many parts of 70%, 60% 40% and 30% alcohol should be mixed to get 50% alcohol.

Calculation

<table>
<tr><td>70</td><td></td><td>20</td><td></td><td>70</td><td></td><td>10</td></tr>
<tr><td>60</td><td></td><td>10</td><td>or</td><td>60</td><td></td><td>2(</td></tr>
<tr><td></td><td>50</td><td></td><td></td><td></td><td>50</td><td></td></tr>
<tr><td>40</td><td></td><td>10</td><td></td><td>40</td><td></td><td>20</td></tr>
<tr><td>30</td><td></td><td>20</td><td></td><td>30</td><td></td><td>10</td></tr>
</table>

Answer

20:10:10:20 or 10:20:20:10

Example 4

In what proportion should 12%, 8% and 3% alcohol be mixed to get 5% alcohol?

Solution

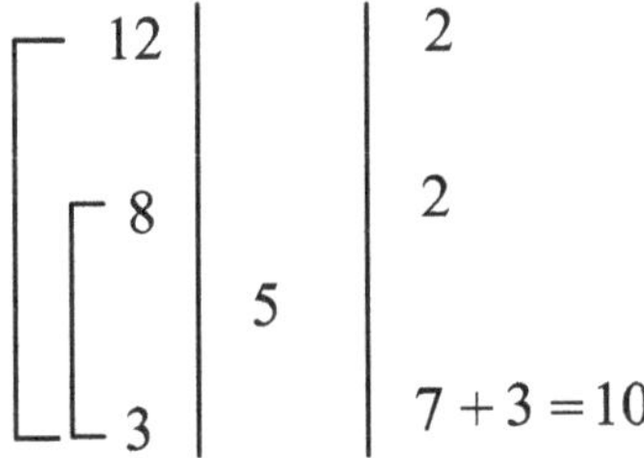

Answer

2 : 2 : 10 (1:1:5)

Practice Exercises

1. What is the percentage of borax in an ointment prepared by mixing 50 grams of 5% ointment 100 grams of 15% ointment and 300 grams of 8% ointment?

2. 500 ml each of 20% dextrose and 50% dextrose solutions are mixed. Calculate the strength of the mixture.

3. In what proportion of alcohol 70% and 40% should be mixed to get 50% alcohol?

4. In what proportion 10%, 6% and 3% alcohol be mixed to make 5% alcohol?

5. 400 g of 20%, 240 g of 43% and 350 g of 66% sulfuric acid are mixed. How much water should be added to make a 10% solution of sulfuric acid?

6. How many parts of 80%, 60%, 40% and 30% alcohol be mixed together to get 50% alcohol?

7. How many ml of water should be mixed with 30 gm. of 40% w/w Sulphuric acid and 50 gm. of 60% w/w sulfuric acid to make 10% w/w acid?

8. How many g. of strong ammonia sp. gr. 0.880 be added to 40 g. of ammonia water sp. gr. 0.97 and 35 g. of ammonia water sp. gr. 0.98 so that the mixture may have sp. gr. 0.95?

9. One pound of a concentrated acid of sp. Gr. is overdiluted with twice its volume of water. What volume of additional acid must be added to yield an acid with sp. Gr. 1.3?

10. How much water has to be added to 700 ml of 92%, 850 ml of 86% and 600 ml of 26% alcohol to bring the strength of the mixture down to 20%?

11. Find out the quantity of pure silver nitrate to be added to a mixture of 125 g. of 8% and 75 g. of 6 % silver nitrate solution so as to make 10% solution.

12. One pound of concentrated acid with sp. gr. 1.62 in over diluted with twice its volume of water. What volume of additional acid must be added to yield an acid with sp. gr. 1.3?

Answers

1.	9.21%	**2.**	35%
3.	10 parts of 70% and 20 parts of 40% (1:2)	**4.**	Proportion 2:2:6 or 1:1:3
5.	3152 g	**6.**	10:20:30:10 or 20:10:10:30
7.	340 ml	**8.** 25.7 grams	**9.**	0.9375 lb
10.	5504 ml	**11.** 6.11 g	**12.**	0.9375 lb.

Isotonic Solutions

Solutions of drugs administered by parenteral and ophthalmic routes enter into the respective body fluids i.e. blood and tears or lachrymal fluid. Hence these solutions must be physiologically acceptable. The greatest determinant of this physiological acceptability is osmotic pressure. Thus a drug solution having osmotic pressure equal to that of blood will be physiologically acceptable. Similarly, a drug solution having the osmotic pressure matching with the lachrymal secretion will also be physiologically acceptable. If the properties of drug solution are not matched with the body fluid in solution, the irritation and cell destruction may occur.

Osmotic pressure and freezing point depression are the colligative properties i.e., they depend on the number of solute particles in the solution irrespective of whether these are large or small or ions or molecules.

Two solutions having the same osmotic pressure are called *iso-osmotic* or *isotonic*. Solutions which do not have the same osmotic pressure are called paratonic. Paratonic solutions can be either hypertonic or hypotonic. *Hypertonic* solutions contain more quantity whereas *hypotonic* solutions contain less quantity of solute(s) than required for making them isotonic. Generally a pharmacist receives prescriptions for isotonic solutions but rarely he may also have to deal with a paratonic prescription. Intravenous solutions should be isotonic with blood while ophthalmic solutions should be isotonic with tears, Blood serum and tears have the same osmotic pressure.

The osmotic pressure of a 1.8% solution of urea and 0.9% sodium chloride solution are same as that of body fluids including blood and lachrymal fluid. Thus 0.9% sodium chloride solution is isotonic with physiological fluids. Isotonic and iso-osmotic are not necessarily equivalent. It is possible that an iso-osmotic solution may cause hydrolysis of RBCs upon injection. This happens because the solutes diffuse through the membranes of the cells.

Adjustment of tonicity calls for the addition of some inert material compatible with drug substance. In practice the following methods are used for calculation of isotonicity.

Methods for Calculating Isotonicity

1. *Freezing Point Method :* The lachrymal secretion contains several solutes in it and has a freezing point of -0.52°C. All solutions, which freeze at -0.52°C, will be isotonic with the

lachrymal fluid. Human blood plasma also freezes at this temperature and hence solutions having freezing point at –0.52^{0}C will be isotonic with blood plasma as well. Adjustment of tonicity is simplified if the freezing points of the medicament and the inert salt (adjusting substance) are known for various strengths of their solutions. Freezing points are usually expressed in terms of 1% solutions and one can calculate the quantity by multiplying the freezing point with the factor.

The following, equation is useful :

Freezing point of tear secretion

or human Blood plasma $\quad = \quad$ Freezing point of drug + freezing point of the adjusting substance

Therefore the amount of adjusting substance required may be calculated from the equation

$$W = \frac{0.52 - a}{b}$$

where

W $=$ the weight, in g, of the added substance in 100 mL of the final solution;

a $=$ the depression of the freezing point produced by the medicament already present in solution, calculated by multiplying the value for the medicament by the strength of the solution expressed as a percentage w/v; and

b $=$ the depression of the freezing point of water produced by 1% of the adjusting substance.

Example 1

Two hundred ml of an eyewash containing 1% boric acid are to be dispensed.

(F.P. of 1% boric acid at $-$ 0.29°C and F.P. of 1% solution of sodium chloride $= -$ 0.58°C).

Applying the above equation-

$$W = \frac{0.52 - 0.29}{0.58} = 0.39 \text{ g/100 ml or } 0.39\%$$

Thus the working formula for for 200 mL of the eyewash will be:

Boric acid (1%, for 200 mL) = 1 g × 2 = 2 g.

Sodium chloride (0.39%, for 200 mL) = 0.39 × 2 = 0.78 g.

Purified water q.s. 200 mL.

Answer

However if the pharmacist has been asked to supply 200 ml of eyewash of boric acid', the calculation will be as follows:

Lowering of 0.29°C in F.P. is caused by 1 g of boric acid

Lowering of 0.52°C in F.P. will be caused by

$$\frac{1.0 \times 0.52}{0.29} = 1.8\,g$$

Therefore 1.8 g of boric acid is required to make 100 ml of eyewash and the working formula will be :

Boric acid (1.8%, for 200 ml) = 1.8 × 2 = 3.6 g. Purified water, q.s. 200 mL.

Answer

The freeing points of common substances used for adjusting the isotonicity are given in the following Table 4.2.

Table 4.2 Freezing Points (°C) of 1 % solution of common substances.

Substance	Freezing Point °C
Amethocaine hydrochloride	−0.109
Atropine sulfate	−0.074
Boric acid, Borax	−0.288, 0.241
Calcium chloride (2H$_2$O)	−0.298
Calcium chloride (6H$_2$O)	−0.200
Calcium gluconate	−0.091
Cinchocaine hydrochloride	−0.074
Cocaine hydrochloride	−0.090
Codeine phosphate	−0.080
Copper sulfate	−0.098
Dexamethasone sodium phosphate	−0.095
Emetine hydrochloride	−0.062
Homatropine hydrobromide	−0.096
Pethidine hydrochloride	−0.124
Pilocarpine hydrochloride	−0.134
Pilocarpine nitrate	−0.131
Potassium chloride	−0.439
Potassium nitrate	−0.323
Procaine hydrochloride	−0.122
Quinine hydrochloride	−0.077
Silver nitrate	−0.190

Table 4.2 *Contd...*

Substance	Freezing Point °C
Silver protein	−0.047
Sodium benzoate	−0.232
Sodium bicarbonate	−0.381
Sodium chloride	−0.576
Sodium nitrite	−0.481
Sodium sulfate	−0.148
Sulfacetamide sodium	−0.133
Sulfadiazine sodium	−0.137
Thiamine hydrochloride	−0.139
Zinc chloride	−0.354
Zmc sulfate	−0.085

2. *Molecular Weight Method* : Freezing point of a solute depends on the concentration of the solute dissolved therein. Greater the concentration of the solute, lower is the freezing point. In other words it depends on the number of ions (more correctly, the number of effective ions), the weight of the substance and its molecular weight. The concentration for 0.9% solution of sodium chloride can be expressed in the following manner:

$$\frac{g \times n}{m} = \text{Isotonic factor or Isotinicty}$$

Where

g = No. of gram of sodium chloride (g)

n = No. of effective ions (n)

m = molecular weight of sodium chloride (m)

i.e. isotonicity factor for sodium chloride is 0.03.

Since 0.9% solution of sodium chloride (normal saline) is isotonic with body fluids, 0.03 will be the isotonicity or tonicity factor for tear secretion and blood plasma as well. Thus quantities for making eye solutions can be calculated by equating the value of 0.03 with the tonicity contributed by the drug and the additive(s).

The following equation is employed for calculating the quantity of the additive(s):

$$0.03 = \frac{g \times n}{m} + \frac{g_1 \times n_1}{m_1} + \frac{g_2 \times n_2}{m_2}$$

where g, n and m denote the weight in gram, effective ion concentration and molecular weight of the medicament, respectively. Values followed by subscript 1 or 2 in the equation above refer to the first additive or the second additive (if present). Effective ionic concentration can be ascertained from the following generalizations;

$n = 1$ for non-ionisable substances, e.g. dextrose

$n = 1.5$ for partially ionisable solutes in two ions, e.g. silver nitrate

$n = 2$ for highly ionisable solutes in two ions e.g. sodium chloride

$n = 2$ for partially ionisable solutes in three ions, e.g. sodium sulfate

Example 2

Send 100 ml of eye drops of silver nitrate.

Solution :

$$0.03 = \frac{0.03 \times m}{n} = \frac{0.03 \times 169.8}{1.5} = 3.4 \text{ g/100 ml}$$

Answer

Suppose the above exercise were to be read differently, 'supply 100 ml of 1% eye drops of silver nitrate' then the calculation will be as follows:

$$0.03 = \frac{g \times n}{m} + \frac{g_1 \times n_1}{m_1}$$

$$0.03 = \frac{1.0 \times 1.5}{169.8} + \frac{g_1 \times 1.5}{85}$$

$$g_1 = 1.26 \text{ g/100 mL}$$

It may be noted that the substance to be used for rendering the solution isotonic is sodium nitrate because it is compatible with silver nitrate and not sodium chloride which, if added, will result into the precipitation of silver nitrate. Thus for making 100 ml of the eye drop solution containing 1% silver nitrate, the working formula will be:

Silver nitrate	1.00 g
Sodium nitrate	1.26 g
Purified water, q.s. ad	100.0 ml

Whereas it is desirable to make solutions isotonic with lachrymal secretion, it may be remembered that paratonic solutions within the range of 0.7 to 15% of sodium chloride or its equivalent in relation to other substances are easily tolerated by the eye.

3. *Sodium Chloride Equivalent Method :* This is the simplest method and is based on the sodium chloride equivalents of various drugs. Sodium chloride equivalent of a drug represents the amount of sodium chloride equivalent to 1 g of the drug. The method avoids tedious calculation. Sodium chloride equivalents of some common drugs are given in the following table.

Table 4.2 Sodium Chloride Equivalents.

1 g (or grain) of drug	Equivalent g (or grain) of sodium chloride
Adrenaline acid tartrate	0.18
Adrenaline hydrochloride	0.29
Aminophylline	0.17
Ampiciilin sodium	0.16
Atropine sulfate	0.13
Bacitracin	0.05
Borax	0.42
Boric acid	0.50
Calcium chloride ($2H_2O$)	0.51
Calcium chloride ($6H_2O$)	0.35
Cephaloridine	0.07
Cephazoline sodium	0.13
Chloramphenicol	0.10
Chlortetracycline hydrochloride	0.10
Cocaine hydrochloride	0.16
Copper sulfate	0.18
Dexamethasone sodium phosphate	0.17
Emetine hydrochloride	0.10
Ephedrine hydrochloride	0.30
Ephedrine sulfate	0.23
Fluorescein sodium	0.31
Fructose	0.18
Gentamycin sulfate	0.05
Homatropine hydrobromide	0.17
Imipramine hydrochloride	0.20
Kanamycin sulfate	0.07
Lignocaine hydrochloride	0.22
Morphine hydrochloride	0.15
Morphine sulfate	0.14
Neomycin sulfate	0.12
Oxvtetracvcline hydrochloride	0.14
Physostigmine salicylate	0.16

Table 4.2 Contd...

1 g (or grain) of drug	Equivalent g (or grain) of sodium chloride
Physostigmine sulfate	0.13
Pilocarpine hydrochlonde	0.24
Pilocarpine nitrate	0.23
Povidone	0.01
Procaine hydrochlride	0.21
Resorcinol	0.28
Silver nitrate	0.33
Sodium borate	0.42
Sodium chloride	1.00
Streptomycin sulfate	0.07
Sulphacetamide sodium	0.23
Terbutaline sulfate	0.14
Tetracycline hydrochloride	0.14
Timolol maleate	0.13
Urea	0.59
Warfarin sodium	0.17
Zinc chloride	0.61
Zinc sulfate	0.15

It can be memorized that 0.27 g of sodium chloride makes 30 mL of a 0.9% solution and that 4.1 grain of sodium chloride makes 1 fl oz. of a 0.9% solution.

Example 3

Calculate the number of g of sodium chloride, which should be added to 120 mL of 0.5% solution of pilocarpine hydrochloride to make it isotonic.

Solution :

Wt. of pilocarpine hydrochloride contained in the prescription = 120 x 0.5% = 0.6 g

Sodium chloride eq. of pilocarpine hydrochloride = 0.22

Hence the amount of sodium chloride represented by pilocarpine hydrochloride contained in the prescription = 0.6 × 0.22 = 0.132 g.

120 mL of 0.9% sodium chloride would contain 120 × 0.9 = 1.08 g of sodium chloride

This is the amount of sodium chloride required to make 120 mL of isotonic solution in absence of pilocarpine hydrochloride.

Hence the no. of g of sodium chloride required = 1.08 g – 0.132 g = 0.948 g   Answer

Example 4

Calculate the no. of g of sodium chloride needed to render 30 mL of physostigmine salicylate solution isotonic.

Solution:

Wt. of physostigmine salicylate contained in the prescription = 30 x 0.5 = 0.15 g

Sodium chloride eq. of Physostigmine salicylate =0.14

Hence Physostigmine salicylate present in the prescription is equivalent to –

$$0.15 \times 0.14 = 0.0210 \text{ of sodium chloride.}$$

30 mL of a solution containing 0.9% sodium chloride will contain 30 x 0.9% = 0.27 g of sodium chloride if sodium chloride alone were present in the prescription.

No. of g of additional sodium chloride needed =0.27 g - 0.0210 g = 0.2490 g Answer

4. ***Isotonic solution V-Values :*** Another method for adjusting tonicity is based on V-values. The isotonic solution V-values for some of the commonly used drugs are given in the following Table. The V-value of a drug is defined as the volume of water in mL to be added to 0.3 g of the drug to make an isotonic solution. The addition of an isotonic vehicle (diluting vehicle) to make 30 ml yields a 1% solution (0.3 g drug in 30 ml). Solutions prepared by this method are iso-osmotic with 0.9% sodium chloride.

Table 4.3 Isotonic Solution V-values.

Drug (0.3 g)	Water (mL) needed for isotonicity
Ammonium chloride	37.3
Ascorbic acid	6.0
Atropine sulfate	4.3
Bacitracin	1.7
Boric acid	16.7
Cocaine hydrochloride	5.3
Ephedrine hydrochloride	10.0
Ephedrine sulfate	7.7
Ephedrine bitartrate	6.0
Epinephrine hydrochloride	9.7
Homatropine hydrobromide	5.7
Neomycin sulfate	3.7
Oxytetracycline hydrochloride	4.3
Pilocarpine hydrochloride	7.0
Pilocarpine nitrate	7.7
Potassium chloride	25.3

Table 4.3 *Contd...*

Drug (0.3 g)	Water (mL) needed for isotonicity
Scopolamine hydrobromide	4.0
Silver nitrate	11.0
Sodium acetate	15.3
Sodium bisulfite	20.3
Sodium borate	14.0
Sodium thiosulfate	10.3
Streptomycin sulfate	2.3
Sulphacetamide sodium	7.7
Tetracaine hydrochloride	6.0
Tetracycline hydrochloride	4.7
Viomycin sulfate	2.7
Zinc chloride	20.3
Zinc sulfate	5.0

Example 5

Calculate the v-value for streptomycin sulfate. Given that sodium chloride equivalent of streptomycin sulfate is 0.07.

Solution

$$\frac{100\,\text{mL}}{0.9\,\text{g NaCl}} \times \frac{0.07\text{g NaCl}}{1\,\text{g drug}} \times 0.3\text{g of drug} = 2.33$$

Answer

$$v = 2.33 \text{ mL water/0.3 g drug}$$

Practice Exercises

1. Give a formula for 1 oz. of 1% solution of silver nitrate made isotonic with lachrymal secretion, using potassium nitrate.

2. Give a formula for 4 fl oz of a 0.25% solution of cocaine hydrochloride containing 0.25% zinc sulfate and 2% boric acid made isotonic with lachrymal secretion

3. Find out the weight of sodium chloride required for 100 mL of solution isotonic with blood serum (Mol, wt. of sodium sulfate = 322, Mol. wt. of sodium chloride = 58.5).

4. Calculate the amount of sodium chloride required for dispensing this prescription

    Rx

Cocaine hydrochloride	0.15
Sodium chloride	q.s.
Purified water ad	15.0
Make Isotonic solution	
Sig. : one drop in left eye.	

5. Send 1 oz. of a solution containing 1/2 gr. of morphine hydrochloride in 20 minims, rendered isotonic with blood serum, using sodium chloride.

6. Calculate the amount of sodium chloride needed to render 4 fl 02 of 1/2 % solution of Procaine hydrochloridc, isotonic with blood serum.

7. Give the formula for 40 mL of a 2% solution of Procaine hydrochloride containing 0.5% phenol. (Molar concentration .of blood serum= 0.030%; Mol. wt. of Procaine HC1 = 272.6; Mol. wt.of phenol = 94; Mol. wt. of sodium chloride = 58.5).

8. How many grams of sodium chloride are needed to make 1 pint of 5% w/v dextrose solution isotonic?

9. Calculate the number of grains of sodium chloride to make 2 fl. oz. of 1% w/v solution of Pilocarpine HC1 isotonic.

10. A solution of anhydrous dextrose contains 20 g in 400 mL of water. Calculate the freezing point of the solution, (Mol. wt. of anhydrous dextrose = 180)

11. If the v value of silver nitrate is 1.0 calculate its sodium chloride equivalent.

12. Rx

> Pilocarpine nitrate   1.75%
>
> Dist-water q.s.   20 ml
>
> Mix and make isotonic buffered solution.
>
> Sig.2 drops in each eye q 4 h.
>
> V-value ofpilocarpine nitrate = 7.7 = 7.7 ml water/0.3 g drug

Answers

1. Silver nitrate- 4.375 gr; Pot nitrate- 4.46 gr; Water q.s.40mL,
2. Cocaine HC1- 4.5 gr.. Zinc sulfate- 45 gr;Boric acid- 3.5 gr.J
3. 231g
4. 0,105 g
5. Morphine HC1- 12 gr.. Sodium chloride- 2 gr, Water q.s 1 oz j
6. 14 gr.
7. Procaine HC1- 0.8 g; Phenol- 0.2 g, Sodium Chloride-0, 116 g. Water to 40 mLJ
8. 0.473 gf
9. 6.22 grj
10. $- 0.52°C$
11. 0.33
12. 8.99 mL

Note : *For calculation of doses for children please refer next chapter.*

CHAPTER 5

Posology

The term posology (Greek *posos*, how much; and logos, science) is the science of doses. All Pharmacopoeias prescribe the doses of drugs for internal use. The dose is usually expressed as a range. The minimum dose or the lower limit of the dose is essential for eliciting an intended therapeutic response whereas the maximum dose or the higher limit of the dose is the amount of the drug substance that can be tolerated by an average individual. These doses are prescribed for the guidance of the prescriber. The pharmacist is much concerned with the maximum limit of the doses which, if exceeded, may cause untoward effects in the patient. The actual dose of a drug is to be decided by the prescriber depending on patient's age, sex, symptoms, his medication history and the factors like tolerance, idiosyncrasy, route of administration etc.

Factors affecting the dose and action of drugs

These factors are discussed below.

1. Age

In general, children require smaller doses than adults. Either Young's formula (based on age) or Clark's formula (based on weight) can be used for calculating the doses for children but the formula based on body surface area is more reliable.

2. Sex

This is particularly important in the case of treatment with sex hormones. Female adults generally require smaller doses than males due to the presence of more body fat.

3. Body weight

The usual doses for drugs are mentioned generally for 70 kg adult. The drug concentration at site of action is based on the ratio between the amount of drug administered and size of the body. The dose calculations for abnormally thin or obese patients are required to calculate on the basis of body weight.

4. Severity of disease

It is a common experience that dull headache may be relieved by a single tablet of aspirin whereas severe headache may necessitate administration of 2-3 tablets of the same drug. But this is no true in all cases. For example, in case of iron deficiency anemia, the dose of iron salt administered orally remains the same irrespective of severity because there is a limit to which iron can be absorbed from the intestine daily and incorporated in haemoglobin.

5. Health and nutrition

Debilitated and anaemic patients are, in general, more sensitive to the toxic effects of drugs and hence they are given smaller doses. Persons with severe anaemia associated with hookworm infestation are more susceptible to the toxic effects of tetrachloroethylene. Myxoedematous patients are known to show less response to drugs like amphetamine because of low cellular metabolism.

6. Pathological state

If the organs, through which biotransformation or excretion takes place, are diseased then smaller dose is indicated. For example, in case of renal insufficiency, phenobarbitone (mainly excreted by the kidneys) should be given in smaller dose and in case of patients suffering from liver diseases, morphine should be given in smaller dose (morphine is mainly inactivated in liver). Aspirin has no effect on normal body temperature but lowers the body temperature in fevered patients. Quinine precipitates black water fever more often with falciparum malaria than otherwise.

7. Tolerance

Some children can tolerate relatively large doses of arsenic, belladonna and calomel. Tolerance can be acquired as a result of repeated administration of some drugs e.g., morphine, heroin and cocaine.

8. Simultaneous administration of two or more drugs

(a) *Addition :* When two or more drugs given together produce the same resulting effect is the algebric sum of their individual effects e.g., carbachol and acetycholine.

(b) *Synergism :* In synergism, the effect produced is greater than the algebric sum of the effects due to individual drugs e.g., adrenaline and cocaine.

(c) *Antagonism :* When two drugs having opposite effect e.g. the use of amphetamine to correct partially the sedation caused by anticonvulsant doses of phenobarbital and the administration of ephedrine to correct hypotension resulting from spinal anesthesia.

9. Route of administration

In general, the rapidity of absorption of a drug decreases with route of administration in the following order:

Intravenous > Intramuscular > Subcutaneous > Oral

Thus, in general, intravenous (intravenous) dose of a drug is smaller than its intramuscular (intramuscular) or subcutaneous or oral dose.

Example : Doses of ergotamine for various routes are as follows.

Oral	: 2 to 5 mg

Intramuscular	: 1 mg (about to 1/2 of oral dose)

Intravenous	: 0.25 mg (about to 1/8 of oral dose and ¼ of IM dose)

10.	**Time and frequency of drug administration**

Biological half-life of a drug i.e. the time required for the blood level to drop down to 50 % of the initial peak level, is the main factor governing frequency of drug administration. For example, if the biological half-life of sulphadiazine is 4 hours, 1 g of the drug has to be given every 4 hours after initial dose of 2 g. But in certain instances e.g., reserpine as a tranquiliser, biological half-life of a drug has no relation to frequency of administration.

11.	**Idiosyncracy**

Morphine normally depresses central nervous system but may produce excitation in some individuals, specially women.

12.	**Allergy**

Penicillin may produce anaphylactic shock (sudden fall of blood pressure) in allergic patients but not in normal patients.

The doses of commonly used drugs are given in the Indian Pharmacopoeia.

Calculation of Dose

Dose represents the amount of a drug to be administered or taken by the patient for therapeutic effect. The dose may be expressed as –

Single dose : The amount of drug is taken one time.

Divided dose : The amount of drug is taken two or more times in a day depending on the characteristics of the drug, types of diseases and severity of diseases.

Total dose : The amount of drug is taken during the complete therapy.

Dose calculation varies with age, weight, sex, surface area, disease condition etc. of the patient. Because of these variables the Pharmacopoeia prescribes the "average adult dose" or the "usual adult dose" for official drugs. Therefore the adult dose as mentioned in the Pharamcopoeia may also vary depending on the various factors to be considered by the prescriber, the physician.

For calculating the doses for children the following methods are used :

I. Methods based on age of child :

A. *Young's Formula :* The formula is most useful for calculating the doses for children under 12 years of age.

Formula :

$$\frac{\text{Age in Years}}{\text{Age}+12} \times \text{Adult dose} = \text{Dose for the child}$$

Example 1 : If the usual adult dose of drug is 60 mg, what is the dose for (a) a child of 6 years (b) a child of 8 years

According to Young's Formula

(a)   Dose of child $= \dfrac{6}{6+12} \times 60 = 20\,\text{mg}$

(b)   Dose of child $= \dfrac{8}{8+12} \times 60 = 16\,\text{mg}$

Answer

(a)   20 mg   (b)   16 mg

B. *Dilling's Formula :* The formula is most useful for the calculating the doses for children in between 4 to 20 years of age.

Formula : $\dfrac{\text{Age in Years}}{20} \times \text{Adult dose} = \text{Dose for the child}$

Example 2 : If the adult dose of Allopurinol is 200 mg, what is the dose for (a) a child of 12 years (b) a child of 16 years

According to Dilling's Formula

(a)   Dose for child $= \dfrac{12}{20} \times 200 = 120\,\text{mg}$

(b)   Dose for child $= \dfrac{16}{20} \times 200 = 160\,\text{mg}$

Answer

(a)   120 mg   (b)   160 mg

C. *Cowling's Formula*

Formula :

Or
$$\frac{\text{Age at next birthday in years}}{24} \times \text{Adult dose} = \text{Dose for the child}$$

Example 3 : The maximum daily dose of a drug is 120mg . How much of it should be given to a child of (a) 11 years (b) 15 years

(a)
$$\text{Dose for the child} = \frac{11+1}{24} \times 120 = 60 \text{ mg}$$

(b)
$$\text{Dose for the child} = \frac{15+1}{24} \times 120 = 80 \text{ mg}$$

Answer

(a)　　60 mg　　　　　(b)　　　80 mg

D. *Fried's Formula* :

The formula is most useful for the calculating the doses for children under 2 years of age.

Formula :
$$\frac{\text{Age in months}}{150} \times \text{Adult dose} = \text{Dose for the child}$$

Example 4 : The adult dose of a drug is 50 mg. How much of it can be to (a) a 6 month old infant (b) a 24 months old infants

(a)
$$\text{Dose for the child} = \frac{6}{150} \times 50 = 2.0 \text{ mg}$$

(b)
$$\text{Dose for the child} = \frac{24}{150} \times 50 = 8.0 \text{ mg}$$

Answer

(a)　　2.0 mg　　　　　(b)　　　8.0 mg

E. **Bastedo's Formula :**

Formula :
$$\frac{\text{Age in years} + 3}{30} \times \text{Adult dose} = \text{Dose for the child}$$

Example 5 : The adult dose of a drug is 100 mg. How much of it can be given to a patient of (a) 9 years　(b) 12 years

According to Bastedo's Formula

(a) $\qquad$ Dose for child $= \dfrac{9+3}{30} \times 100 = 40$ mg

(b) $\qquad$ Dose for the child $= \dfrac{12+3}{30} \times 100 = 50$ mg

Answer

(a) 40 mg (b) 50 mg

II. Method Based on weight of the child

Clark's Formula

Formula : $\qquad \dfrac{\text{Weight in pounds}}{150} \times \text{Adult dose} = \text{Dose for the child}$

Example 6 : The adult dose of nimesulide is 100 mg. How much of it can be administered to a child weighing (a) 12 lbs (b) 15 lbs

According to Clark's Formula

(a) $\qquad$ Dose for the child $= \dfrac{12}{150} \times 100 = 8$ mg

(b) $\qquad$ Dose for the child $= \dfrac{15}{150} \times 100 = 10$ mg

III. Method based on body surface :

The body surface area is widely used in two types of patient groups

(i) Chemotherapy receiving cancer patient

(ii) Pediatric patients of all childhood except premature and full-term newborns

Formula : $\dfrac{\text{Body surface area of a child}}{\text{Body surface area of adult}} \times \text{Adult dose} = \text{Dose for the child}$

In general the adult body surface area of an adult is considered as 1.73 m^2

$$\dfrac{\text{Body surface area of a child}}{1.73} \times \text{Adult dose} = \text{Dose for the child}$$

Table 5.1 Calculation of doses for children on the basis of Body Surface Area.

Weight in kg	Surface area in Square meters	Percent of adult dose
2	0.15	9
3	0.20	11.5
4	0.25	14
5	0.29	16.5
6	0.33	19
7	0.37	21
8	0.40	23
9	0.43	25
10	0.46	27
15	0.63	36
20	0.83	48
25	0.95	55
30	1.08	62
35	1.20	69
40	1.30	75
45	1.40	81
50	1.51	87
55	1.58	91

Problems for Practice

1. If the dose of a drug is 100 mg, how many doses are contained in 2.0 g?

2. A cough syrup is 50 ml. The cough syrup is to be taken two teaspoonful two times a day. How many days are suitable for the given quantity?

3. A liquid medicine is prescribed three times daily by the physician, and if 120 ml are to be taken in 4 days, how many teaspoonfuls should be prescribed for each dose.

4. A liquid medicine is prescribed three times daily by the physician, and if 200 ml are to be taken in 4 days, how many teaspoonfuls should be prescribed for each dose while 5 ml of liquid medicine is lost in a day during handling of product.

5. If a cough syrup contains codeine 0.20 g in 100 ml of product. How many milligrams of codeine are contained in two teaspoonfuls?

6. One teaspoonful of elixir contains 5 mg of drug. How many milligrams of drug are present in 120 ml?

7. If the usual adult dose of drug is 15 mg, what is the dose for (a) a child of 8 years (b) a child weighing 40 lbs.

8. Maximum daily dose of calomel is 250 mg. How much of it should be given to a child of (a) 12 years of age (b) weighing 35 lbs?

9. The dose of drug is 0.25 mg/kg weight/day. How many mg should be prescribed for an adult weighing 145 lbs for three days?

10. How many chloramphenicol capsule each containing 250 mg are needed to provide 25mg/kg/day for a week a patient weighing 175 lbs?

11. The dose of piperazine citrate is 50 mg/kg body weight once daily for seven consecutive days. How many ml of piperazine citrate syrup containing 500 mg/teaspoonful should be prescribed for a child weighing 33 lbs?

12. A drug is to be administrated at the rate of 0.09g /kg body weight as 2% solution. How much of the drug will be required and what quantity of solution of the given strength will be necessary for a single administration for a patient weighing 130 lbs?

13. A cough formula contains diphenhydramine HCl 14.08 mg; ammonium chloride 0.138g; sodium citrate 57.03 mg; menthol 1.14 mg and alcohol 0.0625 ml. Recommended dose for a child is 1 teaspoonful every 4 hours. Calculate the quantity of each ingredient for one-week supply.

14. A nasal solution contains xylometazoline HCl as 1% w/v solution. It is recommended to be used as 3 drops into each nostril 4 times daily. What volume of the solution should be supplied for 15 days and how much xylometazoline HCl will be required?

15. A cough formula contains 14.08 mg diphenhydramine HCl in each teaspoonful dose. How many grams of the drug will be required to prepare 5 litres of the preparation?

16. Each 15 ml (3 teaspoonfuls) of a malt tonic contains 45 mg of niacinamide. How many grains of niacinamide are present in one pound of the tonic if its weight per ml is 1.2?

Answers

1. 20 doses   2. 6 days   3.   2 teaspoonful

4. 4 teaspoonful 5. 0.02 g (20 mg) 6.   120 mg (1teaspoonful = 5 ml)

7. (a) 6 mg   (b) 4 mg

8. (a) 100 mg (b) 47 mg   9.   49.44 mg

10. 55.5 capsules 11. 10.5 teaspoonful 12. 5.03 g; 265 ml

13. Diphenhydramine-591.36 mg, Ammonium chloride-5.796 g, Sodium citrate- 2395.26 mg, Menthol – 43.68 mg and alcohol-2.625 ml

14. 18 ml; 180 mg 15. 14; g 80 mg 16. 17.51 grains

A dispensing pharmacist must remember the doses of important drugs commonly prescribed so as to ensure accuracy in dispensing and avoiding any errors. The doses and uses of commonly prescribed drugs as per Indian Pharmacopoeia are given in the following Table for ready reference.

Table 5.2 Doses and Uses of Different Drugs.

Drug	Dose	Category
Acetazolamide	Initial dose 500 mg, subsequent doses, 250 mg every 6 hours.	Carbonic anhydrase inhibitor used in the treatment of glaucoma
Adrenaline	By s.c. or i.m. injection, 0.2 to 0.5 mg, as a single dose	Sympathomimetic
Adrenaline Bitartareate	By s.c. injection, 0.4 to 1 mg as a single dose	Sympathomimetic
Albendazole	Nematodal infection 400 mg as a single dose and cestodal infection 400 mg daily for three consecutive days	Anthelmintic
Allopurinol	Initial 100 mg daily as a single dose gradually increased to 300 mg daily. Usual maintenance dose 200 to 400 mg daily in divided doses in moderate and severe gout	Gout therapy
Alprazolam	0.25 to 0.50 mg three times daily	Anxiolytic
Aluminium Hydroxide gel	7.5 to 15 ml	Antacid
Dried Aluminium Hydroxide Gel	0.5 to 1 g	Antacid
Amantadine hydrochloride	100 mg daily, increased if necessary to 200 mg daily in divided doses	Antiviral, Antiparkinsonian
Amikacin	By .m. or slow i.v. injection or by infusion upto 1.5 g daily in two divided doses	Antibacterial

Table 5.2 Contd...

Drug	Dose	Category
Amiloride hydrochloride	Initially 5 to 10 mg daily; maximum 20 mg daily	Diuretic
Aminocaproic acid	Orally and slow i.v. infusion, initially 5 g followed by 1 to 1.25 g every hour until bleeding is under control	Haemostatic; Antifibrinolytic
Aminophyline	Orally 100 to 300 mg; by slow i.v. injection, 250 to 500 mg	Bronchodilator
Amitryptiline hydrochloride	50 to 75 mg daily, in divided doses; maintenance dose, 50 to 100mg daily, in divided doses	Antidepressant
Ammonium Chloride	3 to 6 g daily, in divided doses	Expectorant; diuretic; systemic acidifier
Amodiaquine hydrochloride	Suppressive, the equivalent of 400 mg of amodiaquine weekly. Therapeutic, the equivalent of 400 to 600 mg of amodiaquine daily for three days	Antimalarial
Amoxycillin sodium	By i.m. or i.v. injection, the equivalent of 1 to 3 g of amoxycillin daily in divided doses.	Antibacterial
Amoxycillin Trihydrate	The equivalent of 0.75 to 4.5 g of amoxycillin daily, in divided doses	Antibacterial
Amphotericin B	Orally, upto 200 mg every 6 hr. By slow i.v. injection 0.25 mg//kg body weight daily increased to 1mg/kg daily or 1.5 mg/kg on alternate days	Antifungal
Ampicillin	2 to 6 g daily, in divided doses	Antibacterial
Ampicillin Sodium	By .m. or i.v. injection, the equivalent of 1 to 3 g of ampicillin daily, in divided doses	Antibacterial
Ampicillin Trihydrate	The equivalent of 2 to 6 g ampicillin daily, in divided doses	Antibacterial
Alpha Amylase	200 to 500 mg	Digestive enzyme
Amylobarbitone	As hypnotic, 0.1 to 0.2g. As sedative, upto 0.6 g daily, in divided doses	Hypnotic and sedative
Amylobarbitone Sodium	As hypnotic, 0.1 to 0.2 g. As sedative, upto 0.6 g daily, in divided doses	Hypnotic and sedative
Analgin (Metamizol)	0.5 to 3 g daily, in divided doses	Analgesic

Table 5.2 Contd…

Drug	Dose	Category
Ascorbic Acid	Prophylatic, 25 to 75mg daily; therapeutic, not less than 250 mg daily, in divided doses	Vitamin (antiscorbutic)
Aspirin (Acetylsalicylic acid)	An analgestic and antipyretic300 to 600 mg four to six times a day; as antirheumatic –1 to 2 g four to six times a day, upto 10 g daily; as antithrombotic, 75 mg daily.	Analgesic; antipyretic, antirheumatic; antithrombotic
Astemizole	For adult 10 mg once daily upto seven days. For children, 5 mg once daily upto 7 days.	Antihistaminic
Atropine Sulphate	Orally, 0.25 to 2 mg daily in single or divided doses; by s.c., i.m. or i.v. injection, 0.4 to 0.6 mg four to six times a day	Anticholinergic; antidote to cholinesterase inhibitors
BCG (Bacillus Calmette-Guerin) Vaccine	Prophylactic, by intracutaneous injection as a single dose 0.1 ml	Active immunizing agent
Belladonna Dry Extract	15 to 60 mg	Anticholinergic
Benzylpenicillin sodium	By i.m or by slow i.v. injection or by infusion, the equivalent of 1.2 to 2.4 g of benzylpenicillin daily in 4 divided doses	Antibacterial
Bephenium Hydroxynaphthoate	5 g, as a single dose	Anthelmintic (hookworms)
Berberine Chloride	0.1g as a single dose	Bitter stomachic, anti bacterial
Betamethasone	0.5 to 5 mg daily, in divided doses	Adrenocortical steroid (anti-inflammatory)
Bethanide Sulphate	Initial dose, 10 to 20 mg daily, in divided doses	Antihypertensive
Bisacodyl	Orally, 5 to10 mg daily	Laxative
Bismuth subcarbonate	1 to 4 g	Antacid
Bleomycin sulphate	By injection, the equivalent of 15 to 30 units of bleomycin weekly, in divided doses.	Antineoplastic antibiotic
Bromhexine hydrochloride	8 to 16mg three to four times daily	Expectorant
Busulphan	2 to 4 mg daily; maintenance dose, 0.5 to 2.0 mg daily	Antineoplastic (Cytotoxic)
Caffeine	300 to 600 mg	CNS stimulant
Calcium Amino salicylate	10 to 20g daily, in divided doses	Antibacterial (tuberculostatic)
Calcium Carbonate	1 to 5 g	Antacid

Table 5.2 *Contd…*

Drug	Dose	Category
Calcium Chloride	Orally, 1 to 2 g; by slow i.v. injection 5 to 10 ml of 10% w/v solution.	Calcium replenisher
Calcium folinate	Upto 120 mg in divided doses over 12 to 24 hr by i.m. or i.v. injection or infusion	Antidote to folate antagonists
Calcium Gluconate	By i.m. or i.v. injection, 1 to 2 g; orally upto 15 g daily, in divided doses.	Calcium replenisher
Calcium Lactate	Upto 8 g daily, in divided doses.	Calcium replenisher
Calcium Levulinate	By i.m. or i.v. injection 1 g once a day.	Calcium replenisher
Calcium Pantothenate	10 to 100 mg daily, in divided doses	Vitamin B (enzyme co-factor)
Dibasic Calcium Phosphate	1 to 5 g	Calcium Supplement
Captopril	Initially, 12.5 to 50 mg twice; usual maintenance dose, 25 mg twice daily; maximum, 50 mg twice daily.	Antihypertensive
Carbamazepine	200 mg daily, increasing to 1.2 g daily, in divided doses, as per the needs of the patient	Anticonvulsant
Carbenicillin sodium	By i.v. injection, the equivalent of 12 to 30 g of carbenecillin daily in divided doses.	Antibacterial
Carbenoxolone sodium	300 mg daily, in divided doses for 1 week; subsequently, upto 150 mg daily, in divided doses	Ulcer-healing drug in gastric ulcer
Carbidopa	10 to 25 mg in combination with Levodopa	Antiparkinsonian with Levodopa
Castor Oil	5 to 15 ml	Laxative
Cefadroxil	0.5 to 2.0 g daily, in divided doses.	Antibacterial
Cefazolin sodium	By i.m. or i.v. injection or infusion 1 to 4 g daily, in divided doses.	Antibacterial
Cefotaxime sodium	By i.m. or i.v. injection, the equivalent of 1 to 2 g of cefataxime every 8 to 12 hr.	Antibacterial
Ceftazidime	By i.m. or slow i.v. injection or i.v. infusion, 1 to 2 g, every 8 to 12 hr.	Antibacterial
Cefuroxime sodium	Orally, 250 mg twice daily; by i.m. or i.v. injection or i.v. infusion 0.75 to 1.5 g every 6 to 8 hr.	Antibacterial
Cephalexin	1 to 4 g daily, in divided doses	Antibacterial
Cephaloridine	By i.m., i.v. or deep s.c. injection, 1 to 4 g daily in divided doses.	Antibacterial
Chloral Hydrate	0.3 to 2 g	Hypnotic & sedative

Table 5.2 Contd...

Drug	Dose	Category
Chlorambucil	0.10 to 0.20 mg/kg of body weight daily for 4 to 8 weeks	Cytotoxic
Chloramphenicol	For an adult, 1.5 to 3g daily, in divided doses; for a child, 25 to 50mg/kg body weight daily, in divided doses	Antibacterial
Chloramphenicol Palmitae	For an adult, the equivalent of 1.5 to 3.0 g daily, in divided doses; for a child, the equivalent of 25 to 50 mg/kg of body weight daily, in divided doses	Antibacterial
Chloramphenical Sodium Succinate	By i.v. injection, the equivalent of 3 to 4 g of chloramphenicol daily, in divided doses	Antibacterial
Chlordiazepoxide	10 to 100 mg daily, in divided doses	Anxiolytic
Chloroquine Phosphate	In treatment of malaria; suppressive, 500 mg weekly, therapeutic, initial dose 1g subsequent doses, 500 mg daily In treatment of amoebiasis 500mg 3 times a day for 2 week, than 750 mg 2 times a week for several months	Antimalarial, antiprotozoal
Chloroquine Sulphate	In treatment of malaria; suppressive, 400mg weekly; therapeutic, 400mg to 1.2g daily In treatment of amoebiasis; 400 to 800mg daily in divided doses	Antimalarial, antiamoebic
Chlorpheniramine Maleate	Orally, 4 to 16 mg daily, in divided doses. By s.c. or i.m. injection, 10 to 20 mg; maximum 40 mg in 24 hr.	Antihistaminic
Chlorpromazine hydrochloride	Orally, 75 to 300 mg daily, in divided doses; by i.m. injection, 25 to 50 mg. As antiemetic, orally, 10 to 25 mg every four hr; by i.m. injection 25 to 50 mg every 3 to 4 hr.	Antipsychotic; antiemetic
Chlorpropamide	100 to 500 mg daily	Antidiabetic (Hypoglycemic)
Chlorthalidone	50 to 200 mg daily	Diuretic
Cholera Vaccine	Over 10 years Prophylactic. By s.c. injection, initial dose 0.5 ml; second dose, 1.0 ml after an interval of 4 to 6 weeks. For children 2 to 10 years, initial dose 0.3 ml; second dose, 0.3 ml after an interval of 4 to 6 weeks. For 1 to 2 years, initial dose, 0.2 ml; second dose 0.2 ml.	Active immunizing agents

Table 5.2 Contd...

Drug	Dose	Category
Cimetidine	Oral, 200 mg increasing to 400 mg when necessary, 3 times a day, and 400 mg at night; by i.v. injection, 200 mg every 4 to 6 hr. Oral and parenteral dose should not exceed 2 g daily	H₂- receptor antagonist
Ciprofloxacin	Orally, 250 to 750 mg twice daily; by i.v. infusion. 100 mg to 200 mg twice daily.	Antibacterial
Cisplatin	By i.v. infusion, 15 to 20 mg per sq. m. of body surface daily for 5 days	Cytotoxic
Clofazimine	For leprosy, previously untreated patients, 100 mg 3 times weekly; For sulphone-resistant patients 100 mg 6 times weekly. For suppression of lepra reactions, 200 mg daily	antibacterial (Antileprotic)
Clofibrate	Upto 2 g daily, in divided doses	Antihyperlipedemic
Clonidine hydrochloride	Orally 0.50 to 0.10 mg three times daily increased gradually according to the needs and response of the patient maximum daily dose 1.2 mg.	Antihypertensive
Cloxacillin Sodium	The equivalent of 500 mg of cloxacillin every 6 hr, at least 30 minutes before food: by i.m. injection; 250mg every 4 to 6 hr	Antibacterial
Codeine phosphate	30 to 60 mg every 4 hr when necessary, to a maximum of 200 mg daily.	Analgesic; antidiarrhoeal; cough suppressant
Colchicine	Initial dose, 1 mg; subsequent doses, 0.5 mg every 2 hr	Gout suppressant
Cortisone Acetate	Orally, 25 to 37.5 mg daily, in divided doses; by i.m. injection 50 to 400 mg daily in single or divided doses.	Adrenocortical steroid (anti-inflammatory)
Cyanocobalamin	In treatment of megaloblastic anemia by i.m. injection, 1 to 2 mg, in divided doses, in the first week. Subsequent doses, 0.25 mg weekly until the blood count is normal, maintenance dose, 0.25 mg every 3 or 4 weeks	B group vitamin; haematopoietic
Cyclizine hydrochloride	25 to 50 mg	Antiemetic
Cyclophosphamide	Orally or by i.v. injection 100 to 150 mg daily	Antineoplastic immunosuppressive
Cycloserine	0.50 to 1.0 g daily, in divided doses	Antibacterial (tuberculostatic)
Cyproheptadine hydrochloride	4 to 20 mg daily, in divided doses	Antihistaminic

Table 5.2 *Contd…*

Drug	Dose	Category
Danazol	200 to 800 mg daily, in divided doses	Antigonadotrophin
Dapsone	100 mg daily	Antileprotic
Dehydroemetine hydrochloride	By deep i.m. injection, 60 to 90 mg daily	Antiamoebic
Demethylchlortetracy cline hydrochloride	0.6 to 1.8 g daily, in divided doses	Antibacterial
Desoxycortisone Acetate	By i.m. injection, 2 to 5 mg daily	Adrenocortical steroid (Salt regulating)
Dexamethasone	0.5 to 10 mg daily, in divided doses	Adrenocortical steroid (anti-inflammatory)
Dexamethasone Sodium Phosphate	By i.v. or i.m. injection, the equivalent of 12 to 32 mg of dexamethasone phosphate, in treatment of acute adrenal in sufficiently	Adrenocortical steroid (anti-inflammatory)
Diazepam	In anxiety, 2 mg thrice daily, increased if necessary to 15 to 30 mg daily, in divided doses	Anxiolytic; Anticonvulsant, sedative
Diclofenac sodium	Orally or by i.m. injection, 25 to 75 mg	Analgesic; anti-inflammatory
Diethylcarbamazine Citrate	150 to 500 mg daily	antifilarial, anthelmintic
Digitoxin	Initial dose, 1 to 1.5mg, divided over 24 to 48 hr; maintenance dose, 0.05 to 0.2 mg daily	Cardiotonic (Cardiac glycoside)
Digoxin	Initial dose, 1 to 1.5 mg maintenance dose, 0.25 mg once or twice daily. By i.v. injection, initial dose, 0.5 to 1 mg	Cardiotonic (Cardiac glycoside)
Di-iodohydroxyquinoline	1 to 2 g daily, in divided doses	Antiamoebic
Diloxanide Furoate	1.5 g daily, in divided doses	Antiamoebic
Diltiazem hydrochloride	Initially, 30 to 60 mg trice daily; maximum, 480 mg daily	Antianginal; calcium-channel blocker
Dimenhydrinate	25 to 100 mg	Antiemetic
Dimercaprol	By i.m. injection, 2 to 3 mg/kg body weight every 4 hr during first day and subsequently in accordance with the needs of the patient	Antidote in heavy metal poisoning, metal complexing agent
Diphendydramine hydrochloride	50 to 200 mg daily, in divided doses	antihistaminic

Table 5.2 *Contd…*

Drug	Dose	Category
Diphenoxylate hydrochloride	5 to 30 mg daily, in divided doses	Antidiarrhoeal
Diptheria Antioxin	By s.c. or i.m. injection, prophylactic, 500 to 2000 international units; therapeutic, not less than 10,000 international units	Immunising agent
Diptheria and Tetanus Vaccine (Adsorbed)	By deep i.m. injection, two injections of 0.5 ml, 4 to 6 weeks apart, and a third reinforcing dose of 0.5 ml, 6 to 8 months later	Immunising agent
Diptheria, Tetanus and Pertussis Vaccine (Adsorbed)	By i.m. injection, three injections of 0.5 ml, 4 to 6 weeks apart, and a fourth, reinforcing dose of 0.5 ml, 6 to 8 months later	Active immunising agent
Doxycycline hydrochloride	Initial, the equivalent of 0.2 g of doxycycline; subsequent doses, the equivalent of 0.1g of doxycycline daily	antibacterial
Disulfiram	500 mg as a single dose for 1 to 2 weeks; maintenance dose, 125 to 500 mg daily	Used in the treatment of alcoholism
Doxepin hydrochloride	Initially, the equivalent of 75 mg of doxepin daily, in divided doses; increased gradually to a maximum of 300 mg daily, in divided doses.	Antidepressant
Dydrogesterone	10 mg twice daily	Progestogen
Emetine hydrochloride	By s.c. or i.m. injection, 30 to 60 mg daily	antiamoebic
Enalapril maleate	Initial, 2.5 to 5.0 mg daily; maintenance dose, 10 to 20 mg daily; maximum 40 mg daily	Antihypertensive; angiotension-converting enzyme inhibitor
Ephedrine	15 to 60 mg	Sympathomimetic; brochodilator
Ergocalciferol	In prevention of rickets, not more than 20 g (800 Units) daily, allowance being made for Vitamin D obtained from other sources. In treatment of rickets and osteomalacia, 0,125 to 1.25 mg (5000 to 50,000 Units) daily. In treatment of hypoparathyroidism, 1.25 to 5 mg (50,000 to 200,000 Units) daily	Vitamin D (antirachitic)
Ergometrine Maleate	By i.m. injection, 0.25 to 1 mg; by i.v. injection, 0.1 to 0.5 mg	Oxytocic (Uterine stimulant)
Ergotamine Tartrate	1 to 2 mg; by s.c. or i.m. injection, 0.25 to 0.50 mg.	Sympatholytic; antimigraine drug
Erythromycin	1 to 2 g daily, in divided doses	Antibacterial

Table 5.2 Contd…

Drug	Dose	Category
Erythromycin Estolate	The equivalent of 1 to 2 g of erythromycin daily, in divided doses for not more than 10 days	Antibacterial
Erythromycin Stearate	The equivalent of 1 to 2g of erythromycin daily, in divided doses for not more than 10 days	Antibacterial
Ethacrynic Acid	50 to 200 mg daily, in divided doses	Diuretic
Ethambutol hydrochloride	15 to 25 mg/kg body weight daily, for 2 months, followed by 25mg/kg body weight daily	Antitubercular
Ethionamide	0.5 to 1 g daily, in divided doses	Antitubercular
Ethosuximide	500 mg daily, in divided doses increasing to 2 g, as necessary; for a child, 50 to 125 mg twice daily, increasing to 250 mg three to four times daily, as necessay	Anticonvulsant
Ehtyloestrenol	2 to 4 mg daily	Anabolic steroid
Ethylmorphine hydrochloride	6 to 30 mg	Narcotic analgesic
Fenfluramine hydrochloride	Initially, 20 mg morning and evening, increasing to a maximum of 80 mg twice daily, in divided doses	Appetite suppressant
Ferrous Fumerate	0.2 to 0.3 gm	Haematinic
Ferrous Gluconate	Prophylactic, 600 mg daily. Therapeutic, 1.2 to 1.8 g daily, in divided doses	Haematinic
Ferrous Sulphate	0.2 to 0.3g	Haematinic
Dried Ferrous Sulphate	Prophylactic, 200 mg daily; therapeutic, 400 to 600 mg daily, in divided doses	Haematinic
Fluorouracil	By i.v. injection, 3 mg/kg daily for 4 days followed by 6 mg/kg on alternate days, to a maximum of 800 mg daily	Cytotoxic
Fluphenazine hydrochloride	1 to 2 mg daily in single or divided doses (in anxiety states). Upto 15mg daily, in divided doses (for treatment of schizophrenia).	Antipsychotic
Folic Acid	In treatment of megaloblastic anaemia associated with folic acid deficiency, 5 to 20 mg daily. In the prophylaxis of megaloblastic anaemia of pregnancy, 0.2 to 0.5 mg daily	Vitamin B (haematopoietic)
Frusemide	Orally, in oedema, 20 to 40 mg daily; in oliguvria, 250 mg 4 to 6 times daily.	Diuretic

Table 5.2 Contd…

Drug	Dose	Category
Furazolidone	400 mg daily, in divided doses	Antibacterial, antiprotozoal, Antifungal
Gas Gangrene Antioxin (Cedematiens)	By i.v. or i.m. injection, prophylactic, 10,000 International Units; therapeutic, not less than 30,000 International Units	Immunising agent
Gasgangrene Antitoxin (Perfringens)	By i.v. or i.m. injection, prophylactic, 10,000 International Units; therapeutic, not less than 30,000 International Units	Immunising agent
Gas Gangrene antitoxin (Septicum)	By i.v. or i.m. injection, prophylactic, 5,000 International Units; therapeutic, not less than 15,000 International Units	-do-
Mixed Gas-gangrene Antioxin	By i.v. or i.m. injection, prophylactic, 25,000 International Units; thereapeutic, not less than 75,000 International Units	-do-
Gentamycin Sulphate	By i.m. injection, 80 to 240mg of gentamycin (80,000 to 240,000 Units) daily, in divided doses	Antibacterial
Glibanclamide	5 mg daily, adjusted according to response; maximum 15 mg daily, after food	Hypoglycaemic
Glyceryl Trintrate (Nitroglycerin) Tablets	Glyceryl Trinitrate, 0.5 to 1m.g. Usual strengths 0.25mg; 0.3mg; 0.5mg; 0.6mg	Vasodilator (coronary)
Griseofulvin	0.5 to 1 g daily in divided doses	Antifungal
Guanethidine Sulphate	Initial dose, 10 to 20 mg daily; subsequent doses, increasing daily at weekly intervals to a maximum of 300 mg daily, in accordance with the needs of the patient	Antihypertensive
Guaiphenesin	For an adult 200 to 400 mg every hr	Expectorant
Heloperidol	Orally, 1.5 to 20 mg daily, in divided doses; by i.m. or i.v. injection, 2 to 10 mg.	Antipsychotic
Heparin Sodium	For treatment, by i.v. injection, 20,000 to 50,000 units daily, For prophylaxis by s.c. injection, 10,000 to 15,000 units daily, in divided doses	Anticoagulant
Hepatitis B virus vaccine	Single dose of liquid vaccine containing not less than 20 μg of surface antigen per adult dose. The primary immunization schedule employs 3 intramuscular injections at monthly intervals. To maintain good immunity, a booster dose is recommended every 5 years following primary immunization.	Active immunizing agent

Table 5.2 Contd…

Drug	Dose	Category
Hydrallazine hydrochloride	Oral, 10 mg 4 times a day, gradually increased upto 50 mg 4 times a day, by i.v. or i.m. injection, 20 to 40 mg, repeated as necessary.	Antihypertensive
Hydrochlorothiazide	25 to 100 mg	Diuretic
Hydrocortisone	In treatment of adrenocortical insufficiency, 10 to 40mg daily	Adrenocortical steroid (anti-inflammatory)
Hydroxycobalamin	In treatment of megaloblastic anaemia, by i.m. injection, 1 to 2 mg, in divided doses, in the first week; subsequent doses, 250 g weekly until the blood count is normal; maintenance dose, 1mg every two months	Vitamin B_{12} (haematopoietic)
Hydroxyethyithe ophyline	100 to 300mg by mouth or by i.v. or i.m. injection	Smooth muscle relaxant (bronchiolar)
Ibuprofen	0.6 to 1.2 g daily, in divided doses after food	Analgesic and anti-inflammatory
Imipramine hydrochloride	50 to 150 mg daily, in divided doses	Antidepressant
Indomethacin	Orally, 50 to 200 mg daily, in divided doses, with food	Anti-inflammatory and analgesic
Insulin	By s.c., i.m. or i.v. injection, or i.v. infusion, in accordance with the needs of the patient	Hypoglycaemic
Iron and Ammonium Citrate	1 to 3 g	Haematinic
Iron Dextran injection	By deep i.m. injection, 1 to 2ml daily	Haematinic
Isoniazid	300 mg daily or upto 1 g twice weekly	Antibacterial (tubeculostatic)
Isoprenaline hydrochloride	By subcutaneous or i.m. injection, 200 g: by i.v. injection, 10 to 20 g; 2mg by infusion in Dextrose injection according to the needed of the patient	Adrenergic (bronchodilator)
Isoprenaline Sulphate	5 to 20 mg daily	Adrenergic (bronchodilator and cardiac stimulant)
Diluted Isosorbide Dinitrate	20 to 300mg of isosorbide dintrate daily, in divided doses	Anti-anginal (Vasodilator)
Isoxsuprine hydrochloride	Oral, 10 to 20 mg, 3 or 4 times daily; by i.m. injection, 5 to 10mg 3 times daily	Peripheral vasodilator (uterine relaxant)

Table 5.2 *Contd...*

Drug	Dose	Category
Ispagul Husk	3 to 5 g	Laxative
Kanamycin sulphate	By i.m. injection, the equivalent of 0.5 to 1 g (500,000 to 1,000,000 units) to kanamycin base daily in divided doses	Antibacterial
Ketoprofen	100 to 200 mg daily, in 2 to 4 divided doses, with food.	Anti-inflammatory; analgesic
Light Kaolin	15 to 75 g	Adsorbent (in treatment of diarrhoea)
Lanatoside C Laptazol	For rapid digitalisation, 1 to 1.5mg in single or divided doses. For maintenance 0.25 to 0.75 mg daily 50 to100mg	Cardiotonic CNS stimulant
Levodopa	Initial, 125 to 500 mg daily, in divided doses, after meals, increasing gradually in accordance with he needs if the patient, maintenance dose 2.5 to 8 g daily	Antiparkinsonian
Lignocaine hydrochloride	As local anaesthetic, upto 200mg or 500 mg as a single dose, when given with adrenaline. For treatment of cardiac arrhythmias, by intravenous injection, 50 to 100 mg	Local anesthetic; cardiac depressant
Lincomycin hydrochloride	The equivalent of 1.5 g of lincomycin, in divided doses, 30 minutes before food. By i.m. injection, the equivalent of 0.6 to 1.2 g of lincomycin daily, in 2 doses. By i.v. infusion, the equivalent of 600 mg of lincomycin every 8 hr	Antibacterial
Lithium Carbonate	0.25 to 1.6 g daily, in divided doses	Antidepressant
Lomustine	120 to 130 mg per sq. m. body-surface every 6 to 8 weeks	Cytotoxic
Magaldrate	800 mg to 1.6 g	Antacid
Lynestrenol	2.5 to 15 mg daily	Progestin
Milk of Magnesia	As an antacid, 5 to 10ml; as a laxative, 15 to 30ml	Laxative; antacid
Heavy Magnesium Carbonate	As an antacid, 0.3 to 0.6 g; as a laxative, 2 to 4g	Osmotic laxative; antacid
Light Magnesium Carbonate	As antacid, 300 to 600 mg; as laxative, 2 to 4 g	Osmotic laxative; antacid

Table 5.2 *Contd...*

Drug	Dose	Category
Heavy Magnesium Oxide	As gastric antacid, 0.3 to 0.6g; as a laxative, 2 to 4g	Antacid, laxative
Light Magnesium Oxide	As gastric antacid, 0.3 to 0.6g; as a laxative, 2 to 4g	Antacid, laxative
Magnesium Sulphate	2 to 16 g	Cathartic
Magnesium Trislicate	0.5 to 2g repeated in accordance with the needs of the patient	Antacid
Massies Vaccine Live	Pediatric, by s.c. injetion, 0.5 ml of reconstituted vaccine	Active immunising agent
Mebendazole	For threadworm infestation, 100 mg as a single dose; for other infestations, 100 mg twice daily for tow days	Antihypetensive
Mecamylamine hydrochloride	Initial dose, 5mg daily, in divided doses; subsequent doses, in accordance with the needs of the patients.	Antihypertensive
Meclizine hydrochloride	25 to 50 mg	Antihistaminic; anti-emetic
Megestrol acetate	40 to 320 mg daily, in divided doses	Progestogen
Mephenesin	By i.v. infusion 0.1 to 1g	Skeletal muscle relaxant
Meprobamate	0.4 to 1.2g daily, in divided doses	Sedative
Mepyramine Maleate	0.3 to 0.6g daily, in divided doses. By i.m. or i.v. injection, 25 to 50mg	Antihistaminic (H$_1$ receptor antagonist)
Mestranol	0.05 to 0.15mg daily, usually in conjunction with a progestogen	Estrogen
Metformin hydrochloride	0.5 to 2.0 g daily, in divided doses	Oral hypoglycaemic
Methadone hydrochloride	Oral, 5 to 10mg. By s.c. injection, 5 to 10mg	Narcotic analgesic; narcotic abstinence syndrome suppressant
Methandienone	Adults, 5 to 10 mg daily; children, 0.5 to 10mg daily	Anabolic steroid, weak androgen
Methotrexate	5 to 100mg at suitable intervals	Antineoplastic; antipsoriatic
Methylamphytamine hydrochloride	2.5 to 10mg. By i.m. or i.v. injection, 10 to 30 mg	Adrenergic; central stimulant
Methyldopa	The equivalent of 0.5 to 3g of anhydrous methyldopa, daily, in divided doses	Antihypertensive

Table 5.2 Contd...

Drug	Dose	Category
Mehylrgometrine maleate	By s.c., i.m., or .v. injection, 0.1 to 0.2 mg	Uterine stimulant; oxytocic
Metoprolol tartrate	100 to 450 mg daily, in divided doses; the initial dose should not exceed 100 mg daily	Bet-adrenoceptor antagonist
Metronidazole	For trichomoniasis, 200 mg 3 times daily, for 7 days. For amoebiasis, 400mg 3 times daily, for 5 to 10 days. For girardiasis, 2g daily for 3 successive days for adults 1g for children and 400mg daily for infants	Antiamoebic; antitrichomonal; anit-giardial
Mianserin hydrochloride	30 to 90 mg daily, in divided doses	Antidepressant
Morphine hydrochloride	10 to 20 mg	Narcotic, analgesic
Morphine sulphate	10 to 20 mg	Narcotic, analgesic
Nalidixic acid	2 to 4 g daily, in four divided doses	Antibacterial
Nalorphine hydrochloride	By i.v. injection, 5 mg, repeated twice at 3 minutes intervals if necessary	Antidote for narcotic analgesics
Neomycin sulphate	For systemic use, the equivalent of 0.7 to 2.0 g of neomycin base daily in divided doses	Antibacterial (topical and systemic)
Neostigmine bromide	15 to 30 mg, 3 to 6 times a day	Chlonergic
Niclosamide	2 g as a single dose after a light breakfast followed by a purgative 2 hr later	Anthelmintic (teniacide)
Nicotinamide	Prophylatic, 15 to 30mg daily; therapeutic, 50 to 250mg daily. By i.v. injection, 50 to 250mg daily	B-group vitamins;
Nicoumalone	Initial dose, first day, 8 to 12 mg, second day, 4 to 8 mg; maintenance dose, 1 to 8 mg daily.	Anticoagulant
Nifedipine	Initial dose, up to 30 mg daily, in divided doses	Coronary vasodilator, antianginal
Nicotinic Acid	Prophylactic, 15 to 30 mg daily; therapeutic, 50 to 250 mg daily	B-group vitamin; vasodilator
Nikethamide	By s.c., i.m., or i.v. injection, 0.25 to 2 g 50 to 150 mg 4 times daily	Respiratory stimulant Antibacterial (urinary)
Nitrazepam	5 to 10 mg daily, at a bed time	Hypnotic; sedative
Nitrofurantoin	50 to 150 mg four times daily	Antibacterial
Noradrenaline Acid Tartrate	By intravenous infusion, 2 to 20 g per minute, according to the blood pressure of the patient	Adrenergic (vasopressor)

Table 5.2 Contd...

Drug	Dose	Category
Norethisterone	5 to 20mg daily, in single or divided doses	Progestin
Noscapine	15 to 30mg	Antitussive
Novobiocin Sodium	The equivalent of 1 to 2g of novobiocin daily, in divided doses	Antibacterial
Nystatin	In treatment of alimentary moniliasis, 1 to 2 million units daily in divided doses	Antifungal
Omeprazole	20 to 40 mg daily; For Zollinger-Ellison syndrome, initially 60 mg once daily; usual range, 20 to 120 mg daily.	Antiulcerative
Oestradiol Benzoate	By i.m. injection, 1 to 5 mg daily	Oestrogenic hormone
Oestradiol Dipropionate	By i.m. injection, initial 1 to 5 mg every 1 to 2 weeks, maintenance, 1 to 2.5 mg every 10 days to 2 week	Oestrogenic hormone
Opium	25 to 200 mg	Hypnotic, sedative; narcotic; analgesic
Oxyphenbutazone	200 to 400 mg daily, in divided doses	Anti-inflammatory; analgesic
Oxyphenonium	5 to 10mg	Anticholinergic
Oxytracycline	1 to 2 g daily, in divided doses	Antibacterial
Oxytracycline hydrochloride	1 to 2 g daily, in divided doses. By i.v. infusion, in a concentration 0.1% w/v, 1 to 2 g daily	Antibacterial
Pancreatin	0.50 to 1.0 g	Digestive enzyme
Papain	120 to 600 mg	Proteolytic enzyme
Paracetamol	0.5 to 1 g; up to 4 g daily, in divided doses	Analgesic; antipyretic
Paraldehyde	By i.m. injection, 2 to 8 ml. By rectal injection, 15 to 30ml suitably diluted	Hypnotic; sedative; anticonvulsant
Paramethadione	0.9g daily, in divided doses, increasing to 1.8g in accordance with the needs of the patient	Anticonvulsant
Benzylpenicillin	By i.m. or i.v. injection 500,000 to 1,000,000 units daily, in divided doses	Antibacterial
Pentobarbitone Sodium	0.1 to 0.2g	Hypnotic; sedative; narcotic; analgesic
Pepsin	0.3 to 1 g	Proteolytic enzyme
Phenformin hydrochloride	25 to 100 mg. By s.c. or im. injection, 25 to 100 mg; by i.v. injection 25 to 50 mg	Analgesic
Phenformin hydrochloride	50 to 200 mg daily, in divided doses	Oral hypoglycaemic agent

Table 5.2 *Contd...*

Drug	Dose	Category
Phenindamine Tartrate	75 to 150 mg daily, in divided doses	Antihistaminic
Phenindamine Maleate	25 to 50 mg daily, in divided doses	Antihistaminic
Phenobarbitone	Upto 350 mg daily, in divided doses	Hypnotic; sedative; anti-convulsant
Phenobarbitone Sodium	Upto 350 mg daily, in divided doses. By i.v., i.m. or s.c. injection, 50 to 200 mg	Hypnotic; sedative
Phenoxymethyl penicillin Potassium	The equivalent of 0.5 to 1.5g of phenoxymethylpenicillin daily, in divided doses	Antibacterial
Phenylbutazone	100 to 600 mg daily, in divided doses	Anti-inflammatory analgesic
Phenylephrine hydrochloride	By s.c. or i.m. injection, 5mg; by i.v. injection, 0.5mg	Adrenergic (vasopressor)
Phenytoin Sodium	50 mg daily, increasing to 400mg; by i.m. or slow i.v. injection, up to 250 mg in accordance with the needs of the patient	Anticonvulsant
Phthalylsulphathiazole	5 to 10 mg daily, in divided doses	Antibacterial (intestinal)
Physostigmine Salicylate	0.6 to 1.2 mg	Anticholinesterase
Piperazine Citrate	For threadworms 0.6 to 4.5 g daily in divided doses. For roundworms, up to 5 g in a single dose according to the age of the patient	Anthelmintic
Piroxicam	10 to 20 mg daily	Analgesic, Antiinflammatory; antipyretic
Plague Vaccine	By s.c. injection, 1ml (first dose); 1 ml (second dose) after an interval of 7 to 10 days. A single dose of 3 ml may be given in emergency	Active immunizing agent
Potassium Bromide	0.3 to 1.2 g	Sedative; anticonvulsant
Potassium Chloride	1 to 2 g	Electrolyte replenisher
Potassium Citrate	4 to 10 g	Systemic alkaliniser
Potassium Iodide	As expectorant, 250 to 500mg. In pre-operative treatment of thyrotoxicosis, 30 to 60mg	Antifungal; expectorant; source of iodine
Prednisolone	Upto 30 mg daily, in divided doses	Adrencocortical steroid (anti-inflammatory)

Table 5.2 Contd…

Drug	Dose	Category
Prednisolone Acetate	Upto 30 mg daily, in divided doses	Adrencocortical steroid
Prednisone	Upto 30 mg daily, in divided doses	Adrencocortical steroid
Prednisone Acetate	Upto 30 mg daily, in divided doses	Adrencocortical steroid
Primaquine Phosphate	The equivalent of 15 mg of primaquine base, once a day for 14 days	Antimalarial
Primidone	0.5 to 2g daily, in divided doses	Anticonvulsant
Procaine hydrochloride	Epidural, 25ml of a 1.5% solution. Infiltration, upto 200ml of a 0.25 to 0.5% solution. Peripheral nerve block, upto 25ml of a 2% solution. Spinal, 1 to 3ml of a 3.3 to 5% solution	Local anaesthetic
Procaine Penicillin	By intramuscular injection, 0.3 to 0.9g daily	Antibacterial
Proguanil hydrochloride	As suppressant of malaria, 0.1 to 0.3g daily	Antimalarial
Promethazine hydrochloride	20 to 50mg daily, in single or divided doses	Antihistaminic; anti-emetic
Propranolol hydrochloride	20mg to 2g daily, in divided doses, the initial daily dose should not exceed 40mg; by slow i.v. injection 3 to 10mg	Adrenergic, receptor antagonist (anti-hypertensive, anti-anginal; anti-arrhythmic)
Propylthiouracil	300 to 450 mg daily, in divided doses	Antithyroid
Propyphenazone	1.5 to 3.0 g daily, in divided doses	Analgesic, antipyretic
Pyrazinamide	Upto 35 mg/kg body weight daily, in divided doses	Tuberculostatic
Pyridoxine hydrochloride	Prophylactic, 2 mg daily; therapeutic, 10 to 150 mg 1 to 3 times daily	B-group vitamin
Pyrimethamine	Suppressive, 25 mg once a week; therapeutic, 25 to 50 mg once a day for 2 days	Antimalarial
Quindine Sulphate	In prophylaxis of cardiac arrhythmias 0.2g 3 or 4 times daily. In treatment of atrial fibrillation, 0.2 to 04g every 2 to 4 hr to a total dose of 3g daily	Cardiac depressant (anti-arrhythmic)
Quinine Bisulphate	In suppression of malaria, 0.3 to 0.6g daily. In treatment of malaria, 1.2 to 2g daily, in divided doses	Antimalarial
Quinine Sulphate	In suppression of malaria, 0.3 to 0.6g daily. In treatment of malaria, 1.2 to 2g daily, in divided doses	Antimalarial
Quiniodochlor	0.75 to 1.5 g daily, in divided doses	Antiprotozoal; topical and intestinal antiseptic

Table 5.2 Contd…

Drug	Dose	Category
Rabies Vaccine	By s.c. injection, 1 to 2 ml daily, for 7 to 14 days according to the site and severity of the bit and the risk of exposure to infection	Specific immunizing agent
Ranitidine hydrochloride	Orally, the equivalent of 300 to 600 mg of ranitidine daily, in divided doses	Histamine H_2-receptor antagonist
Reserpine	In psychiatric states, 1 to 5mg daily, in divided doses. In treatment of hypertension, 0.5 mg daily	Antihypertensive
Riboflavine	Prophylactic, 1 to 4mg daily; therapeutic, 5 to 10mg daily	B-group vitamin
Rifampicin	450 to 600mg	Antibacterial
Salbutamol Sulphate	The equivalent of 6 to 16mg of salbutamol daily, in divided doses	Adrenergic (bronchodilator)
Scopolamine Hydrobromide	By s.c. injection, 300 to 600g	Anticholinergic
Smallpox Vaccine (Freeze-Dried)	For prophylaxis of smallpox, about 0.02 ml applied to the skin and inoculated by scarification or pressure	Immunizing agent
Sodium Acid Phosphate	2 to 4 g	Urinary acidifier
Sodium Aminosalicylate	10 to 15 g daily, in divided doses	Antibacterial (tuberculostatic)
Sodium Antimony Gluconate	By i.m. or i.v. injection, 0.6 to 2.0 g daily, for 10 to 30 days	Systemic leishmaniacidal
Sodium Ascorbate	The equivalent of up to 1g of ascorbic acid daily	Vitamin C
Sodium Bicarbonate	1 to 4 g	Electrolyte replenisher; systemic alkaliser
Sodium Citrate	1 to 10 g	Systemic alkaliser
Sodium Lactate Injection	By i.v. infusion, as a 1/6 molar solution, at the rate of 5ml or less per minute	Fluid and electrolyte replenisher
Sodium Salicylate	0.6 to 2 g. In treatment of acute rheumatism, 5 to 10g daily, in divided doses	Analgesic, antipyretic
Sodium Thiosulphate	By i.v. or i.m. injection, 25g	Antidote to cyanide poisoning
Snake venom antiserum	Usually 20 to 50 ml, injected i.v. as soon as possible	Passive immunizing agent

Table 5.2 Contd...

Drug	Dose	Category
Streptomycin Sulphate	By i.m. injection, the equivalent of 0.5 to 1g of streptomycin base daily, or at longer intervals. As an intestinal antiseptic, the equivalent of 0.5 g of streptomycin base every 8 hr	Antibacterial (tuberculostatic)
Succinysulphathiazole	10 to 20 g daily, in divided doses	Antibacterial
Sulphadiazine	Initial dose 3 g; subsequent doses, upto 4g daily, in divided doses	Antibacterial
Sodium fusidate	1.5 g daily, in divided doses	Antibacterial
Sodium salicylate	0.50 to 2.0 g with food; in the treatment of acute rheumatism, 5 to 10 g daily, in divided dose	Ant-inflammatory; analgesic
Spironolactone	100 to 200 mg daily, in divided doses	Diuretic
Sulphadimethoxine	Initial dose, 1 to 2 g; subsequent dose, 500mg daily	Antibacterial
Sulphadimidine	Initial dose 3 g; subsequently upto 6 g daily, in divided doses.	Antibacterial
Streptomycin sulphate	By i.m. injection, the equivalent of 500 mg to 1.0 g streptomycin daily, or at longer period	Antitubercular
Sulphadimidine Sodium	By intramuscular or i.v. injection, 1 to 2 g	Antibacterial
Sulphadoxine	Initial, 2 g by mouth; subsequent doses, 1 to 1.5 g weekly. By deep i.m. or slow i.v. injection 2.5 g initially, followed by 1.5 g after 4days	Antibacterial
Sulphamethizole	100 to 200 mg every 4 to 6 hr	Antibacterial
Sulphamethoxazole	Initial, 2g, then 1g 2 or 3 times daily	Antibacterial
Sulphaphenazole	Initial dose, 1g, every 12 hr, for 2 days; subsequent doses, 500mg every 12 hr for 3 to 5 days	Antibacterial
Testosterone Propionate	By i.m. injection, 5 to 25mg, once or twice weekly	Androgen
Tetanus Antitoxin	By s.c. or i.m. injection, prophylactic, not less than 1500 International Units; therapeutic, not less than 50,000 International Units	Immunizing agent
Tetanus Vaccine (adsorbed)	By deep i.m. injection, two injections of 0.5 ml at an interval of 4 to 6 weeks, followed by a third reinforcing dose of 0.5ml, 6 to 8 months later	Active immunizing agent

Table 5.2 Contd...

Drug	Dose	Category
Tetracycline	1 to 3g daily, in divided doses	Antibacterial
Tetracycline hydrochloride	For adults, 1 to 3g daily, in divided doses; for children 10 to 30mg/kg body weight daily, in divided doses	Antibacterial; anti-amoebic
Thiabendazole	1.5g, twice daily for 2 or 3 days, in treatment of nematode infestation	Anthelmintic
Thiacetazone	0.15g, daily	Tuberculostatic
Thiamine hydrochloride	Prophylactic, 2 to 5mg once a day; therapeutic, 25 to 100mg daily	Vitamin B_1 (enzyme co-factor)
Thiamine Mononitrate	---do---	Vitamin B_1
Thiopentone Sodium	By i.v. injection, 0.1 to 0.5g; by rectal injection, 40mg/kg body weight. Maximum dose, 2g	Anticonvulsant; general anaesthetic
Thyroid	30 to 250mg daily	Thyroid hormone
Thyroxine Sodium	0.05 to 0.3mg daily	Thyroid hormone
Tolbutamide	0.5 to 1.5g daily, in divided doses	Antidiabetic
Triamcinolone	4 top 12mg, 1 to 4 times daily	Anti-inflammatory
Triamterene	150 to 250mg daily, in divided doses	Diuretic
Trifluoperazine hydrochloride	Oral, the equivalent of 2 to 30 mg of trifluoperazine daily, in divided doses; by i.m. injection, the equivalent of 1 to 2 mg of trifluoperazine every 4 to 6 hr as required	Antipsychotic agent
Trifluopromazine hydrochloride	Oral, the equivalent of 30 to 150mg of trifluopromazine daily. By intramuscular injection, the equivalent of 5 to 10mg of trifluopromazine repeated every 4 hr, if necessary. By i.v. injection, the equivalent of 1 to 3mg of trifluopromazine repeated every 4 hr, if necessary.	Antipsychotic agent
Troxidone	For adults, 1 to 2g daily, in divided doses; for children, 0.25 to 0.5g daily in divided doses	Anticonvulsant
Tubocurarine hydrochloride	By i.m. or i.v. injection, 0.1 to 0.3mg/ kg body weight, not exceeding 25mg, then 0.025 to 0.1mg/kg repeated as necessary	Skeletal muscle relaxant
Typhoid Vaccine	Prophylactic, by s.c. injection, 0.5ml as initial dose; second dose of 1ml after an interval of 4 to 6 weeks	Active immunising agent

Table 5.2 Contd…

Drug	Dose	Category
Typhus Vaccine	Prophylactic, by s.c. injection, 0.25 to 1ml	Active immunising agent
Urea	5 to 15g	Diuretic
Vitamin A	Prophylactic, 5000 Units of Vitamin A activity, daily; therapeutic, 10,000 to 200,000 Units of Vitamin A activity daily	Antixerophthalmic Vitamin
Yellow Fever Vaccine	Prophylactic, by s.c. injection, not less than 1000 LD_{50} doses	Active immunising agent

CHAPTER 6

Prescription

A prescription is a written communication from a registered medical practitioner or other licensed practitioner to a pharmacist embodying salient instructions regarding the dispensing of prescribed medication. It designates a medication to be administered to a particular patient at a specified time. It is a means through which treatment is provided to a patient by combined skill and services of both the physician and the pharmacist.

The word "prescription" is derived from the Latin term *praescriptus* which is made up of two Latin words – *Prae* - a prefix meaning 'before' and *scribere*- meaning 'to write' .

Putting it all together (Prae + scribere), prescription means 'to write before' which reflects the historical fact that a prescription traditionally had to be written before a drug could be compounded and administered to a patient.

"A prescription is a written order for compounding, dispensing, and administering drugs to a specific client or patient and once it is signed by the physician it becomes a legal document"

Ancient prescriptions were generally noted for their multiple ingredients and complexity of preparation. The importance of the prescription and the need for complete understanding and accuracy made it imperative that a universal and standard language be used. Thus, Latin was adopted, and its use was continued until approximately 50 years ago.

Present day prescriptions are written in English, with doses given in the metric system, but often one still finds contracted Latin words (*Signatura*), Abbreviations (*tid, bid, Sig.*) etc., and Roman numerals intertwined.

Prescriptions are written in a blank of universally accepted format or may be made in pads. A typical prescription consists of the following parts.

1. ***Physician (Prescriber) Information :*** Information about physician is essential so that the doctor could be contacted in emergency to seek clarification and necessary instruction, missing words, confirmation etc. Following information is mentioned on the prescription:

   - Doctor's name, designation and Registration Number
   - Address with phone number and e-mail.

- Date of issue of prescription.

- Prescription number. (required when calling the pharmacy for a refill or for insurance purposes).

2. ***Patient Information :*** The name, address, age and sex of the patient help in identifying the prescription. Date of prescribing and date(s) of presentation for filling are necessary for keeping accurate records and ascertaining the needs of the patient. Age and sex of the patient, if mentioned, help the pharmacist to check the prescribed dose (s) of the medication.

   - *Name of Patient :* The prescribed medication is only for the patient whose name is on the label. Medications should not be given to another patient even if the other patient has similar symptoms.

   - *Sex :* Male / Female

   - *Age and weight :* For calculation of dose, dose frequency and route of administration.

3. ***Superscription :*** The *superscription* which consists of the heading where the symbol Rx (an abbreviation for recipe, the Latin for 'take thou' or 'you take' is found. Rx symbol comes before the inscription. The sign at the foot of the letter R is believed to represent the sign of Jupiter, the God of Healing. Some historians believe that the symbol Rx originated from the sign of Jupiter.

4. ***Inscription :*** The inscription (body of prescription) comprises an important part of prescription containing-

   - Name(s) of drug(s) and their quantities,

   - Other chief ingredients of the prescription with quantity,

   - Instruction regarding dosage form like tablet, capsule, suspension, mixture, etc., and

   - Dose and quantity of prescription

5. ***Subscription :*** The subscription gives specific directions for the pharmacist on how to compound the medication. Most of direction is usually expressed in contracted Latin or in the form of abbreviation. Instructions for preparation are also given such as: 'make a mixture', 'mix and make 10 tablets', or 'dispense 10 capsules'.

6. ***Transcription or Signatura :*** The signatura which gives instructions to the patient –

   - How, how much, When, and how long the drug is to be taken.

These instructions are preceded by abbreviation 'Sig.' from the Latin, meaning 'mark.' The signatura should always be written in English; however, physicians continue to insert Latin abbreviations, e.g., '1 cap t.i.d. pc' which the pharmacist translates into

English as 'take one capsule three times daily after meals'. It may also contain special instructions, warnings, followed by the signature of the prescriber.

7. ***Renewal :*** The number of times a prescription is to be repeated, is written by the physician under renewal instructions.

8. ***Signature :*** Finally the prescription must bear the signature of the prescriber to impart it the legal validity.

9. **Other Important Instructions**

   (a) Refills — the label will show the number of refills permitted /no refills

   (b) *Qty :* "quantity" or how much is in the package.

   (c) *Mfg. :* "manufacturer" or who makes the medication.

   (d) *Expiry date :* do not use the medication past this date. Do not save unused prescription. If same patient gets sick again, prescriber should be consulted.

   (e) *Take complete /full course :* means that patient should finish taking the entire contents of the prescription even if feeling better especially patient taking antibiotics. This is to avoid recurrence of infection and development of resistance.

   (f) *Take with / without food :* means whether the medication is to be taken after a meal or empty stomach. Some medications work better when the stomach is full while some medications work better when the stomach is empty.

   (g) *Take four times a day :* means to take the medication four times in 24 hours with equal spacing of time. It is different than 'Take every four hours'. If any confusion occurs when to give the medications, one should consult doctor or pharmacist. Most medications do not have to be precisely timed to be effective, but some do.

   (h) *Take as needed as symptoms persist :* means the medication can be taken when symptoms are present, without consulting the prescriber.

   (i) The package may also have bright colored warning labels with additional information. The following are examples:

      (i) Safe storage instructions, such as 'keep refrigerated'.

      (ii) Instructions for use, such as 'shake well before use'.

      (iii) Possible side effects, such as 'may cause drowsiness'.

Prescription are known to be difficult to decipher and understood by a lay man. Initially, even a pharmacist requires effort and it is only after considerable experience that he can read the prescription. There are two reasons for it. Firstly, the busy physician always writes very swiftly and uses too many abbreviations, sometimes coined by himself, which a pharmacist alone can decipher. Somehow the physicians are known for a bad, illegible handwriting. The process of swiftness at times crosses all limits and physicians writing a letter or two only for the name of a drug are not too uncommon. Secondly, the use of Latin in prescription writing is traditional. Although teaching of Latin has slowly gone out of the curricula of medicine and pharmacy, some of the words and abbreviations have very deep roots and physicians still use them frequently. In earlier days, a prescription was a secret between the physician and the pharmacist and a mystery for the patient. With the increasing awareness about drugs no secrecy is now warranted. As such the patient has a right to know what medication has been prescribed and his interest is protected under the Consumer Protection Act. Some of the common Latin abbreviations are given below.

Latin Terms Commonly Used in Prescription

Table 6.1 Terms Related to Dosage Forms.

Latin terms	Abbreviation	English meaning
Aurinarium	aurin.	An ear cone
Auristillae	auristill.	Ear drops
Buginarium	buginar.	Nasal drops
Capsula	caps.	A capsule
Casula amylacea	caps. amylac.	A cachet
Capsula gelatina	caps. gelat.	A gelatin capsule
Cataplasma	cataplasm.	A poultice
Cereolus	cereol.	An urethral bougie
Collunarium	collun.	A nose wash
Collutorium	collut.	A mouth wash
Collyrium	collyr.	An eye lotion
Cremor	crem.	A cream
Emulsio	emul.	An emulsion
Gargarisma	garg.	A gargle
Gelatina	gelat.	A jelly
Guttae	gtt.	Drops
Haustus	ht.	A draught
Inhalatio	inhal.	An inhalation
Injectio	inj.	An injection
Insufflatio	insuff.	An insufflation
Linctus	linct.	A lictus
Linimentum	lin.	A liniment
Lotio	lot.	A lotion
Mistura	m., mist.	A mixture
Nebula	neb.	A spray solution
Oblatum	oblat.	A cachet
Pasta	past.	A paste

Table 6.1 *Contd...*

Latin terms	Abbreviation	English meaning
pastillus	pastill.	A pastille
Pessus	pess.	A pessary
Pigmentum	pigm.	A paint
Pilula	pil.	A pill
Pulvis	pulv.	A powder
Conspersus	consper.	A dusting powder
Sternutamentum	sternut.	A snuff
suppositorium	suppos.	A suppository
Tabletta	tab.	A tablet
Trochiscus	troch.	A lozenge
Unguentum	ung.	An ointment
Nomen Proprium	n.p.	Proper name

Table 6.2 Terms used in preparation of dosage Forms

Latin terms	Abbreviation	English meaning
Fiat	ft.	Let (it) be made
Fiant	ft.	Let (them) be made
Misce/misceatur	m.	Mix
Misce fiat mistura	m.ft.m.	Mix to make a mixture
Misce secundum artem	m.s.a.	Mix pharmaceutically, Mix according to the art
Divide/dividatur	div.	Divided
Dividatur in partes aequales	div. in pt. aeq.	Divide into equal parts
Fiat pulvis subtilis	ft.pulv subtil.	Make a fine powder
Tere / teratur	ter.	Rubbed
Tere bene simul	ter. bene simul	Rubb well together
Duplum	duplum	Twice the quantity
Mitte	mitt.	Send
In phiala		In a bottle
Phiala prius agitata	p.p.a.	The bottle being first shaken
Quantitas duplex	qt. dx.	Twice the quantity
Talis/Tales/Talia	tal.	Such
Capiendus	capiend.	To be taken
Dandus	dand.	To be given

Table 6.2 Contd...

Latin terms	Abbreviation	English meaning
Deglutiendus	degult.	To be swallowed
Infricandus	infricand.	To be rubbed in
Inhaletur	inhal.	Let be inhaled
Instillandus	instilland.	To be dropped in
Miscendus	miscend.	To be mixed
Sugendus	sugend.	To be sucked
Sumendus	sum.	To be taken
Ut antea	u.a.	As before
Utendus	utend.	To be used

Table 6.3 Common Terms Used in Dose, Administration and Parts.

Latin terms	Abbreviation	English meaning
Bis in die / bis die	b.i.d./b.d.	Twice a day
Ter in die / Ter die	t.i.d. / t.d.	Three times a day
Qauter in die /Quarter die	q.i.d. / q.d.	Four times a day
Bis terve in die	b.t.i.d.	Two or three times a day
Ter quaterve die	t.q.d.	Three or four times a day
Quotidie / indies	quot./indies	Daily
Prima luce / primo mane	prim. luc. / prim. m.	Early in the morning
Mane	m.	In the morning
Omni mane	o.m.	Every morning
Jentaculum	jentac.	Breakfast
Omni nocte	o.n.	Every night
Hora decubitus	h.d.	At bedtime
Nocte maneque	n.m.	Night and morning
Hac nocte	hac noct.	To-night
Omni hora / omni singula	o.h. /o.s.	Every hour
Omni altena hora / Quaque alterna hora	o. alt.h. / qq. alt. h.	Every alternate hour
Omni quarta hora	o.q.h.	Every fourth hour
Anti cibos	a.c.	Before meals
Ante cibum	a.c.	Before food
Post cibos	p.c.	After meals
Post cibum	p.c.	After food
Inter cibos	i.c.	Between meals

Table 6.3 Contd...

Latin terms	Abbreviation	English meaning
Lente		Slowly
More dicto / modo dicto	m.d.	As directed
Pro re nata	p.r.n.	Occasionally
Si opis sit	s.o.s.	When required; when necessary
Tussi urgente	tuss.urg.	When the cough is troublesome
Parti affectae / Partibus affectis	p.a.	To the affected part
Parti affectae applicandus	p.a.a.	To be applied to the affected part
Sinister / Laevus	sinist. / laev.	Left
Oculis	ocul.	For the eyes

A Model Prescription :

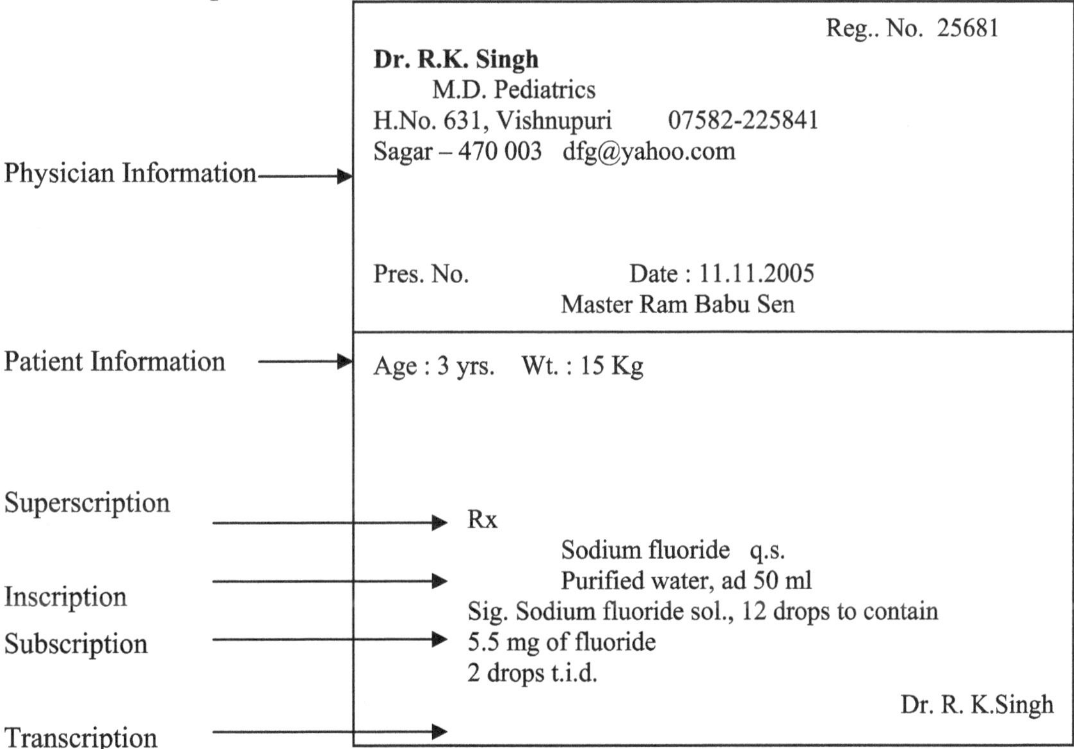

A practising pharmacist is expected to be thoroughly conversant with common systems of weight and measures, their inter-conversions and household equivalents; besides he ought to be well versed with such calculations as are applicable in his professional work.

The increasing use of manufactured dosage forms has gradually reduced the quantum of compounding to be handled by the pharmacist. However, he is ultimately responsible for dispensing the correct drug and accurate compounding. Whatever be the role of the pharmacist, he has to be constantly aware of the degree-of-accuracy due to absent mindedness, or negligence. A wrong drug may be dispensed on the one hand or mistakes in calculations or equivalents may occur. Such errors are inexcusable. To guard against them, it is desirable to check the labels of the ingredients at different stages of dispensing; while removing the container from the shelf, before weighing or measuring the drugs and at the time of replacing the container calculations must be thoroughly understood and doubly checked. If units are to be transferred from one system to the other, one should exercise great caution. Finally, care should be taken in writing and deciphering *decimal places*. Ultimate error in compounding is an outcome of the ± errors of weighing and measuring each ingredient and the final dilution. Dispensing balances are available for varying degrees of accuracy and varying quantities that can be weighed with their help. Usually, the selection of a balance depends on the degree of its accuracy desired. Also it is useful to ascertain the degree of sensitivity of the balance. Suppose the balance shows movement from the rest point only after a weight of 10 mg is placed on the pan, it is obvious that quantity less than 10 mg in weight can not be weighed by that balance. Secondly, one ought to fix the per cent error that can be tolerated. Suppose the sensitivity of a balance is 10 mg and the permissible error is ± 5%. The minimum quantity that can be weighed with such a balance will be $100 \times 10/5 = 200$ mg. In other words, the quantity by weight less than 200 mg should not be weighed with such a balance. If very small weights are to be taken, one may adopt solid : solid dilution by triturating the potent medicament with an inert diluent, both in suitable proportions; or a solid : liquid dilution by dissolving the drug in a solvent and making up to a volume. Appropriate quantity of such dilutions will represent the required quantity of the drug.

The following example may illustrate the point.

Rx

Atropine sulphate   0.5 mg

Send such 10 powders. To be used as directed.

The quantity of atropine sulphate required for 10 powders each of 0.5 mg shall be 5 mg. However the minimum quantity that can be weighed on the balance which is available is 10 mg. Therefore, a 10 mg : 10 mg dilution of atropine sulphate and lactose can be prepared. 10 mg of this triturate representing 5 mg of atropine sulphate should be weighed and thoroughly mixed with 90 mg of lactose, in geometric proportion, yielding a total weight of 100 mg (5mg of atropine sulphate and 95 mg of lactose). 10 powders each weighing 10 mg dispensed from the triturate will contain 0.5 mg of atropine sulphate and 9.5 mg of lactose each.

The equipment commonly used for measuring small volumes of liquids consists of either pipets or droppers. Larger volumes are measured with volumetric graduates. The measures may be graduated in milliliters, ounces, drachms or minims. The shapes differ from cylindrical to conical with a flat bottom. Volumetric apparatus may be meant either for delivering or containing desired volumes. The former class includes burettes, pipets and measuring glasses and the latter includes volumetric flasks and measures. Measuring glasses or graduated measures are used both 'to contain' (TC) and 'to deliver', (TD) liquids. However, household measures for food etc., are not suitable for pharmaceutical compounding as these are likely to be inaccurate. Transference of highly viscous liquids leads to errors as some of the liquid is bound to remain sticking to the measure. Bottles bearing graduations should not be used to make up volumes as these graduations are not always reliable and may result into erroneous content. In general, one should use only such apparatus and appliances which are reliable for compounding accuracy.

The main purpose of correct weighing and measuring is to provide accurate dosage of the medication. The object stands defeated if the patient does not take quantities which represent accurate doses of the medicaments. It is desirable that proper guidance is provided to the patient and instructions given to withdraw proper volumes for administration. For solid dosage forms, the problems are limited as the medication is supplied in unit dosage form. For accurate delivery of liquid preparations, either dose marks should be affixed to the container or a plastic measure or dropper of appropriate size should be provided. Household measures are sometimes recommended e.g., tea, dessert and tablespoons; and tumblers of different sizes and nomenclature to deliver liquid medication. Unless these are available in standard sizes, it is not a good practice to use them. Use of droppers also needs care. Serious errors are possible due to difference in the construction of droppers, viscosity, density and surface tension of liquids in addition to personal factor. Polythene and glass droppers of the same aperture produce drops that are not uniform in size. A graduated dropper is the best answer in such cases.

The scheme of dispensing may be considered from its beginning-receiving of the prescription-to the end delivery of the medication to the patient. Several steps are involved, some of them being procedural while others requiring compounding operations. The sum total of the scheme where compounding is not required can be briefly summarized as consisting of:

1. Receiving the prescription.
2. Reading and checking the prescription.
3. Packaging and labelling; if necessary.
4. Filing, pricing and delivery of the medication to the patient.

For compounded prescriptions the process is more elaborate and consists of:

1. Receiving the prescription.
2. Reading and checking the prescription.
3. Compounding, labelling and packaging.
    (i)   weighing and measuring
    (ii) grinding and size reduction
    (iii) solution
    (iv) mixing
    (v)   filtering
    (vi) finishing
    (vii) checking and recording
4. Filing, pricing and delivery of the medication to the patient.

Receiving the Prescription

A prescription should always be received by a pharmacist himself. The waiting area for the patients should be easily accessible, comfortable and clean, reflecting professional environment. Some magazines and other literature on health matters and current topics should be available to the patient during the waiting time. The patient should be informed about the likely waiting period. In large dispensaries, it is advisable to adopt some system of identification of the prescription like slip or token as practiced in banks. While receiving the prescription, a pharmacist should not make any comments or gesture either approving or disapproving it. A pharmacist should not even give a physiognomic expression to the patient that he is surprised or confused on seeing the prescription.

Reading and Checking the Prescription

A proper scrutiny of the prescription should not be attempted in the presence of the patient; it should be examined behind the counter. Any difficulty in reading or ambiguity in the prescription may be solved by consulting senior pharmacists and if the solution is difficult to find, reference made to the prescriber. Problems of prescription reading and checking may be varied. With the increasing number of proprietary products and very little differences in the spelling of several drug names, a pharmacist's job has become very difficult. The illegible handwriting may make the situation worse. Prescription writing errors and omissions may range from missing quantities of the ingredients, units of weights and measures, strengths of solutions, vehicle, quantity to be supplied, directions for use etc., to errors in dosage of individual drugs and dosage regimen. Then, one frequently encounters incompatibilities in prescriptions. Although it falls under the domain of the pharmacist to detect and remedy the incompatibility yet there may be situations when reference to the physician may have to be made. In no circumstances should a pharmacist take liberties in situations of indecision or lend oneself in guesswork. This does not mean that the pharmacist should not take decisions at all but every issue must be judiciously looked into. In modern therapeutic practice, it is common to prescribe very high doses of medicaments in specific conditions. Calculation of doses of medicaments meant for children have to be done by the pharmacist and he should maintain standard tables and charts which may be referred to whenever necessary. At times a pharmacist has to receive prescriptions on telephone. It requires some experience and therefore it is desirable that a senior person receives the prescription as it may have to be taken down swiftly and in abbreviated form.

To guard against any error arising out of this practice, it is advisable that the prescription be repeated in parts or in full to the prescriber. A pharmacist sometimes comes across prescriptions written in foreign countries. In order to fill such prescriptions, he is expected to have knowledge of Latin and deciphering numerals in other scripts. Reference may be made to standard texts in foreign language maintained in the library.

Compounding, Labelling and Packaging

After reading and checking a prescription, the pharmacist proceeds to dispense it. Compounding, labelling and packaging should be carried out in a neat place. All the equipment etc. should be thoroughly cleaned and washed. In case a prepackaged medicine is to be dispensed under a manufacturer's label, the pharmacist may have to only wrap it and deliver to the patient. Sometimes, a smaller number or volume may have to be dispensed from a larger package. In such cases, he chooses a suitable container with a closure, or a package, and packs the requisite number or volume, affixes a label and delivers it duly wrapped. When compounding is to be done, a pharmacist has to perform a series of operations depending on the nature of the preparation he handles. This is the main area where his professional competence is required.

General Aspects of Compounding

Compounding should be done on a proper work table with suitable fittings. The pharmacist puts on his professional dress, a white overall, while engaged in his professional duties. Ingredients are arranged alphabetically on shelves to which he has an easy access. All equipment and apparatus necessary for compounding is within easy reach, properly arranged, duly cleaned and dried. More than one prescription should not be compounded at a time by a pharmacist. Since he has to work with concentration of mind, he should not be disturbed. But if it is inevitable, he should suspend compounding temporarily and restart only when he can pay undivided attention to his work. Labeling should be done immediately and under no circumstances two unlabeled containers of medication kept side by side to one another. Bottles of all the ingredients to be compounded should be assembled on the left hand side of the table with the dispensing balance in the centre. Labels should be read while removing the bottles from the shelf. Ingredients should be accurately weighed/measured and checked preferably by another pharmacist. The labels are read a second time while removing the quantity for weighing/measuring. After all the ingredients have been taken from the bottles, they should be kept on the right hand side of the balance in the order of their disposal after use. All the ingredients should then be compounded according to the directions of the prescriber or according to the pharmaceutical art. After compounding is over, the bottles should be replaced back on the shelf, again the label is read a third time. While removing and handling the containers and the ingredients, due care should be exercised not to soil the labels of the containers or spill the ingredients on the table or the floor.

The preparation, during processing, is expected to remain untouched by hand. The product is then filled in a suitable container and securely closed. Label of a suitable size is written or typed giving all the desired information in a clear-cut manner. Dropper or measure, when necessary, should be enclosed in the final package. Checking, recording and pricing should be done before delivery of the prescription. While delivering the prescription to the patient, the pharmacist should explain the mode of administration, storage etc. and repeat directions for use.

Labelling

Labelling is an important operation in dispensing practice. Information stated on the label is the only link between the patient and the pharmacist after the prescription has been delivered. It has to be interpreted by the patient who is not an expert and hence the direction should be stated in writing in simple and unambiguous words. Further, the label gives a face-lift to the prescription container and contributes to its elegance. Therefore the label design should be in artistic taste with regard to shape and size of the container, in quality and colour of the paper and printing thereupon. The label should be affixed with a strong adhesive so that it holds firmly in handing. Besides the information to the patient, the label bears other essential details so that on production of the container the prescription could be identified and its filling traced wherever necessary. A specimen label is written below, special labels if required for a product are affixed separately and prominently so that they do not miss attention of the patient.

Specimen label

<table>
<tr><td colspan="2">Serial number   Date</td></tr>
<tr><td>Name of the patient</td><td>...........................</td></tr>
<tr><td>Name of the prescriber</td><td>...........................</td></tr>
<tr><td>Directions for use</td><td>...........................</td></tr>
<tr><td colspan="2">Name and full address of the Pharmacy with its telephone number</td></tr>
</table>

A label should be typed preferably with a machine having clear, narrow letters using computer so that the patient has no difficulty in reading it. A pharmacist is expected to type it himself. In case the label has to be written by hand it should be in clear print letters. While affixing it, the moistening should be done with a moistener and in no case with saliva. Use of saliva is both unhygienic and a non-professional practice. After affixing the label wrinkles, if any should be removed by smoothening with a soft paper. Affixing adhesive labels/stickers on glass surface is an easy operation but plastic and metallic surfaces are problematic in this respect. Special adhesives or lacquers may be needed for such surfaces. If the container is small to hold a label bearing all the directions, one may affix a small number on the container and enclose the container in a larger container with the same number and bearing all the information. Labels are sometimes intended to give a warning to the patient and taking special care while handling and using the medication. Such labels may be affixed separately to give prominence. Common examples of such labels are: 'Shake well before use', 'Do not use after.........days', 'Store in a cool place', 'Keep tightly closed', 'Not to be used internally', 'For external use only' etc. It is a good practice to avoid the use of word 'Poison' on the main or auxiliary label. The product should be finally checked at this stage from all angles - scientific such as colour, gas formation etc., safety and legal requirements etc. It should be on record that it has been checked and must bear the initials of the pharmacist who did the checking. During and after compounding a pharmacist makes a note of some important information which may be useful later for refilling the prescription or other reasons. These may include full words for illegible words, calculation if any, colour of the product, size of the capsule and its colour, procedure etc. The price charged should also find a place on the prescription so that the same price may be charged on a subsequent occasion. Some pharmacists maintain a record of their clients including the ailment and the medication supplied. This is a very desirable practice as it enables him to render a better service to his clients. The drug profile is readily available by a suitable filing system which should be consulted whenever necessary. Commonly the indexing is done on cards and preserved in cabinets for ready consultation.

Packaging

Final packaging of the container is done in a neat carton or bag which tightly hugs the container in proper shape. Sometimes corrugated paper is used to provide padding between the container and the carton. Loose paper bags are not suitable for packaging. Gaudy paper with dark colors should be avoided for external wrapping. Good quality paper in light colors or a paper bearing advertisement of the Pharmacy may encase the packet. A sticking tape is employed for affixing the wrapper in proper position.

Pricing, Filing and Delivery of the Prescription

Pricing a prescription is a very difficult task. The public in general feels that the price charged is high. When the pharmacist is alleged or interrogated in this regard, he finds himself in an embarrassing situation. He should be extremely polite and truthful when confronted with allegations of excessive profit making. The reasons for the price charged should be convincing. One of the reasons for a differing price structure is due to constant change in the prices of the ingredients and drugs as well as services. The society ignores such facts and looks at the pharmacist at times with extreme feelings of disfavour and unfriendliness. Remarks at times amount to accusing him as a profiteer and exploiter. The main reason for this unsympathetic attitude is great variation in the prices charged by different pharmacies for the same prescription particularly if it happens to be a compounded one. It is not true that the price charged is always high but may be lower at times when dispensing has been done by the same pharmacy. A pharmacist while pricing should have a clear policy and work within a framework of rules and rationalize the prescription price. By so doing, he is in a strong position to justify the price and convince the patient. There are several inputs that govern the price of prescriptions. These include cost of ingredients, labour cost, cost of containers, cost of professional services and other overhead expenses and lastly the profit. Cost of ingredients should be calculated without profit and tables stating the price of small quantities of each substance should be maintained and consulted to save time of the pharmacist. Container cost should be calculated taking into consideration the damage or breakage in storage and handling as well as rejections. Usually the cost of labour involved in compounding is dependent on the time required for the purpose. In western countries where the profession of pharmacy is highly developed, norms have been computed for compounding or dispensing prescriptions of different classes. According to an estimate the average time required for dispensing of a non-compounded prescription is 8 minutes and the dispensing of a compounded prescription requires 14 minutes. In India, such norms do not exist and it would be well worth if the profession works out the time-cost schedule of different types of prescriptions. Public is also likely to disregard the professional fee which is included in the prescription price. There has to be a charge for professional service rendered apart from the dispensing time. In addition to the price of knowledge and skill, the advantage derived from the advice by the pharmacist has to be compensated for and not expected to be free. Overhead expenses differ from pharmacy to pharmacy and establishment to establishment. These charges embody all such payments that are unavoidable to run an establishment e.g. rent of the premises, electricity bills, insurance, advertising, interest on the capital invested, furniture and fittings etc. In the aforesaid charges profit is not included and has to be charged extra. Profit calculation is dependent on the profit philosophy of the Pharmacy. Net profit expected for each prescription is added to arrive at the price chargeable for a prescription. Following example may illustrate the calculation of price chargeable from the patient:

Cost of ingredients	Rs. 15/-
Cost of container	Rs. 1/-
Labour	Rs. 3/-
Overhead charges	Rs, 1/-
Professional service charges	Rs. 1/-
Profit	Rs. 3/-
Total price	Rs. 24/-

Filing of prescription in some way or the other is an essential requirement for a variety of reasons e.g. future service to the patient, calculating statistics and for situations legal in nature should complications arise as a result of dispensing the prescription. It has been pointed out earlier that all pharmacists should fully understand the implications of legal requirements prevailing in the country. Filing systems are adopted or evolved by the Pharmacy taking into consideration the nature of the establishment. Filing and maintaining the record depends upon how frequently and expediently one has to refer to it. At present three systems prevail in India. In some Pharmacies and Government hospitals, the original prescriptions are not retained by the pharmacist. The patient is allowed to take it with him. On authorization by the physician the patient presents it for refilling, with modifications if need be. A register is maintained in which all prescriptions dispensed are date wise and serially recorded in the order these prescriptions are presented to the pharmacist. The register has the requisite number of columns for recording the salient features. These columns are usually for serial number, date, name of the patient and the inscription. Tracing back a prescription after the lapse of a long time is difficult unless the original prescription or a reference regarding the date or serial number is available. It is possible to trace the same if the container bearing the date or serial number is presented. Another method is to retain the original prescription. This practice is prevalent in private dispensaries which are attached to a consulting physician. Larger establishments maintain a record of the prescription by photocopying or microfilming, the original prescription being returned to the patient. Whichever be the system, the object is to preserve bonafide information as a record in the hospital or retail pharmacies.

Even for proprietary preparations dispensed in the manufacturer's package, it is necessary that a record is maintained by the pharmacist. Pharmacies and pharmacists would be immensely benefited by the use of computers in keeping records of prescriptions and data retrieval.

For delivering the medication to the patient, two systems prevail - the direct and the indirect. In the direct system of delivery the pharmacist is able to establish a direct contact with the patient or his agent and thus while delivering the medication he can answer questions or at his own initiative explain the salient directions etc., and make certain that the patient has understood "the manner in which the drug is to be administered and the precautions if any, that he has to take. This minimizes the possibilities of error in drug administration. The indirect system does not provide for a dialogue between the pharmacist and the patient. It can be classified in three categories. The delivery can be affected at a window where the patient collects the medication. Secondly, the medication is delivered at the residence of the patient i.e. home delivery. Thirdly, the medication can be sent to the patient by post. In all the three forms of indirect delivery the patient gets the directions and guidance through written information only and is not in a position to make enquiries from the pharmacist. Finally, in the process of compounding, dispensing and sale of medication, a pharmacist is to be guided by ethics of his profession and a sense of service to the sufferer and his approach is expected to be in the best interest of his clients.

Legal Provisions

Supply of drugs to a patient on prescription is the exclusive domain of a pharmacist which also has a legal sanction. Provisions of the Drugs and Cosmetics Rules, 1945 relating to dispensing and supply of medication are briefly summarized below.

In context with the supply of drugs the Rules provide as follows.

(i) The description 'Drug Store' shall be displayed by such licensees who do not require

(ii) The services of a 'qualified person.'

(iii) The description 'Chemists and Druggists' shall be displayed by such licensees who employ the services of a **qualified person** but who do not maintain a 'Pharmacy' for compounding against prescription.

(iv) The description 'Pharmacy', 'Pharmacist', 'Dispensing Chemist' or 'Pharmaceutical Chemist' shall be displayed by such licensees who employ the services of a 'qualified person' and maintain a 'Pharmacy' for compounding against prescription.

['Qualified person' means a person who i) holds a diploma or degree in pharmacy or pharmaceutical chemistry of an approved institution, or ii) is a registered pharmacist under the Pharmacy Act, 1948]

Following licenses are provided to sell, stock or exhibit for sale or distribution of drugs by **Retail :**

(a) drugs specified in Schedule C, C(1), and X;

(b) drugs specified in Schedule C and C(1) excluding those specified in Schedule X; and

(c) drugs specified in Schedule X.

Those holding the licenses for retail sale of drugs must satisfy the following conditions :

1. If any drug is compounded or made on the licensee's premises such operation should be conducted by or under the direct and personal supervision of a 'qualified person'.

2. The supply of any drug on the prescription of any Registered Medical Practitioner (RMP) shall be affected only by or under the personal supervision of a 'qualified person'.

3. The supply of any drug (other than those specified in Schedule X) on a prescription of a RMP shall be recorded at the time of supply in a prescription register specially maintained for the purpose and the serial number of entry in the register be entered on the prescription. The following particulars shall be entered in the register :

    (a)   serial number of the entry;

    (b)   the date of supply;

    (c)   the name and address of the prescriber;

    (d)   the name and address of the patient (or the owner of the animal);

    (e)   the name of the drug or preparation and the quantity or in the case of a medicine made up by the licensee the ingredients and their quantities;

    (f)   in the case of a drug specified in Schedule C or Schedule H the name of the

    (g)   manufacturer of the drug; its batch number and the date of expiry of potency, if any;

    (h)   the signature of the qualified person.

    In the case of drugs which are not compounded in the premises and which are supplied from or in the original containers the particulars specified in items (a) to (g) above may be entered in a cash or credit memo book maintained for this purpose.

    In the case of **refill prescriptions**, it shall be sufficient if the new entry in the prescription register includes a serial number, the date of supply, the quantity supplied and a reference to the earlier entry in the register. It shall not be necessary to record the above details in the register or cash or credit memo, particulars in respect of:

    (i)   drugs supplied against prescription under the Employee's State Insurance Scheme if all the above particulars are given in that prescription, and

    (ii) any drugs other than those specified in Schedule C or Schedule H if it is supplied in the original unopened container of the manufacturer and if the prescription is duly stamped at the time of supply with the name of the supplier and the date on which the supply was made.

    The option to maintain a prescription register or a cash or credit memo book in respect of drugs and medicines supplied from or in original container, should be made in writing to the Licensing Authority. However, the Licensing Authority may require records to be maintained only in prescription register.

1. The supply by retail, otherwise than on a prescription of a drug specified in Schedule C shall be recorded at the time of supply either;

    (i)   in a register specially maintained for the purpose in which the following particulars shall be entered :

(a) serial number of the entry,

(b) the date of supply,

(c) the name and address of the purchaser,

(d) the name and quantity of the drug,

(e) in the case of a drug specified in Schedule C, the name of the manufacturer, the batch number and the expiry date; or

(ii) in a cash or credit memo book, serially numbered and containing all the particulars specified in items (b) to (e) under (i) above,

The supply by retail of any drug shall be made against a cash or credit memo which shall contain the following particulars :

(a) name and address and sale number of the order;

(b) serial number of the cash/credit memo;

(c) the name and quantity of the drug supplied,

The licensee should also maintain carbon copies of cash/credit memos as record.

Records of purchase of a drug intended for sale or sold by retail shall be maintained by the licensee and such records shall show the following particulars :

(a) the date of purchases,

(b) the name and address of the person from whom purchased and the number of relevant license held by him,

(c) the name of the drug, the quantity and the batch number, and

(d) the name of the manufacturer of the drug.

Purchase bills including cash or credit memos should be serially numbered by licensee and maintained in a chronological order.

1. All registers and records are open to inspection by Inspector and should be preserved for a period of not less than two years from the date of the last entry therein.

2. It shall not be necessary to record any particulars in a register specially maintained for the purpose if the particulars are recorded in any other register specially maintained for the purpose under any other Act for the time being in force.

3. Substances specified in Schedule H or Schedule X **shall not be sold by retail except** on the prescription of a RMP and in the case of substances specified in Schedule X, prescriptions shall be in duplicate, one copy of which shall be retained by the licensee for a period of two years.

The supply of drugs specified in Schedule M or Schedule X to RMPs, hospitals, dispensaries and nursing homes shall be made only against the signed order in writing, which shall be preserved by the licensee for a period of two years.

A prescription for Schedule H or Schedule X drugs shall :

  (i) be in writing and be signed by the person giving it with his usual signature and be dated by him;

  (ii) specify the name and address of the person for whose treatment it is given, or the name and address of the owner of the animal if the drug is meant for veterinary use;

  (iii) indicate the total amount of the medicine to be supplied and the dose to be taken.

1. The person dispensing a prescription containing a drug specified in Schedule H and Schedule X shall comply with the following requirements in addition to other requirements of the Rules :

  (a) the prescription must not be dispensed more than once unless the prescriber has specified otherwise:

  (b) at the time of dispensing there must be noted on the prescription above the signature of the prescriber the name and address of the seller and the date on which the prescription is dispensed.

2. No person dispensing a prescription containing substances specified in Schedule H or X may supply any other preparation whether containing the same substance or not in lieu thereof.

Substances specified in Schedule X kept in retail shop or premises used in connection therewith shall be stored –

  (a) under lock and key in cupboard or drawer reserved solely for the storage of these substances; or

  (b) in a part of the premises separated from the remainder of the premises and to which only responsible persons have access.

3. A substance specified in Schedule E sold by retail shall be labelled with word "Poison" in such language or languages as the State Government may prescribe by notification in the Official Gazette.

4. The licensee shall maintain an Inspection Book in Form 35 to enable an Inspector to record his impressions and the defects noticed.

5. No drug shall be sold or stocked by the licensee after the date of expiration recorded on its container, label or wrapper, or in violation of any statement or direction recorded on such container, label or wrapper.

6. The supply by retail of any drug in a container other than the one in which the manufacturer has marketed the drug, shall be made only by dealers who employ the services of a 'qualified person' under the direct supervision of the 'qualified person' in an envelope or other suitable container showing the following particulars on the label :

    (a) *name* of the drug,

    (b) quantity supplied and

    (c) name and address of the dealer,

7. The supply of drugs specified in Schedule X shall be recorded at the time of supply in a register specially maintained for the purpose and separate pages shall be allotted for each drug. The following particulars shall be entered in the said register:

    - date of transaction;
    - quantity received; if any, the name and address of the supplier and the number of the relevant license held by the supplier;
    - name of the drug;
    - quantity supplied;
    - manufacturer's name;
    - Batch No. or Lot No.;
    - name and address of the patient/purchaser;
    - reference number of the prescription against which supplies were made;
    - Bill No. and date in respect of purchases and supplies made by him;
    - signature of the person under whose supervision the drugs have been supplied.

Medication Errors

Mistakes in the use of a medication are sometimes serious problem. Problems can include adverse reactions and interactions with other medications, and also basic administrative errors such as patients being given the wrong medication or wrong dosage. A less studied aspect of mistakes involving medications is the misdiagnosis of a disease when the real cause is a side effect of a medication. Children and infants are particularly at risk of medication errors mainly due to incorrect dosage, because of the need to modify dosages based on age and weight. The dosage modification may be either overlooked or miscalculated. Various studies have shown high error rates in doctors and nurses in calculating weight-dependent dosages in infants and especially neonates. Errors with medication can occur in hospitals, at the pharmacy, in the doctor's office, and even due to the patient.

The dispensing of prescription medications at the pharmacy can have various errors. The wrong medication can be given particularly when medications are named or packaged similarly. There are particular drugs that are known to have problems because their names are very similar. The pharmacy can also give out the wrong dosage of the drug in some cases.

Most studies of medication errors only analyzed hospital medication usage, and there is a large volume of medications prescribed in doctor's offices and dispensed by pharmacies.

The medications causing most problems are cytotoxics, cardiovascular drugs, antihypertensives, anticoagulants, and NSAIDs.

An **adverse drug reaction** (ADR) occurs when a patient suffers a reaction, side effect, or other injury from a medication. This can occur without an error, such as when a patient has an allergy to a medicine, but has never shown any signs or risk factors for this allergy previously. On the other hand, an error would occur if a previous allergy was known but the medication was still given to the patient.

The list of medications most frequently causing adverse reactions in order of incidence is given below.

- antibiotics,
- chemotherapeutic agents,
- anticoagulants,
- cardiovascular agents,
- anticonvulsants,
- antidiabetic agents,
- antihypertensives,
- analgesics,
- antiasthma agents,
- sedative-hypnotic agents,
- antidepressants,
- antipsychotic agents, and
- antiulcer agents.

Following types of errors are generally found in the dispensing of prescription.

- misdiagnosis (40%),
- medication error (28%),

- medical procedure error (22%),
- administrative error (4%),
- communication error (2%),
- incorrect laboratory results (2%),
- equipment malfunction (1%), and
- other error (7%).

Medication errors generally occur in following locations.

- hospital (48%),
- doctor's office (22%),
- operating room (7%),
- clinic (5%),
- emergency room (5%),
- pharmacy (4%),
- home (3%),
- medical laboratory (1%),
- nursing home (1%), and
- other (5%).

About 70% of all errors are believed to be preventable. The remainder are presumably non-preventable errors such as a patient reacting to a drug who had no previous history of an allergy to the drug.

Mistakes Occur

There are numerous ways that an error can occur in medical treatment.

- Self-treatment mistakes: Mistakes are very commonly when a patient tries to treat him/her self. Always professional medical advice should be sought.
- Wrong condition treated: i.e., from a *misdiagnosis* of the condition.
- Wrong choice of treatment plan: the overall strategy used to treat condition might not be the best one.
- Wrong type of treatment given.
- Delayed treatment: there must not be an undesirable delay in treatment, by choice or through non-diagnosis.
- Wrongly performed procedures: all medical events such as surgeries and tests performed wrongly can make things worse.
- Wrong medications.

Prevention mistakes: The failure to prevent a condition is another type of medical failing. In certain cases, it is clear that preventive actions should be taken and failure to do so is a medical mistake.

- Failure to prevent known complications of a diagnosed disease.
- Failure to treat family members or others exposed to an infectious disease.
- Failure to address clear risk factors for various conditions.

Surgery mistakes: Surgical procedures are often complex and subject to various errors. Administration of surgery can also lead to errors. In some cases, there are known complications or risks of surgery that are often unavoidable.

- Surgery administration mistakes: wrong-patient, wrong-site, wrong-organ, equipment left inside.
- Surgical mistakes: the surgeon might make a wrong cut or other mistake.
- Anaesthesia mistakes: too much, too little (waking up).
- Complications from surgery .
- Infections from surgery: called **iatrogenic infections.**
- Wrong blood type transfusion.

Hospital mistakes: A hospital can make errors in any of its varied activities. There are many staff who can make human mistakes and overall system problems can also lead to errors.

- Hospital-caused infections: called ***nosocomial infections***.
- *Medication errors in hospitals :* ordered medication not given, wrong medication, wrong dosage, wrong combinations, wrong patient given medication, and so on.
- *Wrong procedures :* failure to do ordered tests, wrong procedures or tests.

Medication mistakes : Errors in medication are a major source of medical mistakes. *Medication errors* can occur in hospitals or pharmacies, and the error may be made by any of the staff involved with choosing or dispensing medication.

- Inappropriate medication: the wrong medication given for a disease.
- Wrong medication: the patient gets the wrong medication despite the doctor prescribing the correct one.
- Drug name mix-ups: several medications have similar-sounding names and can be mixed up by doctors or pharmacists.
- Wrong medication combinations: there are numerous types of medications that should not be mixed, because of side effects and cross-reactions when combined.
- Adverse reactions to medication: Some people have allergic or other adverse reactions to certain medications. These are risks and not necessarily avoidable mistakes if the person has no previous history of a particular adverse reaction.

- Side effects of medication: Almost all medications have some types of side effects. Some are mild, some nasty. It is almost impossible to know up front whether a person will have side effects from a medication.

- *Non-compliance* : the failure to follow prescribed medication regimen can be a mistake made usually by the patient.

Pharmacist errors: The dispensing of drugs by the pharmacy is a complex and busy activity. Various errors can made by the pharmacist.

- Wrongly filled prescriptions

- Wrong drug supplied

- Wrong dosage supplied

- Drug name mix-ups: various drugs have similar names.

Pathology lab errors *:* Diagnostic testing done by a pathology laboratory can be subjected to various errors. Some are administrative or human mistakes; other mistakes are inherent to the limitations of the type of test.

- Wrong biopsy results: visual inspection of cellular slides

- Administrative errors: mixing samples, etc.

- Known test errors and risks: almost all tests have a small percentage of unavoidable errors (false positives, false negatives).

- Known limitations of tests

Equipment failure errors *:* Physical failures with medical equipment can occur.

- IV drips dislodged

- Dead batteries in equipment

Unnecessary medical treatment *:* Excessive medical care can be a form of mistake for medical professionals and institutions. This can occur with good intentions (to ensure correctness) or for cynical reasons (to increase income).

- Unnecessary procedures

- Unnecessary tests

CHAPTER 7

Solid Dosage Forms

Powders

Powder is a term generally applied to solid substances in small particle size. The particles may be crystalline or amorphous or a resultant of larger particles rendered to a fine state of subdivision. In the context of dispensing, powders is a class of solid preparations meant for internal or external use containing one or more drugs intimately mixed with each other in a fine state of subdivision. If necessary, an inert diluent may be added to the potent medicament. Small proportions of volatile constituents- solids or essential oils may also be present.

Historically, powders are the oldest form of presenting a medication. It is perhaps the simplest too, where comparatively little processing and manipulation are involved because most of the basic drugs are marketed in powder form. Powders are dispensed in bulk or as individual doses. In the former case, the patient uses sufficient quantity at a time as directed from the bulk supplied to him. Powders for internal use are dispensed both in bulk as well as in individual doses; however external powders are generally dispensed in bulk excepting sterile powders, which may be dispensed in separate packets. The packet after opening should be used immediately and another sterile packet is opened when required next time. Sometimes, powders for internal use are not dispensed in fine state of subdivision but are rendered to a granular form by moistening, passing the mass through a sieve and drying. This form of medication is called **granules**. The granules are free-flowing and convenient to handle and are generally dispensed in bulk form.   Before use, the granules which contain ingredients that react to evolve a gas, when added to water, are called **effervescent granules**.

Powders for internal use, in course of time, have been partially replaced by tablets and capsules; however in hospitals powders are still very commonly used.

Advantages of powders :

- Powder form is the most versatile and convenient to prescribe, compound and administer.
- A physician has the option to deviate from the conventional dose of a medicament according to the requirement of the patient.

- Powders are stable and do not enter into reaction in solid state, lesser difficulties are experienced in compounding them together.

- It is possible to reduce them in the desired particle size range and thus facilitate rapid absorption.

- Less incompatibility as compared to liquid dosage form.

- Powders are in the form of small particles; they offer a large surface area and are rapidly dissolved in the gastrointestinal (GI) tract minimizing the problems of local irritation. Drugs that have to be given in bulk can be best administered in powder form by mixing them with foods or drinks.

- Whenever effervescence is desired, accurate quantities of the two reacting powders are mixed with water.

- It is difficult for children and infants to swallow tablets and capsules and under such circumstances drugs may be administered in powder form making them palatable by mixing with milk, fruit juice or honey.

- Manufacturing of powder is economic hence product cost is quite economic as compare to other dosage form.

Disadvantages of Powder

- As compared to other dosage forms, powders are time consuming to compound.

- Volatile, hygroscopic, oxidizing and deliquescent drugs create obvious difficulties when dispensed as powders.

- Dose inaccuracy.

The degree of coarseness or fineness of a powder is differentiated and expressed by reference to the nominal mesh aperture size of the sieves used. The terms used in the classification of powders are –

1. *Coarse powder (10/44)* : A powder all particles of which pass through a 10 no. sieve and not more than 40% by weight through 44 no. sieve.

2. *Moderately coarse powder (22/60)* : A powder all particles of which pass through a 22 no. sieve and not more than 40% by weight through 44 no. sieve.

3. *Moderately fine powder (44/85)* : A powder all particles of which pass through a 44 no. sieve and not more than 40% by weight through a 85 no. sieve.

4. *Fine powder (85/120)* : A powder all particles of which pass through a 85 no. sieve and not more than 40% by weight through a 120 no. sieve.

5. *Very fine powder (120/350)* : A powder all particles of which pass through a 120 no. sieve and not more than 40% by weight through a 350 no. sieve.

6. *Microfine powder (350)* : A powder of which not less than 90% by weight of the particles pass through a no. 350 mesh.

7. *Superfine powder* : A powder of which not less than 90% by number of the particles are less than 10 μm in size.

General compounding methods :

The dispensing process, irrespective of the powder being in bulk or divided doses, for internal or external use or in a granular form, consists of grinding (if necessary), weighing, mixing (to provide homogeneous admixture) and wrapping.

A. Grinding (Milling)

It is presumed that a student is familiar with the process of grinding and its importance particularly the fact that the size of the particles of a drug influences its physico-chemical properties due to increase in its specific surface affecting rate of absorption. The milling operation is usually done by the manufacturer of the drug. However, at the compounding stage a pharmacist may have to grind crystalline substances or particles that tend to form lumps. This can be done with the help of mortar and pestle. This process of size reduction can be performed behind the counter in advance and drugs put on the dispensing shelves duly powdered to save time at the compounding stage. While grinding, excessive pressure need not be applied to the pestle as it leads to sticking of the mortar or to each other. The drug adhering to the pestle or mortar should be scrapped during the operation with the help of spatula. Generally, it is not necessary to sift the powder unless the drug is required to be in smaller size than particular sieve range.

B. Weighing

The pulverized drug is weighed to the required accuracy with the help of a suitable balance as described earlier. A watch glass or a paper with a suitable counterpoise is used for placing the drug while weighing. All ingredients are weighed one after another and kept separately. It may be reemphasized that the drug should be placed either directly from the container on the watch glass or paper or with the help of a spatula. At no stage the drug is to be touched with hands. Similarly the weights should be removed from the box and replaced using forceps. Due care should be exercised to avoid any contact between the weights and the drugs.

C. Mixing

Mixing is an important operation and the quality of mixing determines the even and uniform distribution of each ingredient in the powders and thereby the accuracy of dosage of each drug. Mixing at the dispensing counter is not done by mechanical devices such as blenders or mixers. Four alternative methods are available for hand mixing of the medicaments. These methods are trituration, sifting, tumbling or spatulation. The nature of the finished product is to be borne in mind before deciding upon the method. Sometimes it becomes necessary to dissolve an ingredient in a volatile solvent for even distribution e.g., iodine in alcohol using a glass mortar and pestle.

(i) *Trituration*

Trituration is the most common method using Wedgwood or porcelain mortar and pestle. A mortar which is large enough to hold all the ingredients leaving sufficient space above is selected for the purpose. While handling substances that are likely to react with porcelain, a glass mortar and pestle are to be used. The ingredients are transferred to the mortar beginning with the one present in smallest quantity and mixed with the pestle with equal proportion of the drug in next higher quantity. This process of mixing is known as **geometric dilution**. Geometrical mixing is suitable when potent substances are to be mixed a large amount of diluent. The potent dug is placed upon an approximately equal volume of the diluent in mortar and mixed by trituration. A second portion of diluent equal in volume to the powder mixture in mortar is added, and trituration is repeated. (e.g., 1g potent drug and 15 g diluent should be mixed in such a way : **1** + 1 = 2; 2 + 2 = 4; 4 + 4 = 8; 8 + 8 = 16 where **1** is the quantity of potent drug and other quantities represent diluent). The geometrical dilution is essential to achieve uniform admixture resulting in a homogeneous product. This process of mixing equal quantity of two lots ensures better mixing and is referred to as trituration. If a coloured ingredient is present in the mixture, uniformity in mixing is visually apparent. Homogeneity in colour of the powder indicates even mixing. Sometimes an edible dye in minute quantity dissolved in a volatile solvent is added to provide a tint to the product to ascertain uniform mixing. Dispensing of potent medicaments warrants dilution with an inert solid by trituration to minimize error in dosage.

(ii) *Sifting*

Sifting is another method used for mixing. It controls the particle size and brings about homogeneity in distribution of each ingredient. Particle agglomerates, if any, get broken by this method. The ingredients after simple mixing are sifted through a sieve with the help of a brush or one may use standard sieves for the purpose. Household sieves of fine grade are good enough for this work.

(iii) *Tumbling*

Tumbling is an extremely simple and expedient method of mixing. However it is useful for sticky particles only. All the drugs are kept in a wide mouth bottle with a tight-fitting cap; taking care that the bottle is large enough to fill up to not more than half of its height with the medicaments. The bottle is closed and tumbled up and down allowing the particles to fall freely. The process brings about an even randomization of particles of different densities after the bottle is tumbled 8 to 10 times.

(iv) *Spatulation*

Spatulation or mixing with the help of a spatula is an effective and expedient method when powdered drugs of similar densities are to be mixed. Perfect mixing can be achieved if the particle size range is also similar. The powdered drugs are kept on a tile or a sheet of glazed paper and mixing done with the blade of a spatula.

Most powders are dispensed in divided doses and therefore the mixed ingredients have to be divided in requisite number of doses, each powder representing uniform quantity of each ingredient. This can be achieved by any one of the three methods-

    (i)   using powder measures e.g., spoons, boxes, cups etc;

    (ii)   making a block of the mixture and cutting it in desired number of parts and;

    (iii)   weighing each powder.

The measure method is the least accurate of the three methods because a measure will never hold the same weight of different powders of different compositions due to differences in bulk densities of the ingredients or the mixture. Variation is inherent by this method unless one uses a calibrated measure for the same powder over and over again. Blocking and cutting is a fairly dependable method of dividing powders. The mixed ingredients are transferred to a smooth tile or glazed paper and built to a solid rectangular block with a spatula having a long blade. When the rectangle looks uniform it is cut with a knife or a spatula in as many blocks of equal size as the number of powders required. Thus each block is expected to represent equal weight and uniformity of content of each ingredient. Each block is transferred to a paper in which it is to be wrapped. Since blocking is done by approximation, there is likelihood of some error in the uniformity of weight of each power. Wherever accuracy is required, each power should be weighed in a balance and then wrapped.

(v)　Levigation

Particle size is reduced by adding a suitable nonsolvent known as levigating agent to form a paste and then mixed in mortar with pestle. This method is used to incorporate solids into ointments and suspension to remove gritty feel.

(vi)　Pulverization by intervention

Particle size is reduced by adding a suitable material that can be removed easily after pulverization. This method is most suitable for gummy substances.

Calculation in Powder Dispensing

During mixing etc., there is always a chance of loss of some of the powder and therefore on weighing, the last powder is likely to be lesser in weight. This can not be allowed to happen. A pharmacist therefore weighs each medicament for an additional powder over the number to be dispensed. Thus if 10 powders are to be dispensed quantities of each ingredient are weighed for 11 powders. The first ten are dispensed, the last one being rejected. It is a good practice to weigh the extra powder also which should be less in weight. If it is not so, it establishes an error in weighing at some stage. It is often felt that weighing is time consuming but an experienced pharmacist should be able to weigh quickly without any difficulty. Using a powder measure or **blocking** should be avoided when small powders containing potent medicaments are to be dispensed.

D. Wrapping

Bulk powders are dispensed in bulk containers. Divided powders are packed in powder papers. Powder papers are of four types:

1. Vegetable parchment, a thin semi-opaque moisture resistant paper.
2. White bond, an opaque paper with no moisture-resistant properties.
3. Glassine, a glazed, transparent moisture-resistant paper.
4. Waxed, a transparent waterproof paper.

Wrapping or enclosing the powder in a suitable paper is the last stage in dispensing divided powders. Special papers are available for enclosing powders with or without lining. The quality of the paper is important because the wrapper has to provide protection to the contents without cracking at the folds or springing back in its position on folding. It should also be reasonably impervious to atmospheric moisture etc. It should be light in weight and preserve pharmaceutical elegance of the finished wrapping. A water repellent paper is preferable to a paper that absorbs water. Powder papers of special grades are available ready cut in different sizes. Alternatively a pharmacist may cut the sheets in suitable sizes and preserve them or cut to a desired size whenever needed. Hygroscopic materials are best enclosed in double wrapping, the inner wrapping being of waxed or parchment paper or glassine. Powders containing volatile substances are also provided with double wrapping.

Selection of Paper and box

- The shape of the paper is rectangular.
- The size depends on the quantity to be enclosed and on the size of the powder box in which the powders are to be packed.
- The size of the paper should neither be too large nor too small in which case the medicament bulges excessively from the folds or there is a possibility of the powder spilling out in handling.
- A box of suitable dimensions in first selected and it should hold the requisite number of powders with a tight fit.
- The length of the wrapping paper ought to be 40 to 50mm less than double the inside length of the box so that the powder can be conveniently placed in the box after a double fold lengthwise.
- The powders are placed either vertically or horizontally in the box and width of the paper after folding should confirm either to the width or depth of the box, after three folds i.e., it ought to be three times as wide as the height or depth of the box as the case may be.

Wrapping in paper

The requisite number of papers of the proper size are taken and three to six of them may be folded lengthwise at one time at one of the ends to about 1/7th of the width of the paper.

They are kept on the bench with the folded ends away from the pharmacist or towards the pan of the balance if the powders are to be divided by weighing.

The papers should be as much in number as the total number of powders to be dispensed. Each paper should slightly overlap the other ususally a little more than the folded portion of the paper.

The whole operation of weighing and wrapping should be done over a clean sheet of paper to avoid soiling of the powder wrappers.

The proper quantity of the powder to be wrapped is placed in the centre of the paper.

The lower edge of the length is brought under the folded edge at the top and creased.

The paper is further folded in a manner that the height of the paper after folding is a little more than the powder box.

The powder paper in this position is put over powder folder of the proper size (in little smaller than the length of the powder box).

The position of the paper ought to be such that folds of equal size are possible on both sides.

After the crease mark is made, it is carefully folded back, one fold under the other, so that the final crease is neat.

The wrapped powders are then arranged in the powder box placing one after the other with the folds up. Sometimes the powders are enclosed in envelopes of a suitable size.

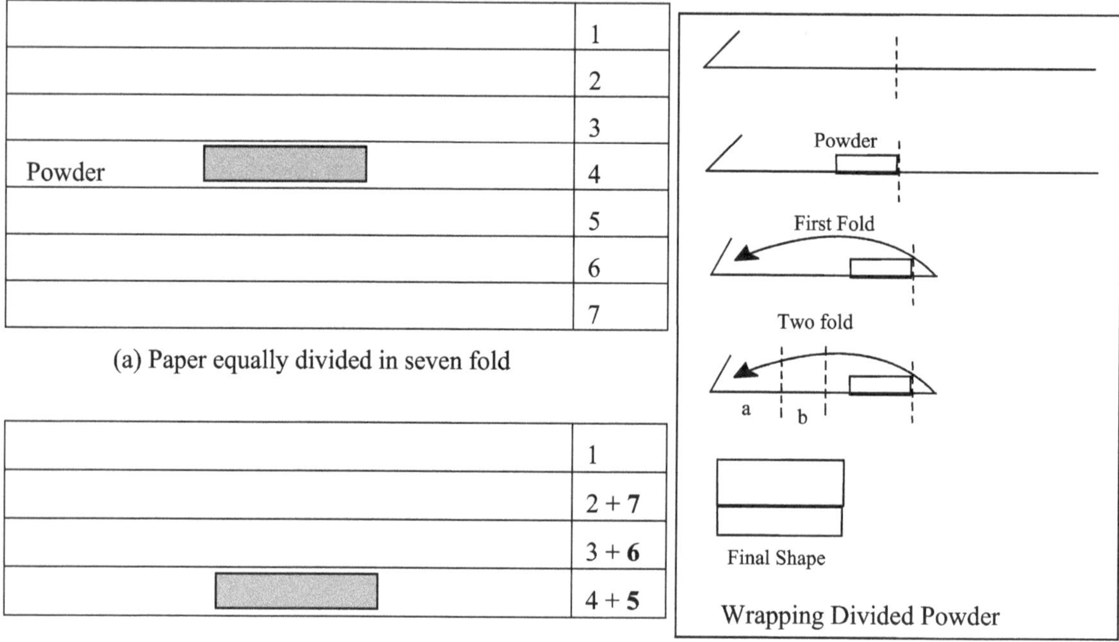

(a) Paper equally divided in seven fold

(b) In centre on forth fold placed the powder and overlap as given fold number

(c) Overlap as given fold number

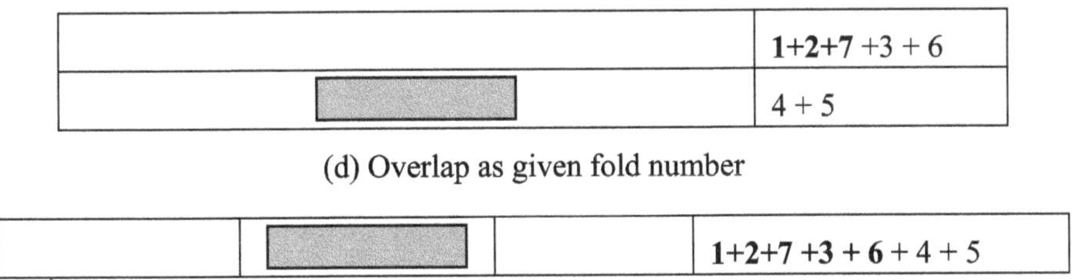

(d) Overlap as given fold number

(e) Final position of power in the paper rapping in side the box

Fig. 7.1 Powder rapping in papers.

There is another method of enclosing powders. The drug is placed in a small envelope of a suitable size and sealed. Such envelopes are provided with lining of a water impervious material and made of superior paper. This provides an elegant wrapping to the drug. Bulk powders are usually supplied in cylindrical boxes made of cardboard with a metallic rim both for the upper and lower edges.

Granules are an interesting form of dispensing solid medication. When the dose of a medicament is large it is convenient to present it as granules. Granules are aggregates of particles of the drugs and can be compounded with colours and flavours to make the product attractive and tasteful so that the patient accepts even a large quantity as a single dose. Drugs that are unstable in liquid form can also be dispensed as granules to be mixed with water or another liquid before use. Sometimes the pharmacist himself may mix granules in a liquid before use if there is the possibility of a drug relating its potency till it is consumed. In such cases the pharmacist states in the directions the period after which the medicament should not be administered. Sometimes the granules provide effervescence on mixing with water which yields a sparkling liquid giving it a palatable appearance. Ordinary granules do not require special precautions in compounding. The process includes weighing the ingredients, making due allowance for the loss in granulation; making a cohesive mass with a suitable liquid which evaporates in air or on heating; passing the mass through a suitable sieve; and drying the granules. Effervescent granules however, require special care and the method is described under special procedures for powders and granules in the following text.

Classification of Powders

Powders are subdivided solids which are classified in the BP according to the size of their constituent particles of range from 1.25 μm to 1.7 mm in diameter. Another classification of powders is based on the manner of their dispensing.

1. Bulk powders for external use :
   (a) Dusting powders (b) Snuffs (c) Dental powder (d) Insufflations
2. Bulk powders for internal use.
3. Simple and compound powders for internal use.
4. Effervescent granules
5. Cachets

1.   Bulk powders for external use

External bulk powders contain non-potent substances for external applications. These powders are dispensed in glass, plastic wide mouth bottles and also in cardboard with specific method of application. Bulk powders for external used are of four types.

(a) Dusting powders (b) Snuffs (c) Douche powders (d) Dental powder (e) Insufflation

(a) *Dusting powders*

These are used externally for local application not intended for systemic action. The desired characteristics of powders include- (a) homogeneity, (b) non-irritability, (c) free flow, (d) good spreadability and covering capability, (e) adsorption and absorption capacity, (f) very fine state of subdivision, and (g) capacity to protect the skin against irritation caused by friction, moisture or chemical irritants.

Dusting powders usually contain substances such as zinc oxide, starch and boric acid or natural mineral substances such as kaolin or talc.

Talc may be contaminated with pathogenic microorganisms such as – *Clostridium tetani* etc., and hence it should be sterilized by dry heat. Dusting powders should not be applied to broken skin. If desired, powders should be micronised or passed through a sieve # 80 or 100. Dusting powders should preferably be dispensed in sifter-top containers. Such containers provide the protection from air, moisture and contamination as well as convenience of application. Currently some foot powders and talcum powders have been marketed as pressure aerosols.

Dusting powders are employed chiefly as lubricants, protectives, absorbents, antiseptics, antipruritics, astringents and antiperspirants.

Rx

Zinc oxide	20 parts
Salicylic acid	2 parts
Starch powder	78 parts

(b) *Snuffs*

These are finely divided solid dosage forms of medicaments dispensed in flat metal boxes with hinged lid. These powders are inhaled into nostrils for decongestion, antiseptic, and bronchodilator action.

(c) *Douche powders*

These powders are intended to be used as antiseptics or cleansing agents for a body cavity; most commonly for vaginal use although they may be formulated for nasal, otic or ophthalmic use also. As douche powder formulation often include aromatic oils, it becomes necessary to pass them through a # 40 or 60 sieve to eliminate agglomeration and to ensure complete mixing. They can be dispensed either in wide mouth glass bottles or in powder boxes but the former are preferred because of protection afforded against air and moisture.

Rx

Zinc sulphate	0.25%
Magnesium sulphate	20.0%
Boric acid	3.0%
Oil of lemon	0.02%
Water	q.s.

(d) *Dental powders*

Dental powders are rarely prescribed. However this class of powders is interesting from the compounding angle. This preparation is a type of dentifrice meant for cleaning the teeth. As such, dental powders contain detergents, abrasives, antiseptics and colouring and flavouring agents incorporated in a suitable base. Generally the base is calcium carbonate. The detergent is in the form of soap and the abrasive action is provided by finely powdered pumice stone. Essential oils are added to provide flavour and freshness to the mouth as well as antiseptic action. Essential oils, if present in smaller quantity, are easily absorbed by calcium carbonate and pumice. This makes the uniform distribution of the oil difficult. Best results are obtained if the oil is triturated in the solids taking considerable care to distribute it uniformly.

(e) *Insufflation*

Insufflations are a class of powders meant for application to the body cavities e.g., ear, nose, vagina etc. The powder has to be extremely fine and must find an entry to the cavity deep enough to bring about its action at the site. It is delivered to the affected part in a stream with the help of a device called an insufflator, which blows the powder to the site. Some of the insufflations contain volatile liquid ingredients which may require uniform distribution in the powder. If these liquid ingredients are present in large quantity, the liquid portion may have to be evaporated. Generally evaporation is brought about slowly in a china dish which is heated on a water bath. The resultant product is re-powdered and sifted through a sieve of a suitable size. However, active volatile liquids present in small portions should not be removed by evaporation but only incorporated by trituration in the powder. The pharmaceutical industry packages the insufflations in pressurized form i.e., aerosols. Aerosols contain the medication in a stout container with a suitable valve, the delivery of the powder being accomplished by a liquefied or compressed gas propellant of very low boiling point. On pressing the actuator of the valve the propellant delivers the medication in a stream.

2. Bulk powders for internal use

Bulk powders contain many doses in a wide-mouth container that is suitable to remove the powder by a teaspoon. The non-potent substances are used in bulk powder form such as antacid, laxative, purgative, etc.

Rx

Rhubarb powder	25%
Light magnesium carbonate	32.5%
Heavy magnesium carbonate	32.5%
Ginger powder	10.0%

Make a powder.

3. Simple and compound powders for internal use.

These are unit dose powders normally packed in properly folded papers and dispensed in envelopes, metal foil, small heat-sealed plastic bags or other containers.

Usually for the preparation of simple powders, the ingredients are weighed correctly and blended by geometrical mixing in ascending order of weights. The mixture is then either divided into blocks of equal size, numbers of blocks representing the number of powders to be dispensed or each dose is weighed separately and placed on a powder paper. The paper is then folded according to the pharmaceutical art and placed in either an envelope or a powder box.

4. Effervescent granules

This class of preparations can be supplied either by compounding the ingredients as granules or dispensed in the form of salts. The ingredients whether in granular form or present as salts, react in presence of water evolving carbon dioxide gas. For evolution of the gas two constituents are essential, a soluble carbonate such as sodium bicarbonate and an organic acid such as citric or tartaric acid. The preparation can be supplied either as a bulk powder or distributed in individual powders.

There are three alternative methods of dispensing depending upon the nature of prescription.

(i)   If the effervescent salts are prescribed to be dispensed in bulk form, no granulation is necessary. The ingredients are mixed uniformly and directions stated on the label to add the prescribed quantity to water, before use.

(ii) If the effervescent salt is prescribed in divided doses, the ingredients which cause effervescence on mixing with water are enclosed separately in papers of different colour. The patient is advised to take one powder of each colour and add to water, before use. Quantities of the sodium bicarbonate and the organic acid, citric or tartaric, are equimolecular in proportion.

(iii) In the third case the product contains all the ingredients mixed together in a granular form. Preparation of granular products requires pharmaceutical technique. If sodium bicarbonate and citric acid are taken in equimolecular proportion and mixed to make granules, the quantity of water of crystallization liberated from the citric acid is large enough to make the mass wet and carbon dioxide may be liberated during the preparation itself. If one tries to substitute citric acid by tartaric acid, which contains no water of crystallization; it may not be possible to form a mass necessary for granulation. Therefore both citric and tartaric acids are taken in suitable proportions leaving a little acid in surplus than the quantity required to neutralize sodium bicarbonate. This surplus is necessary to give the final preparation an acidic taste that is more palatable. There is a certain loss in weight of such a preparation due to the loss of water in drying the granules and partial loss of carbon dioxide due to its release during preparation. Heating is done on a water bath keeping all the ingredients thoroughly mixed in a porcelain dish. Gentle application of heat liberates the water of crystallization from citric acid and the mass tends to be coherent. Prolonged heating may result in complete evaporation of the released water leaving the product in the form of a dry lump which can not be rendered into granules. The coherent mass is transferred from the porcelain dish to an inverted sieve of suitable aperture size kept over a glazed paper. The mass is pressed through the sieve taking care to change the position of the sieve over the paper to prevent the formation of a lump of the sieved granules. The granules are dried in an oven taking care to regulate the temperature which should be generally kept below 80°C. The operation requires considerable skill and experience to obtain granules of uniform size and an elegant product. If necessary, the dry granules are passed through a sieve of appropriate size to break larger granules which result due to sticking of the sieved wet granules.

The water of crystallization of the citric acid and the water from the reactions make the material coherent. Loss of weight occurs during granulation due to (a) evaporation from the damp mixture, and (b) loss of carbon dioxide. The losses constitute approximately one-seventh of the weight of powder used and must be allowed for when calculating the amount to be prepared.

Chemical reaction

$$3\ NaHCO_3\ +\ C_6H_8O_7.H_2O\ =\ C_6H_5Na_3O_7\ +\ 3\ CO_2\ +\ 3\ H_2O$$

(Sodium bicarbonate)   (Citric acid)

$$2\ NaHCO_3\ +\ C_4H_6O_6\ \ \ \ \ =\ C_4H_4Na_2O_6\ +\ 2\ CO_2\ +\ 2\ H_2O$$

(Sodium bicarbonate)   (Tartaric acid)

5. Cachets

Cachet as a unit dosage form was very popular sometime back. Presently cachets are seldom used and have been replaced by capsules. Cachets, like capsules, can be easily filled and sealed at the dispensing counter. This dosage form holds larger quantity of the medication as compared to capsules. Since the cachets are made of flour and water they are easily damaged in handling. Further this dosage form offers little protection against light and moisture. Due to its size and shape a cachet is difficult to swallow. The process of filling is similar to that of capsules. The drug is placed in one of the two halves of the cachet, the upper half is then placed over it and pressed with the help of a suitable device.

The flange of the upper plate is moistened carefully taking care not to wet it, with the help of a dampener. The sealing takes place due to the moisture between the flanges of the upper and the lower half and the pressure over the flanges. About 15 minutes are allowed for drying of the seal. After this time the middle portion of the cachet is slightly pressed to ensure complete sealing. In absence of a machine a pharmacist can improvise and use two bottles the mouths of which are broad enough so that flanges of the plates – upper and lower, when kept over the mouths of the bottles, just rest over them. The drug is transferred to one of the plates resting over the mouth of the bottle kept vertically on the working bench. The flange of the empty half resting over the mouth of another bottle is moistened with the help of a damp camel hair brush. The empty half of the cachet is then placed over the other half in which the medication is kept so that the flanges of the two halves are perfectly superimposed. The second bottle is then inverted and brought over the superimposed cachet and carefully put over the flange and pressed in position without disturbing the resting place of the cachet. This provides a good seal. Cachets can be dry-sealed also. These cachets however are of a different shape where the cap is pressed over the body of the cachet. A protruded stud is also provided to hold the upper and lower halves together. Like capsules, cachets are also expected to remain untouched by hand and one should use gloves while handling them. Since there are inherent losses of the drug in this operation also like that of powders and capsules, the quantities of each ingredient should be weighed for an extra powder over the number to be dispensed. The cachets are dispensed in wide-mouthed bottles of glass or plastic with a perfectly fitting cap. The patient should be instructed to keep the bottle securely closed.

Rx

Phenolphthalein	1 grain
Rhubarb powder	5 grain
Magnesium sulph.	15 grain

M.Ft.cachet. Mitte tales sex.

Special Powders

Ordinarily the powders can be prepared by the general method stated above. However, special procedure may have to be adopted under the following condition:

(a)	medicaments liquefying on mixing;

(b)	hygroscopic and deliquescent substances;

(c)	efflorescent materials;

(d)	volatile substances;

(e)	liquids;

(f)	explosive mixtures and incompatible salts.

(a) *Medicaments liquefying on mixing*

Some of the drugs which tend to liquefy on mixing include Camphor, Thymol, Menthol, Phenol, Aminopyrine, Chloral hydrate, Acetylsalicylic acid, Antipyrine, Salol and Acetanilide. Mixtures of these drugs liquefy and create problems in compounding. Their mixtures have a melting point below room temperature. Such mixtures are called **eutectic mixtures**. There are two alternatives in overcoming this difficulty. Firstly, one may add an absorbent e.g. talc, calcium phosphate, lactose or starch in sufficient quantity to each ingredient and then mix them. Alternately, one may allow the eutectic mixture to form and add sufficient quantity of the absorbent to the liquid. Second method is that each of the substances is dispensed separately as a powder with directions to take one powder of each one of these at a time.

(b) *Hygroscopic and deliquescent substances*

Substances which absorb moisture from the air are called **hygroscopic.** If the content of water absorbed is so much that the material becomes a liquid it is called a **deliquescent** solid. It is difficult to dispense such substances. However the situation can be partly met by taking the crystalline form without powdering and thus minimizing the surface area available for absorption of water. Secondly, such substances should be dispensed in double wrapping taking due care to provide maximum protection from the air. In highly humid climate one may use aluminium foil or plastic packets for preventing the access of air. Commonly used drugs under this category include Pepsin; Ephedrine sulphate; Hyoscine hydrobromide; Iron and ammonium citrate; Bromide, Iodide and Nitrate of sodium; Potassium citrate; Physostigmine salts; Phenobartibone sodium; Halides of ammonium; and Pilocarpine.

(c) *Efflorescent substances*

Substances that are crystalline and contain water of crystallization tend to lose it. Such substances are called **efflorescent**. This usually occurs due to change in humidity and solid powder may become pasty in course of time. The only way out is to use the anhydrous salt in place of the crystalline substance. However allowance should be made for the water of crystallization associated with the material while calculating the quantity of the anydrous salt. Efflorescent substances met in dispensing practice include Morphine acetate; Ferrous sulphate; Sodium carbonate; Sodium phosphate; Sodium acetate; Quinine bisulphate, hydrobromide and hydrochloride; Alum; Atropine sulphate; Caffeine; Terpin hydrate; Scopolamine hydrobromide; Cocaine; Codeine phosphate and sulphate; and Citric acid.

(d) *Volatile substances*

Volatilization of substances like menthol, camphor and essential oils may take place on incorporation in powders. This is prevented or minimized by use of double wrapping with an inner waxed paper and outer bond paper cover or by using heat-sealed plastic bags.

(e) *Liquids*

For the incorporation of a relatively small portion of liquid into a powder, the liquid can be triturated with an equal weight of powder followed by the addition of the remaining powder in several portions with trituration.

Large portions of liquids such as tinctures or fluid extracts are evaporated on a water bath to a syrupy consistency to reduce the volume. Addition of lactose during process enhances the rate of evaporation by increasing the evaporating surface. Substitution of a liquid extract by a dry extract, wherever possible, is another alternative.

(f) *Explosive mixtures and incompatible salts*

Trituration of an oxidizing agent such as potassium chloride in a mortar with a reducing agent such as tannic acid may result in a violent explosion. Other potentially explosive materials include potassium dichromate, potassium nitrate, sodium peroxide etc., as oxidizing agents; and sulphur, charcoal and sulfides as reducing agents. Such materials should be mixed by employing minimum force and preferably by tumbling in a jar or on a paper. Alternatively they can be dispensed separately with appropriate directions to the patient.

Practice Exercises

Rx,

Aspirin   600 mg

Send 8 powders. 1 s.o.s.

(Simple individual powder for internal use)

Rx

Sodium bicarbonate   gr v

Heavy mag. oxide   gr ii

Al. hydroxide dried   gr iii

M.ft.pulv.Mitte 10 tales. Mode dicto utenda.

(Compound individual powder for internal use)

Rx

Phenolphthalein   2 mg

Atropine   1 mg

Mitte tales 8.

(Compound individual powder containing small quantity of potent medicament)

Rx

Thymol		10 mg
Menthol		
Camphor	aa	20 mg

M.ft. pulv. Mittle xv.

(Compound individual powder containing liquefiable substances)

Rx

Calcium lactate 200 mg

One tablespoonful to be taken with water.

(Bulk powder for internal use)

Rx

Sod. bicard. 10 mg

Pot bromide 20 mg

Phenobarbitone sodium 2 mg

D.T.D. # 6

(Compound individual powder containing hygroscopic substances)

Rx

Codeine sulphate 60 mg

Caffeine 20 mg

D.T.D. chart numero 16.

(Compound individual powder containing efflorescent substances)

Rx

Precipitated chalk 80

Soap 10

Pumice 9

Ol. menth. pip. 1

Ol. caryophylli 1

M.ft.dental powder. Mitte 100 gm. Tint suitably.

(Dental powder. Alcoholic solution of an edible dye in small quantity may be used for tinting. Preferred colours are pink or cream.)

Rx

Tr.Benz. Co.	fl dr ii
Starch	oz i

M.ft. insufflatio. Mode Dict. Ut.

(Insufflation containing a liquid which should be slowly evaporated on a water bath after thoroughly mixing with starch)

Rx

Talcum	100 gm
Precipitated chalk	50 gm
Peppermint oil	10 minims

M.ft. Conspergio. Sprinkle when irritation occurs.

(Dusting powder)

Rx

ASA	200 mg
Mag. sulph.	80 mg
Citric acid	100 mg
Sod.bicarb.	200 mg

D.T.D. 8. One every 4 hours with water during effervescence.

(Effervescent powder)

Rx

Rhubarb	gr xxxxv
Sodium bicarbonate	oz i
Citric and tartaric acids	q.s.

Prepare an effervescent powder. Use as directed.

(Effervescent granules may require calculating the quantities of citric and tartaric acids required to neutralize sod.bicarb.)

Pills

Pill is an old dosage form of presenting solid medication. Inconvenience associated with the administration of powders led to the use of pills by converting the powder into a spherical shape with the help of a liquid and excipients. Historically, the pills have been into use for the last 200 years and till the advent of compressed tablets, pills were a very popular dosage form. Almost 60% of the prescriptions at one time comprised of pills. The word 'pill' has become so deep-rooted in medical practice that today when pills are seldom used and prepared in dispensing practice or by the industry, the term 'pill' is at times used for a tablet. However pills continue to be popular as homeopathic and ayurvedic medicine. A century ago, making good pills was considered to be a great pharmaceutical art and only experienced pharmacists were known to be able to roll attractive looking pills. At one stage the pharmacist was considered to be a pill maker. The pills were provided with coatings of a variety of substances e.g., sugar, salol, talc, silver and gold leaf, and varnish. From the dispensing counter, the pill reached the pharmaceutical industry and machinery was designed to manufacture pills on large scale prior to the introduction of compressed tablets.

Pills are generally spherical in shape, sometimes oval. The only positive aspect of this dosage form was its shape that facilitated swallowing. A large pill meant for veterinary use is called a **bolus**. Freshly made pills provided rapid disintegration in the gastro-intestinal (GI) tract but manufactured, particularly coated pills were most unpredictable as regards their disintegration time. Further, variation in the weight of individual pills is more than that in the tablets and capsules. The pills were kneaded to make a mass with hand which from modern standards is considered an unhygienic practice.

It is interesting that the basic principles of pill making and coating are presently being applied to tablet making and coating and fabrication of sustained release dosage forms. In the process of evolution of unit dosage forms of medicaments, pills may be considered as predecessors of tablets.

In compounding pills the drug(s) and excipients are taken for two additional pills than the number of pills that are to be supplied. The excipients used in pills are many and include diluents e.g., glycyrrhiza, lactose and gums or their combinations. The quantity of the diluent to be used is a matter of experience, the object being to produce a pill of reasonable size. Although no norms are prescribed, yet the average weight of a pill is expected to be within 120 to 150 mg. The drug, the diluent and other excipients are made into a suitable mass which should be plastic, firm and adhesive. These properties are essential to keep the mass cohesive to enable the pill to retain its shape. Liquid excipients also called moistening agents include mucilages, honey, syrup, syrup of liquid glucose, water, alcohol and glycerin. Water alone is not used as it does not assist coherence on drying. This is also true with alcohol and the pills tend to be hard on drying. Sometimes solid excipients that are absorbents are used e.g., glycurrhiza, calcium phosphate, acacia and oxides and carbonates of magnesium. Oleaginous substances like waxes and oils are used as excipients in some preparations. After a mass of proper consistency is obtained, it is rolled on a pill tile to yield a pill pipe in the shape of a pencil. Dusting Powders e.g., lycopodium, magnesium carbonate or starch may be used to prevent sticking of the tile or the roller. The choice of the dusting material depends upon the colour of the pill. The dusting powders are expected not to show themselves conspicuously over the surface of the pill. The pipe is rolled in uniform diameter to a length of two more cutters than the number of pills to be prepared. It may be remembered that the ingredients were also taken for two extra pills. The pipe so rolled is placed next to the edge of the pill cutter and pressed with the roller to cut it in small pieces. The cut mass at the two ends will be lesser in weight as compared to others and hence it is rejected. The rest of them are removed one by one from the cutter and rolled round in the palm of one hand with the help of the index finger of the other hand. Appropriate quantity of the dusting powder may be applied to the palm and the finger to prevent sticking. Sometime, pill rounders are also used for the purpose to provide a perfectly round shape. Pearl, silver or gold coating may be provided to the pills by adding a small quantity of talcum powder or a silver or a gold leaf, respectively, keeping the pills in the rounder. A drop or two of water may be sprinkled, if necessary. The lid is placed in position and the rounder gently rotated to provide a uniform coating. Two to three of such coats yield a good finish to the product. At the dispensing counter varnish, sugar or enteric coating can be provided by dipping individual pills attached to a pin in the solution of these materials, the pills and sealing the pin hole with the solution applied with a thin brush. Pills are supplied in cylindrical paper board boxes or wide-mouthed plastic or glass containers of a proper size and a tight-fitting lid.

Practice Exercises

Rx

Aloe	3 gr
Excipient	q.s.
Mitte tales pilula numero	xii.

Rx

Calomel	1 gm
Pulv. Ipecac.	100 gm

Make a pill mass and divide in 10 pills

Rx

Belladona extract	½ grain
Opium	½ grain

Supply 8 pills. To be used as directed.

Pastilles

Pastilles are preparations which are kept in the mouth and slowly allowed to dissolve thus gradually releasing the medication for local action generally in the throat. The base is composed of glycerin and gelatin. The drug may be either in solution or in suspension form in the base. In extemporaneous dispensing the pastilles are prepared by pouring hot molten mass in moulds and allowing to cool when it sets in a soft mass. They can be scooped out of the mould easily because the mould is previously wiped with a cloth moistened with liquid paraffin, which prevents sticking to the mould surface. They are then wrapped in a waxed or cellophane paper. Pastilles manufactured by the pharmaceutical industry are relatively harder as they contain a greater proportion of gelatin. As they are harder, a longer time is required for dissolution in the mouth. Since the pastilles are designed to remain in the mouth for a long time, they are sweetened and flavoured to make them agreeable in taste and partially mask the taste of the medicament(s). The pastilles are packed in air-tight containers and stored in cool, dry place since they are liable to absorb moisture and become damp which, in absence of a preservative, may encourage mould growth.

Rx

Penicillin	100,000 I.U.
Menthol	0.001 gm
Glycerin	
Gelatin	
Water	aa q. s.

Send 12 such pastilles. Keep in mouth and let dissolve slowly.

Lozenges

Lozenges resemble tablets and provide a prolonged effect of the drug. They are sucked in the mouth to disintegrate slowly releasing the medication for local action. The base however is different than that for the pastilles and consists of gum, starch and sugar along with a suitable liquid excipient which dries. In industry, the lozenges are formulated like tablets using higher proportion of gum and compressing them harder. The traditional method of compounding is by moulding the lozenge mass in suitable shape and size. A hard dough is prepared using appropriate quantity of the drugs and excipients providing for losses, water or alcohol are used for moistening which provides rapid drying. The mass is rolled flat on a tile using a dusting power, if necessary. The lozenges are then cut from the flat mass with the help of a lozenge cutter. Lozenge cutters are available that provide different shapes and sizes. They are allowed to dry and packed in containers similar to those employed for pastilles.

For making pastilles, the moulds are calibrated for the weight of the base they can hold when filled to the brim. The quantities of the medicaments and the excipients are accordingly weighed, providing for losses. Similarly for moulded lozenges, the mass should be spread over an area from which lozenges in required number may be cut to provide correct quantity of medication in each lozenge.

Rx

Sulphadiazine	200 mg
Ol. menth. pip.	0.01 ml
Gum Tragacanth	
Sucrose	
Water	aa q.s.

Mitte tales 20 lozenges. Label: Suck occasionally.

CHAPTER 8

Tablets

Tablets are a solid, unit dosage form prepared by compression using tablet compression machine. Tablet can be defined as solid, flat or biconcave disc (also available in various shapes) prepared by compressing a drug or a mixture of drugs with or without suitable diluents. About 90% of drugs are available in the form of tablets to produce a therapeutic effect when administered by the oral route. They vary in shape and differ greatly in size and weight, depending on the amount of medicinal substances and the intended mode of administration.

Tablet fabrication by compression was initiated in 1843 by Brockedon. Since then the popularity of this dosage form has been increasing and today tablets remain the most popular of all the dosage forms, intended for oral use. This may be attributed in part to the availability of variety of compression machines and advances in tablet technology.

Common Abbreviations of Tablets

- Sugar Coated Tablets   [SCT]
- Multiple Compressed Tablets   [MCT]
- Film Coated Tablets   [FCT]
- Enteric Coated Tablets   [ECT]
- Chocolate Coated Tablets   [CCT]
- Multiple Compressed Tablets   [MCT]
- Buccal Tablets   [BT]
- Sublingual Tablets   [ST]
- Effervescent Tablets   [ET]
- Dispensing Tablets   [DT]
- Hypodermic Tablets   [HT]

Advantages

Tablet dosage form has number of potential advantages over the other solid dosage forms as well as liquid dosage forms such as :

1. Unit dosage form (dosage accuracy). 2. Compactness of dosage. 3. Easy to swallow. 4. Highly soluble. 4. Flexibility of dosage form. 5. Easy to prepare. 6. Economic for packaging, shipping and storage.

Disadvantages

1. Highly amorphous substances are very difficult to compress.
2. Poor wetting and slow dissolution drugs can not be placed in the form of tablets.
3. Objectionable odor, bitter tasting and humectant substances need special treatment for compression.

Classification of Tablets

Tablets are classified on the basis of shape and size, process involved in its preparation and route and other characteristics.

I. Shape and size	II. Process
· Round tablets : (a) flat surface, (b) concave surface, (c) convex surface · Oval tablet : (a) oral route, (b) other than oral route tablets · Oblong tablet : suppositories · Cylindrical tablet : suppositories · Triangular tablets (a) Lozenges, (b) chewable tablets	· Compressed Uncoated tablets · Compressed Coated tablets (a) sugar coated, (b) film coated, (c) enteric coated

III Route and other special characteristics

1. Oral tablets for ingestion	2. Tablets used in oral cavity
(a) Compressed tablets (CT)	(a) Buccal tablets
(b) Multiple compressed tablets (MCT)	(b) Sublingual tablets
(c) Prolonged action tablets	(c) Troches and Lozenges
(d) Sustained release tablets	(d) Dental cones
(e) Delayed action tablets	
(f) Chewable tablets	
(g) Coated tablets	

Table Contd...

3. Tablets administered by other than oral route	4. Special tablets
(a) Suppositories	(a) Effervescent tablets
(b) Implant	(b) Dispersible tablets
	(c) Dispensing tablets
	(d) Hypodermic tablets
	(e) Tablet triturates (TT)
	(f) Soluble tablets

Compounding

Compounding of tablets requires following additives, in addition to the drug substance.

Diluents : Diluents are substances to increase bulk and convert in the compressible form, when drug material is potent or inadequate to provide a suitable shape and size to tablet. A tablet diluent must be compatible, inert, economic, easily available and organoleptically acceptable. It should not affect the bioavailability of a drug adversely.

Examples of tablet diluents include dibasic calcium phosphate, calcium sulphate, lactose, lactose anhydrous, lactose spray dried, mannitol, sorbitol, sucrose, dextrose etc. Examples of directly compressible diluents include Sta-Rx-1500, Emdex (contains dextrose 90 to 92% and maltose 3 to 5%), Celutab (dextrose & maltose), Avicel (Microcrystalline cellulose), Di-Cal (Dicalcium phosphate dihydrate), Cab-O-Sil (Colloidal silica).

Binders and Adhesive : These materials are used in dry or liquid form to reduce the amorphous nature of substance and convert into compressible form (wet granulation).

Example include acacia, tragacanth, gelatin, alginates, methylcellulose, hydroxypropyl-methylcellulose, hydroxypropylcellulose, PVP, Starch, sorbiol, ethylcellulose, pregelatinized starch, glucose, iris moss, ghatti gum, arabogalactan, waxes, etc.

Disintegrants : Most of the tablets contain disintegrating agent. Disintegrating agents facilitate the disintegration of the tablet in small particles in the gastrointestinal tract. Breaking of tablet is based on the swellability, adsorption of water or chemical reaction. Examples include soluble starch, pre-gelatinized starch (PGS), veegum HV, bentonite, microcrystalline cellulose, sodium carboxy methylcellulose, PVP, guar gum, Isapgul, primogel, explotab, aerosil, natural sponge citrus pulp, Alginic acid and alginates, Ion exchange resin, magnesium aluminium silicate, modified corn starch, sodium dodecyl sulphate, sodium starch glycollate, etc.

Glidants : Glidants act as a flow promoter and reduce the friction between particles. It improves the flow properties of granules or powder through hopper to die. It is not deformed by compression pressure of the tablet machine. Examples include talc, starch, magnesium stearate, calcium stearate, boric acid, sugar, lycopodium and sodium chloride.

Lubricants : Lubricants reduce inter-particular friction. It improves the ejection of tablet from die wall and reduces the sticking problems and smooth tablets are produced. Examples include Talc, magnesium stearate, calcium stearate, stearic acid, polyethyleneglycols, starch derivatives.

Antiadhesives or Antisticking agents : These materials are used to reduce the adhesion of the tablet surface to dies and punches during the compression of tablets. The pressure of the machine deforms these materials. It reduces sticking, picking and chipping problems. Examples include paraffin, stearic acid, cocoa butter, soaps, starch derivatives.

Coloring agent : Colours are selected from 'permitted' list and are added to promote elegance and also to mask differences in colour or speckling when either the drug or an additive is off white. Pastel shades are commonly used as these shades help in achieving uniform colour distribution. Coloring materials or dyes are used in tablet formulation mainly for three purposes; disguising of off color drugs, product identification and production of more elegant products. Colours may be added either to the vehicle used for granulation or to the mixture of powders prior to granulation. The first approach is known to give better results provided migration of dye to the top of granules along with solvent during drying does not occur. When wet granulation is not to be employed, lake dyes (dyes adsorbed on alumina or aluminium hydroxide) are recommended. Fading of the colour on standing and exposure to light leading to mottling of tablets is the common problem with dyes. Examples include water soluble dyes and many other FD&C approved colors or dyes.

Flavoring agent : These substances are not necessary for the formulation of compressed tablets. The proportion of flavours should generally be limited to 0.5% because excessive amounts may interfere with the free flow or cohesion of the granules. Special tablets require flavoring agents such as chewable tablet, lozenges, etc. Examples include flavoring oils like cinnamon, coriander, and caraway etc.

Sweeteners : Chewable tablets have sweetening agents because such tablets remain in the mouth and are not swallowed. Examples include saccharin sodium, aspartame, sugar, etc.

Compressed Tablets

For making compressed tablets, it is necessary to prepare the material in a dry, granular form to render it suitable for passing through a compression machine. Following general processes are employed for this purpose.

I. Wet granulation

1. The drug or a mixture of drugs in powder form is mixed; diluent and half quantity of disintegrating agent are added. The material in the desired degree of fineness is mixed and damped with a suitable moistening agent selected with regard to its effect on the chemical and physical nature of the material.

2. The moistened material is made into granules by passing it through a sieve # 12, 16, 22 etc.

3. The granules are dried in a current of air, at a suitable temperature generally not exceeding 60 °C.

4. The dry granules are passed through suitable sieve to get uniform granules and half quantity of disintegrant, lubricant, antiadhesive and glidant are added.

5. These granules are mixed well and are suitable for compression to get the desired type of tablets.

II. Dry granulation

1. The drug or a mixture of drugs in powder form is mixed. If necessary, add a suitable inert substance to act as diluent along with half quantity of disintegrating agent and lubricant.

2. Compress the powder materials in the form of large tablets.

3. These large tablets are broken up into granules of a suitable size.

4. These granules are passed through set of sieves to get granules of uniform size.

5. The remaining quantities of disintegrant, lubricant and glidant are added and mixed well. The granules can be compressed using tablet machine.

III. Direct compression

1. The drug or a mixture of drugs in powder form is mixed. If necessary, add a suitable inert substance to act as diluent, direct compressible disintegrating agent, glidant and lubricant.

2. Pass the powder material through a suitable sieve.

3. Compress the powder materials in the form of tablets.

Table 8.1 Stages involved in various granulation methods.

Wet granulation	Dry granulation	Direct compression
Raw material (drug)	Raw material (drug)	Raw material (drug)
Weighing and measuring	Weighing and measuring	Weighing and measuring
Screening	Screening	Screening
Manual feeding	Blending (slow-speed planetary mixer)	Manual feeding
		-
Blending (slow-speed planetary mixer)	Compress slug	-
		-
Wetting (hand addition)	-	-
Subdivision (comminutor)	Subdivision (comminutor)	-
Drying (fluid bed dryer)	-	-
Subdivision (comminutor)	-	-
Premixing (barrel roller)	Premixing (barrel roller)	-
Lubrication (ribbon blinder)	Lubrication (ribbon blinder)	-
Manual feeding	Manual feeding	-
Compression	Compression	Compression

Development of Formulae

Considerations involved in developing formulae of different kinds of tablets are discussed below.

Soluble tablets : Soluble tablets have become much popular for administering antibiotics specially for paediatric patients. All the components of a soluble tablet base must be completely soluble, inert, nontoxic and should not contribute any taste of their own. Lactose and glucose are generally preferred as diluents. A mixture of 4% sodium benzoate and 1% sodium acetate is suitable as lubricant. The materials employed as diluents and lubricants being water-soluble, the moisture level should be carefully controlled. Relative humidity (RH) in the working room should be maintained between 35 and 45%.

Effervescent tablets : Effervescent tablets are based on a chemical reaction to generate carbon dioxide when a dry mixture is added to water. Thus the formula includes alkali carbonates/bicarbonates and citric/tartaric acids, which evolve carbon dioxide in presence of water. Besides these ingredients the formula may also include sweeteners such as saccharin sodium, flavours such as citrus and berry flavours, and colourants.

A formula for effervescent aspirin tablets is given below.

Aspirin	5.00 parts
Sodium bicarbonate	26.50 parts
Citric acid anhydrous	10.25 parts
Glycine	0-75 parts
Calcium phosphate, monobasic	0.50 parts

Lozenge tablets : Lozenges or troches are intended to be held in the mouth for slow dissolution and release of drug, which provides prolonged (up to 30 minutes) contact for drug with the mouth and throat. As lozenges are not intended for disintegration but slow dissolution in the oral cavity, no disintegrant is needed in the formula but the proportion of binder should be more. Drugs administered as lozenges are primarily local anaesthetics, antiseptics, astringents or antitussives. They may also contain antihistaminics, analgesics and decongestants. Such tablets must have a very agreeable taste and flavour. The compression of lozenges is also of higher degree as compared with tablets.

A formula for penicillin lozenges is given below.

Penicillin sodium	1,00,000 units
Gelatin	50 g
Syrup	70 ml
Water	75 ml
Saccharin sodium	0.50 g
Oil of lemon	0.50 ml
Paraben	0.50 g

Vaginal tablets : These are ovoid or pear shaped tablets made by compression. They are also known as inserts and are intended for insertion into the vagina where dissolution and release of the medicament take place. They may contain organic iodine such as iodochlor or iodohydroxyquinoline compounds or other antiseptics, astringents or steroids in a soluble base of lactose or sodium bicarbonate. The tablets are usually buffered to produce the desired pH. Such tablets are usually inserted by means of a plastic tube inserter with a plunger. The tablet should be placed in the upper region of the vaginal tract. Vaginal tablets are commonly used in the treatment of *Trichomonas vaginitis.* Flagyl and Floraquin Vaginal Inserts (Searle) are examples of such tablets.

Chewable tablets : These tablets have a smooth, rapid disintegration and are designed to be sucked or chewed before swallowing. Mannitol is most commonly used as the tablet base. Disintegrants are needed in such tablets. The sweetener, flavouring agents and lubricant should always be added to the dried granules. Lubricants are usually selected on the basis of their taste. Chewable tablets are commonly employed in the preparation of muitivitamin, antacid and antibiotic tablets.

A formula for a chewable antacid tablet is given below.

Magnesium trisilicate	500 mg
Dried aluminium hydroxide	250 mg
Mannitol	300 mg
Sodium saccharin	2 mg
Starch paste (5%)	q.s.
Oil of peppermint	1 mg
Magnesium stearate	10 mg
Corn starch	10 mg

Buccal and sublingual tablets : These are generally flat and oval in shape intended to be dissolved in the buccal pouch (buccal tablets) or beneath the tongue (sublingual tablets). These tablets contain drugs that are often destroyed, inactivated or not absorbed in the gastrointestinal tract but are absorbed through the oral mucosa. These tablets should not disintegrate but dissolve slowly over a period of 15 to 30 minutes. However, nitrogtycerin and mannitol hexanitrate tablets should dissolve in 2 minutes beneath the tongue for providing fast relief to treat patients of angina pectoris. Steroidal hormones are generally formulated as buccal or sublingual tablets.

A formula for a sublingual tablet is given below.

Methyl testosterone	10 mg
Lactose	85 mg
Sucrose	85 mg
Acacia	10 mg
Talc	6 mg
Purified water	q.s.

Hypodermic tablets : These are not much used in modern practice. Hypodermic tablets were popular amongst physicians who used to prepare extemporaneous injection by dissolving the tablet in 'sterile water for injection' and the resulting solution was injected hypodermically. The tablets are prepared either by moulding or compression. The base used should be water-soluble.

Evaluation Parameters

Shape and size : Thickness of the tablets should be controlled within $\pm 5\%$ variation with a standard value. It may change with die-wall, particle size, distribution, packing of particles and compressive load. The crown thickness of tablets may be measured by micrometer (sliding caliper scale). This test is necessary for packaging of tablets as well as drug content uniformly.

1. *Organoleptic properties :* Some tablets may contain organoleptic substances such as flavoring agent, coloring agent and sweetener. Color uniformity of the tablet can be evaluated by reflectance spectrophotometry, tristimulus colorimetry or microreflectance photometery.

2. *Hardness :* Suitable hardness is necessary for handling during manufacturing, packaging and shipping. Hardness of the tablets can be measured by Monsanto tester, Strong-cobb-tester, Pfizer tester and Erweka tester.

3. *Friability :* Friability is another measurement of tablet strength as tablet hardness is not an absolute indicator of strength. Roche friabilator is used as laboratory equipment for the determination of friability. It has a plastic chamber that revolves at 25 rpm, tablet drops a distance of six inches with each revolution and operated for 100 revolutions. Compressed should not lose more than 1.0% of their weight.

4. *Weight variations :* It is measured to ensure that tablet contains the proper amount of drug and is a satisfactory test for determination of content uniformity of tablets. Usually ten tablets are taken for this test. In USP, 20 tablets are weighed individually and average weight of tablets is calculated.

USP limit		IP limit	
Average weight of tablets (mg)	Maximum variation	Average weight of tablets (mg)	Maximum variation
130 or less	$\pm 10.0\%$	80 or less	$\pm 10.0\%$
130 to 324	$\pm 7.5\%$	80 to 300	$\pm 7.5\%$
More than 324	$\pm 5.0\%$	More than 300	$\pm 5.0\%$

5. *Disintegration :* Breaking of tablets into smaller particles or granules is known as disintegration and time taken for breaking of tablets in a suitable medium is called disintegration time (DT). IP apparatus consists of 6 glass tubes each 3 inches long, open at top and has 10 mesh screen at the bottom end of basket rack. One tablet is placed in each tube and placed in a one litre beaker of water, simulated gastric fluid or simulated intestinal fluid at $37 \pm 2°C$. It moves up and down through a distance of 5 to 6 cm at 28 to 32 cpm. Uncoated tablets have disintegration times as low as 5 minutes. Majority of

tablets have DT of 30 minutes. Disintegration time of enteric coated tablet is one hour in simulated gastric fluid and two hours in simulated intestinal fluid.

6. *Dissolution :* The rate of absorption depends on the dissolution of the product. It is directly proportional to the bioavailability of the products. For dissolution study two types of apparatus are used, basket assembly and paddle assembly. It consists of a hemispherical flask of 1000 ml capacity, temperature is maintained at $37 \pm 0.5°C$, $t_{90\%}$ obtained within 30 min. is satisfactory.

7. *Drug content :* Drug uniformity in tablet is determined by assay. It is calculated on batch to batch or lot to lot basis. It is estimated by the titration, spectrophotometer and HPLC.

Tablet Defects

Defect	Description	Causes	Remedy
Capping	Partial or complete separation of top or bottom surface of the tablet from the main body is called capping. This type of problem is generally found after compression.	(a) Entrapment of air, (b) deformational problems (c) incorrect set up of tablet press	(a) Reduce the speed of press (b) increase percentage of moisture
Lamination	Separation of a tablet into two or three layers is called as lamination	(a) entrapment of air (b) deformational properties of formulations (c) direct compression (d) low moisture content (less than 5%).	(a) Reduce the speed of press (b) Increase percentage of moisture.
Picking	Removal of surface material from the punch surface is called picking	(a) Embossing or engraving of punch tips (b) Convex type of punch (c) insufficient anti-adhesive	(a) Reduce convex curve of punch (b) uniform distribution of anti-adhesive (c) Reduce letters like A, O, Welcome, etc. on punch.
Sticking	Some material of tablet adhering inside the die wall, is called sticking.	(a) insufficient lubricant (b) Excessive moisture content	(a) mix sufficient lubricant (b) Reduce moisture content

Defect	Description	Causes	Remedy
Chipping	Serious problem of sticking is called chipping. The tablet produced has rough surface due to this problem. It creates difficulty in free movement of punches	Low melting point substances	Add higher melting point substances e.g., stearic acid.
Mottling	Unequal distribution of color in tablet is called mottling.	a. Migration of dye b. Unequal distribution of color c. large particle size	Add anti-leaching dye substances in the product such as acacia, tragacanth etc.
Poor flow	Incomplete filling of dies by the powder material due to poor flow of material from hopper to die wall.	a. speed of tablet machine b. Different density of powder material as well as additives.	Addition of glidant e.g., talcum, colloidal silica.
Double Impression	One dark and one lighter impression on tablet surface are called double impression.	Uncontrolled movement of lower punch.	Regulation of the punch movement as well as speed of the machine.

Coating and Polishing

Purpose of Coating

The tablets are coated for the following purposes:

1. To mask unpleasant taste.
2. To control site of dissolution.
3. To protect components from atmospheric degradation such as oxidation, absorption or evolution of moisture, light etc.
4. To separate incompatible ingredients and prevent their interaction.
5. To provide a controlled rate of absorption and pattern of action.
6. To produce a pharmaceutically superior product.
7. To convert liquids into free flowing solids.

Coating materials largely comprise of sucrose, water-soluble film-forming polymers of substances which are soluble in the intestinal secretions but resist stomach fluids. Examples include sugar, waxes, shellac, cellulose derivatives, gelatin, organic acids, aminoalkyl aryl polymers, polyvinylstyrene compounds etc. Coating is normally applied by spray pan method, air suspension method or by compression.

Basic types of tablet coating are described below.

Sugar Coating

This is one of the oldest processes known in the field of pharmacy. Sugar coating is an art that imparts smooth, rounded, elegant appearance to the tablet. It comprises of the following steps :

(a) *Sealing* : The basic object of sealing is to prevent the core tablet from water during subsequent steps in sugar coating. Sealing is performed on dust free tablets for depositing a thin layer of water impervious material such as shellac or cellulose acetate phthalate. Sealing is affected by applying a dilute, nonaqueous solution of the coating material and 2 or 3 coats are sufficient to seal the tablets. It is generally done in a coating pan. Sealing can also be done by spraying or fluidized bed coating techniques. Process of sealing is exactly similar to film coaling. Application of excessive quantity of sealing material leads to prolongation of disintegration time.

(b) *Sub-coating* : This process is also called tablet rounding. The sub-coat is applied by wetting the tablets with an adhesive solution, dusting with filler and drying to remove moisture. The purpose of sub-coating is to round the tablet contours and provide a bond between the seal coat and the sugar coat. The adhesive solution consists of aqueous solution of sucrose; or sucrose, corn syrup and acacia; or gelatin, acacia and corn syrup. Usually 3 to 4 sub-coats are applied in succession allowing the previous coat to dry off before the subsequent coat is applied. A gap of 15 to 20 minutes between the applications of two coats is sufficient. Talc and precipitated calcium carbonate are commonly used as sub-coat fillers together with some sucrose and a small proportion of acacia. Sub-coating is carried out in a sugar coating pan. The process is continued till the tablets have a rounded appearance and the edges are completely covered.

(c) *Syrup coating* : Syrup coating can be divided into (a) grossing, and (b) heavy syrup coating. Grossing smoothens and rounds the tablet contours rapidly and builds the tablets to the desired size. Several coats of grossing syrup with or without colouring materials and opacifying agents are applied.

For initial colouring, a combination of 1 part of coloured grossing syrup and 3 parts of colourless grossing syrup is satisfactory. Concentration of coloured syrup may be increased once the tablet is of uniform colour. If this pattern is not followed then spotting or mottling may be seen in final coated tablets.

Heavy syrup coating is performed after the tablets are grossed. Heavy syrup contains a higher proportion of sugar. This application of a syrup concentrate builds up a solid colour rapidly. Regular syrup coat utilizes dilute syrup. Regular syrup coating represents the finishing step in the syrup coating process. It is critical in producing a tablet with optimum elegance.

(d) *Finishing :* It consists of applying 3 to 4 coats of syrup in rapid succession without allowing tablets from becoming dusty. A final coat is applied while the tablets are still damp. After this the tablets are left overnight in the coating pan with lid closed so that they may retain high moisture content.

(e) *Polishing :* The tablets obtained after finishing are smooth and evenly coloured but have a dull surface appearance. Polishing is carried out in canvas lined coating pans and the process consists of applying thin layer of waxy materials to impart shine to the finished tablets. A solution of waxy material such as beeswax, carnauba wax or a synthetic chlorinated wax is applied. Three coats may be necessary. Polished tablets will have high luster of an elegant sugar coated tablet.

Successful sugar coating depends upon the composition of various applications as well as the skill of the operator. Sugar coating can also be employed to expedite the process and to improve the mechanical properties of the coating.

Film coating

Film coating has many advantages over sugar coating. Sugar coating is tedious, time consuming, requires expertise of a highly skilled operator and increases the size of the original compressed tablet considerably. Film coating fulfils all the objects of coating without significantly altering the tablet weight or size. It is applied successfully not only to tablets but also to capsules, granules, pills etc. It was first employed in 1930 and now the film coating technique is fully developed. Film forming agents are mainly polymers including -

1. vinyl polymers such as polyvinylpyrrolidone, poly vinyl alcohol and acetate and carboxyviny derivatives;
2. celluloses such as carboxymethylcellulose, hydroxypropycellulose; methylcellulose, ethylcellulose and cellulose;
3. acrylates and methacrylates;
4. copolymers such as vinyl-maleic acid and styrene-maleic acid types; and
5. natural gums and resins such as acacia, gelatin, shellac and zein.

Solvents are usually nonaqueous. A plasticizing agent such as diethyl phthalate in relatively low concentration or waxy material such as high molecular weight polyethylene glycols in higher concentration, are also included to impart flexibility to the film. They are used in the range of 1 to 50% of the total weight of film forming substances. Colouring agents are generally incorporated in film coating solutions. Colourants are used to provide elegance and product distinction. Normally, permitted coal tar colours are used, but occasionally insoluble dyes and lakes are employed in conjunction with opaqueness extenders to overcome problems of mottled colouring.

Opacifying agents increase the covering power of the film coats. Titanium dioxide, carbonate and oxide of magnesium, calcium sulfate, aluminium hydroxide, silicates etc. are commonly used to improve the organoleptic properties of the film coated tablets. Film coating may be achieved either by spray-pan or air-suspension method.

Spray-pan coating : The process comprises of spraying polymer solution into conventional wall mushroom shaped pan or into a side vented coating pan. Coating solutions are prepared in tanks. The side vented coating pan has thousands of holes in the periphery. An exhaust plenum is located near the portion of the pan where tablets tumble. Coating solution is atomized at the nozzles by the fluid pressure alone.

Air suspension method : The tablets are placed into a coating chamber and hot air is introduced through bottom of the chamber. Solids within the air stream rotate both vertically and horizontally. Coating solution is applied through an atomizing nozzle from the upper end of the chamber.

Drying of the tablets begins immediately as they travel upward in the air stream. Coated tablets descend along the perimeter of the coating chamber and are ultimately replaced by additional tablets. Thus the operation is continuous. However, as the velocity at which tablets travel up to the centre of column in the main stream of air is high, the tablets are subjected to great deal of attrition and hence may break.

In yet another method called **dip coating** the tablets are placed in coating solutions and wet tablets are transferred to coating pan to avoid their adhering to one another. This operation is repeated several times allowing each coat to dry sufficiently before the subsequent coat is applied.

Film Defects

These defects occur due to improper formulation of coating solution, application of coating solution and processing of the coated product.

Blistering	An unsmooth film surface shows a number of uneven spots called blisters. Blistering is mainly due to improper curing conditions. The problem can be overcome by drying at low temperatures for prolonged time.
Wrinkling	Presence of wrinkles indicates improper drying or natural tendencies of the film forming agents, wrinkles are magnified when the film is too thick.
Bridging	This may occur with monogrammed or bisected tablets. The problem is usually due to a lack of adhesion of the film to the tablet surface. Inclusion of a tackifier in the formula may be helpful.
Sweating	It occurs due to exclusion of plasticizers and surfactants from the film due to strong cohesive forces of the polymers or severe drying temperature. Adjustment of coating compositions and proper drying conditions may solve the problem.
Orange peel	It implies the appearance of the surface of the coat resembling the peel of an orange. It is due to improper distribution of coating solution or a too rapid drying. Application of additional coats and control of evaporation rate may help solve the problem

Table Contd...

Flaking	It refers to the easy removal of coating material from the product in sheets or large flakes, after coating. Flaking is due to inadequate adhesion between the film coat and the tablet surface. Flaking occurs due to concentration of solids in the film, which prevents the formation of a continuous film of the material and the material flakes off. The remedy lies in reducing the solvents in coating solution.
Bloom	Development of a dull film or bloom is called blooming. It is due to processing of the product under humid conditions and also due to migration of plasticizers to the surface of the coat.
Spotting	It occurs due to migration of plasticizers, dyes or other additives in the coating formula, to the coat. It also occurs when the solvent carries soluble materials to the surface during the process of drying. Drying the tablets in air-conditioned areas at slow speed is the possible remedy.

Compression Coating

It is also known as **dry coating**. The process consists of making tablet and compressing a second tablet around it. Thus two incompatible ingredients can be separated by placing one in the core and the other in the coating. Tablets can be sugar coated by compression. The coating material in the form of granules or powder is compressed on to a tablet core of drug. Manesty Drycota machine is widely used for compression coating. The process is also useful in making sustained release tablets by providing the coated granules in the core and simple drug in the coat. In a simple manner compression coating may be produced by coupling two or three tablet presses together. The first press produces the core tablets which are transferred to the second press. Coating material is pressed on the core tablet in the second press. Second coating on coated tablets can be applied by transferring the tablets to a third press. Granules of the coat should have enough fluidity so that they flow around the core quickly. This may be achieved by inclusion of polyethylene glycols.

Enteric coating

An enteric coated tablet does not release a significant quantity of drug in the stomach but releases the drug rapidly and completely when the tablet passes into the intestine. Enteric coating is necessary (i) to prevent gastric decomposition of drugs such as certain antibiotics and glandular products, and (ii) to inhibit interaction of the drug in the stomach *e.g.,* mucosal irritation and bleeding may be induced by aspirin. The process generally consists of water proofing the tablet by coating with shellac in a coating pan and then the enteric coating material is added to the rotating tablets to form a coat. Enteric coating may also be applied by spray-pan or air-suspension method. Materials which are commonly used for enteric coating include shellac, cellulose acetate phthalate, lipids and synthetic resins. One convenient method employs n-butyl stearate (45 parts), carnauba wax (30 parts), and stearic acid (25 parts). The mixture is heated to 75°C on a water bath. The tablet is held with one end of the tweezer and dropped into the liquid. Coating solidifies rapidly when the object is withdrawn. Then the uncoated end is dipped in the melted mixture to a depth sufficient to overlap the coating material over the previously coated end. Two coats are sufficient. The method can be applied for enteric coating of capsules and pills, in a similar manner.

Formulae of some tablets are given below-

Example 01

Chewable laxative tablets prepared
by wet granulation

Rx	
Phenolphthalein	64 mg
Sugar, in powder	750 mg
Cocoa, in powder	350 mg
Calcium stearate	12 mg
Talc	60 mg
Gelatin (10% solution)	qs

Dose : 1 to 2 tablets for adults

Example 02

Soluble acetylsalicylic acid tablets prepared
by wet granulation / dry granulation

Rx	
Acetylsalicylic acid	300 mg
Citric acid	30 mg
Calcium carbonate	100 mg
Saccharin sodium	3 mg

Dose : 1 to 3 tablets

Example 03

Pediatric dispersible aspirin tablets
prepared by dry granulation

Rx	
Aspirin	75.0 mg
Citric acid	7.5 mg
Calcium carbonate	25.0 mg
Saccharin sodium	0.75 mg

Dose : as directed by physician

Example 04

Chewable antacid tablets prepared
by wet granulation

Rx	
Aluminium hydroxide, dried gel	400.0 mg
Magnesium hydroxide, fine powder	80.0 mg
Sucrose	20.0 mg
Mannitol, fine powder	180.0 mg
Polyvinylpyrollidine (10%) solution	30.0 mg

Dose : 1 or 2 tablets, repeated in accordance
with the needs of the patient.

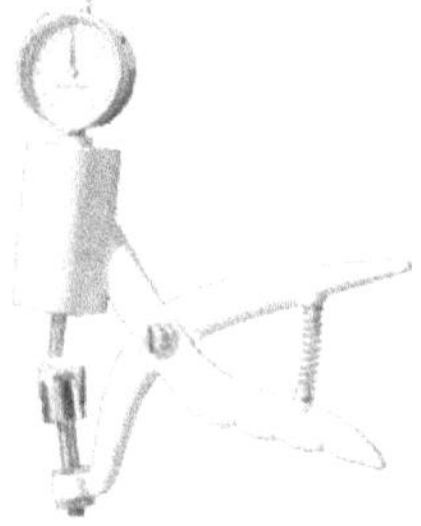

Fig. 8.1(a) Pfizer Tablet Hardness Tester.

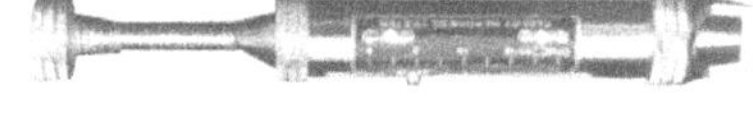

Fig. 8.1(b) Monsanto Tablet Hardness Tester.

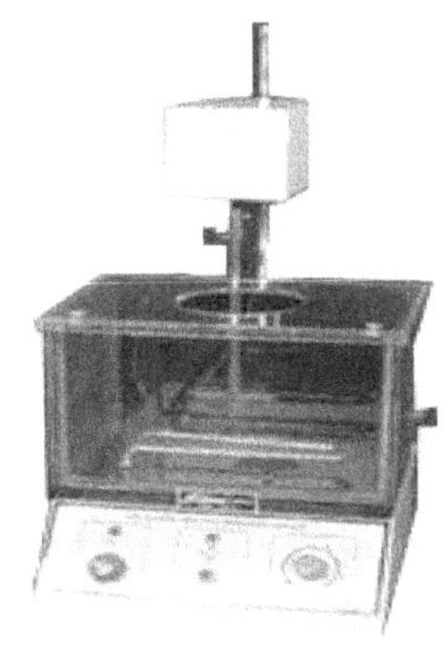

Fig. 8.1 (c) Dissolution Test Apparatus.

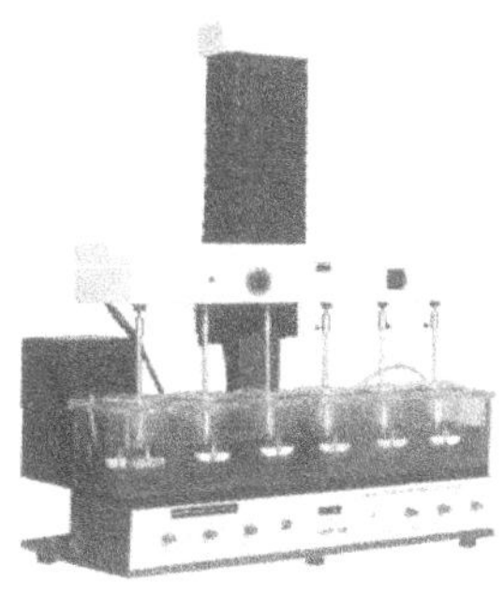

Fig. 8.1(d) Dissolution Test Apparatus (Six basket).

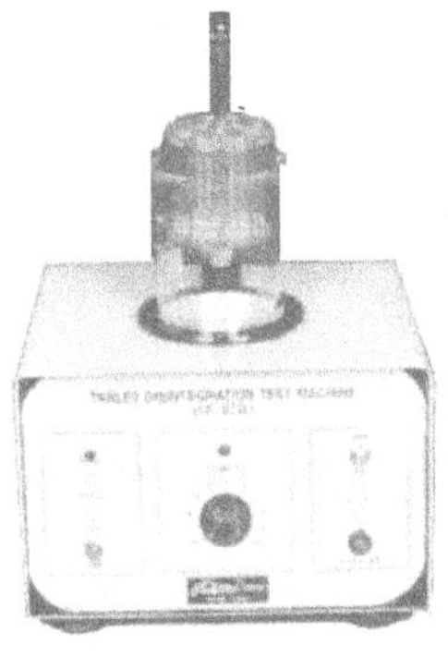

Fig. 8.1(e) Disintegration Test Apparatus (Digital).

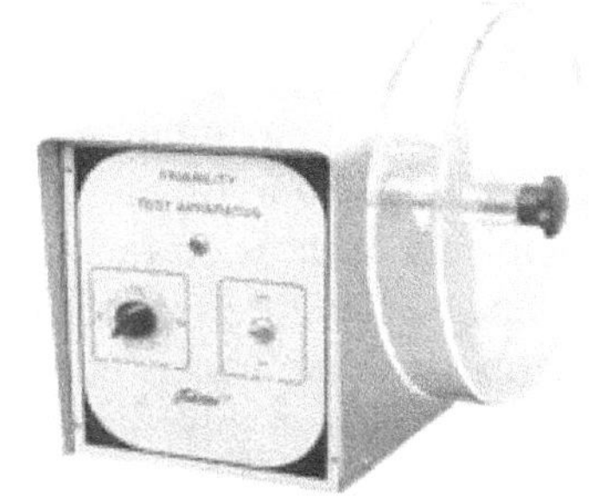

Fig. (f) Friabilator (Single drum digital).

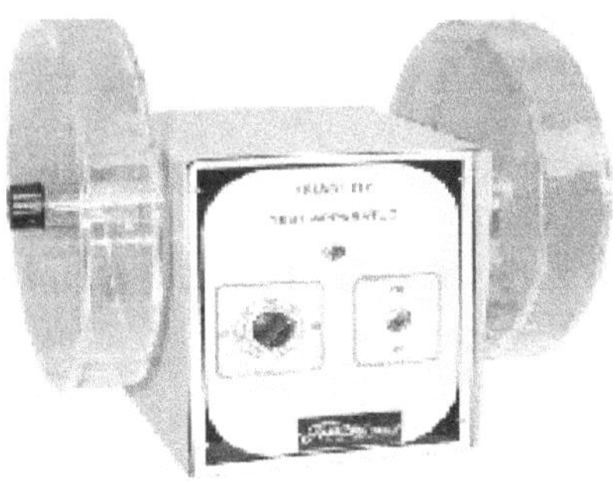

Fig. 8.1(g) Friabilator (Double drum digital).

CHAPTER 9

Capsules

The word capsule is derived from the Latin *capsula* meaning a small box. The word is used to describe an edible package made from gelatin that is filled with medicines to produce a unit dose mainly for oral use. Capsules are defined as solid dosage form in which one or more medicament with or without inert substances are enclosed within a small gelatin shell.

The capsule shells are composed of gelatin or other materials, the consistency of which may be adjusted by the addition of substances such as glycerol and sorbitol or a mixture of both. It contains excipients such as surface-active agents, opaque fillers, anti-microbial preservatives, sweetening agents, flavoring agents and coloring agents. The contents of capsules may be of solid, liquid or paste-like consistency. Capsules consist of one or more medicaments, with or without excipients such as solvents, diluents, lubricants or disintegration of the shell.

There are two types of capsules

I. Hard Gelatin Capsules

It consists of mainly two pieces, a cap and a body that fit inside the other. It is manufactured from a mixture of gelatin, colorants and sometimes may contain opacifying agents and is filled in separate operation. Empty capsules are sold by sizes from 000 the largest, to size 5, the smallest. The most popular sizes in practice are size 0 to 5 for human use.

Table 9.1 Different Size of capsules and volume filled in ml.

S.No.	Capsule No.	Volume in ml
1.	000 Largest size	1.36
2.	00	0.95
3.	0	0.67
4.	1	0.48
5.	2	0.37
6.	3	0.27
7.	4	0.20
8.	5 Smallest size	0.13

In dispensing practice it is advised that the pharmacist should note down the size of the capsule on the prescription so that he would use the same size in case the prescription is refilled. Number 10,11 and 12 capsules are also manufactured for veterinary use only.

Hard gelatin capsules contain about 12 to 16% water and require storage under controlled conditions of temperature and humidity. Capsules become flaccid and lose their shape if stored under high humidity whereas under low humidity they become brittle.

Capsule shells are prepared by two methods:

1. Plate Process, and 2. Rotary Die Process

Following materials are filled in hard gelatin capsules:

1. *Dry solids* : Powder, granules, pellets, tablets

2. *Semisolid* : Thixotropic mixture, thermo-softening mixtures, pastes, etc.

Advantages of Capsules

1. Ease of use due to the fact that it is smooth, slippery and easy to swallow.
2. Suitable for substances having bitter taste and unpleasant odor.
3. As produced in large quantities it is economic, attractive and available in wide range of colors.
4. Minimum excipients required.
5. Little pressure required to compact the material.
6. Unit dosage form.
7. Easy to store and transport.

Disadvantages of Capsules

1. Not suitable for highly soluble substances like potassium chloride, potassium bromide, ammonium chloride, etc.
2. Not suitable for highly efflorescent or deliquescent materials.
3. Special conditions are required for storage.

Determination of Capsule Fill Weight

Capsule fill weight is determined applying following formula

Capsule fill weight = Tapped bulk density of substance × capsule volume

Example 9.1

A formulation has a theoretical fill weight of 325 mg and tapped bulk density of the substance is 0.75 g/ml while bulk density of inert substance is 0.80 g/ml.

Given

1. Weight of substance in each capsule = 325.0 mg

2. Bulk density of substance   = 0.75 g/ml

3. Bulk density of inert substance   = 0.80 g/ml

$$\text{Volume occupied by fill weight} = \frac{\text{Weight of substance in each capsule}}{\text{Bulk density of substance}}$$

$$\text{Volume occupied by fill weight} = \frac{0.325}{0.325} = 0.43 \text{ ml}$$

Volume of size '1' capsule = 0.48 ml (from Table.)

Volume occupied by drug = 0.43 ml (by calculation)

Volume unoccupied = 0.48 − 0.43 = 0.05 ml

Weight of diluent or inert substances = volume × bulk density

$$= 0.05 \times 0.80 = 0.040 \text{ g} = 40.0 \text{ mg}$$

Send ten capsules of the given materials (Always weigh substance for one extra capsule as material is lost during powdering, mixing, and handling of the substance)

Weight for 11 capsule of substance = 325 × 11 = 3.575 g

Weight of diluent or inert substance = 40 × 11 = 0.440 g

Total weight of filling substance in the hard empty shell = 4.015 g

Example 9.2

Fill the substance containing drug in each capsule, of size '1' capsule 280 mg of bulk density 0.70 g/ml. Determine how much amount of inert substance is required to fill 10 capsules while bulk density of inert substance is 0.85.

Solution

Similar problem as in example I.

Example 9.3

Which number of capsule is to be used for 375 mg material having bulk density 0.75 g/ml. Bulk density of inert substance is 0.68. Calculate the total g/ml required for 10 capsules.

Given

Weight of substance in each capsule = 375.0 mg

Bulk density of substance   = 0.75 g/ml

Bulk density of inert substance   = 0.68 g/ml

$$\text{Volume occupied by fill weight} = \frac{\text{Weight of substance in each capsule}}{\text{Bulk density of substance}}$$

For filling this volume of substance '1' number capsule is most appropriate because

Volume of size '1' capsule = 0.48 ml (from Table 9.1.)

Volume occupied by drug = 0.466 ml (by calculation)

Volume unoccupied = 0.48 – 0.466 = 0.014 ml

Weight of diluent or inert substances = volume × bulk density

$$= 0.68 \ = 0.040 \text{ g} \ = \ 0.00952 \text{ g} = 9.52 \text{ mg}$$

Send ten capsules of the given materials

Weight for 11 capsule of substance = 375 × 11 = 4.125 g

Weight of diluent or inert substance = 9.52 × 11 = 0.105 g

Total weight of filling substance in the hard empty shell = 4.230 g

Evaluation of Capsules

1. *Drug content :* Determine by assay process for the drug.
2. *Weight variations :* Determine by simple weighing of 20 capsules using digital balance, should be within the limit of 90% to 110% in weight.
3. *Disintegration :* Disintegration test is usually not required for capsules unless it is treated to resist solution in gastric fluid. In such cases it must meet the requirements for disintegration of enteric-coated tablets.
4. *Dissolution test :* Use dissolution apparatus basket assembly for determination of dissolution test.

Storage

Capsules should be kept in well-closed containers at a temperature not exceeding 30°C.

Filing Equipments

1. Eli Lilly Co., Indianapolis, IN.
2. Farmatic SNC, Bologna, Itlay
3. Hoflinger and Karg, Waiblingen, Germany
4. mG$_2$ S.P.A., Bologna, Itlay
5. Osaka, Osaka, Japan
6. Macofar SAS, Bologna, Itlay
7. Perry Industries, Green Bay, WI
8. Zanasi Nigris, S.P.A., Bologna, Itlay
9. Parke-Davis and Company, Detroit, MI

Other Machines

1. Rotoweigh   : Capsule weighing machine
2. Rotosort   : Filled capsule sorting machine
3. Seidenader Model PM 60   : Unfilled capsules cleansing and polishing machine
4. Erweka KEA   : Capsule deducting and polishing machine
5. Hartnett Model B   : Capsule imprinting machine
6. Markem Model 280 A   : Capsule imprinting machine

Most of these machines are suitable for large scale manufacturing of capsules. For dispensing, hand operated capsule filling machines are available in various sizes.

II. Soft Gelatin Capsules

The shells of soft capsules are thicker than those of hard capsules. It consists of a single part and may be of various shapes. The shells are usually formed, filled and sealed in a combined operation but in some cases, shells for extemporaneous use may be performed. The shell material may contain medicament. It may be used for enclosing liquid material while solids are usually dissolved or dispersed in a suitable excipient to give a paste like consistency. Soft gelatin capsule are also known as **soluble elastic** or **soft elastic capsule**. Their composition differs from hard gelatin capsules in that the sugar is replaced by a plasticizer like glycerin, sorbitol or a similar polyol. Soft gelatin can be modified to impart enteric, chewable and with some drugs sustained release properties. They have also been employed as a suppository dosage form for rectal or vaginal administration. Single dose application of topical and ophthalmic preparations, rectal ointments and medications for ear and nose can be packaged in soft capsules. In cosmetic industry these capsules may be used for the packaging of perfumes, shampoos, various skin creams, suntan oils etc. Soft capsules provide an attractive, odourless and tasteless form for prescribing the medication.

Soft gelatin capsules are available in oblong, spherical, elliptical and other shapes. Spherical or oval capsules are also known as **pearls** or **globules**. They are also available in different sizes to contain from 0.1 to 30 ml volume.

Following types of liquids are encapsulated in soft gelatin capsules-

1. Water-immiscible, volatile and nonvolatile liquids e.g. vegetable and animal oils, aliphatic hydrocarbons, chlorinated hydrocarbons, ethers, esters, alcohols and organic acids.

2. Water-miscible, nonvolatile liquids e.g. polyethylene glycols and non-ionic surfactants such as tween-80.

3. Water–miscible and relatively nonvolatile compounds e.g. propylene glycol, isopropyl alcohol.

Example 1 :   Amoxycillin capsule

Rx	
Amoxycillin trihydrate	250 mg
Diluent	q.s.

Dose : 2 to 3 capsule daily

Example 2 :   Ibuprofen capsule

Rx	
Ibuprofen	300 mg
Diluent	q.s.

Dose : Ibuprofen 200-600 mg twice daily

Example 3 :   Chlortetracycline capsule

Rx	
Chlortetracycline	250 mg
Diluent	q.s.

Dose : 1 to 3 capsules daily in divided doses.

Example 4 :   Paracetamol capsule

Rx	
Paracetamol	250 mg
Diluent	q.s.

Dose : 1 to 3 tablets

CHAPTER 10

Liquid Dosage Forms

Liquid dosage forms commonly encountered in pharmaceutical practice are either monophasic or biphasic. Monophasic systems are characterized by the presence of a single homogeneous phase e.g., solution, mixtures, elixirs, tinctures, syrups, ear drops, nasal drops, etc., whereas biphasic liquid dosage forms consist of two distinct phases e.g., emulsions and suspensions. Liquid preparations may be broadly classified under two categories -

I. Internal Liquid Preparations

(A) Monophasic liquid preparations

    (a) Syrups   (b) Elixirs   (c) Solutions   (d) Linctuses

(B) Biphasic liquid preparations

    (a) Suspension (Mixture)   (b) Emulsion

II. External Liquid Preparations

(A) Applied on the skin

    (a) Lotions   (b) Liniments (c) Throat paints (d) Collodions

(B) Instilled into body cavities

    (a) Douches (b) Enemas   (c) Ear Drops   (d) Nasal Drops

    (e) Nasal Sprays   (f) Inhalations

(C) Used in the mouth

    (a) Gargles   (b) Mouthwashes

(a) ***Syrups***

Syrups are concentrated oral solutions of sugar or nearly saturated solutions of sucrose in water or other aqueous liquids. Syrups containing 85% *w/v* or 66.7% *w/w* sucrose will retard the growth of microorganisms. It is important to note that sucrose concentration should not reach the saturation point as a saturated solution may lead to crystallization of a small amount of sucrose due to change of physical condition viz. temperature. Dilute solution of sucrose provides an excellent nutritional source for yeast, moulds and other microorganisms. When heat is employed for the preparation of syrups, a small portion of sucrose changes to dextrose and levulose. This phenomenon is called as inversion. Sucrose solution is optically active and rotates polarized light to right while on heating optical activity decreases, rotates the light to left due to formation of other compounds (dextrose ad levulose). The rate of inversion is enhanced by the presence of acids and hydrogen ions, which act as catalyst.

Syrups are mainly of three types :

Simple syrup : It contains sucrose in purified water alone or in combination of other polyols such as glycerin or sorbitol. These substances are added in syrups to reduce the crystallization of sucrose or enhance the solubility of excipients. (e.g., simple syrup etc.)

Medicated syrups : It contains some added medicinal substances in the syrups and used for therapeutic purpose (e.g., ephedrine sulphate syrup, chlorphineramine maleate syrup)

Flavored syrup : It contains various aromatic or pleasantly flavored substances but are non-medicated and generally used as vehicle or as a flavoring agent or for preservation. (e.g., cherry syrups, tolu balsam syrup, cocoa syrup etc.)

Methods of Preparation

Preparation of syrup depends on the physical and chemical characteristics of the substance employed for its preparation. Four methods are commonly used for preparation of syrups.

1. ***Agitation without heat :*** This method is used for the preparation of syrups containing volatile substances. In this process active substance is added in solution and agitated in a glass-stoppered bottle. Closing of bottle is necessary to protect the syrup from contamination and loss of solution during the process. For preparation of large quantities, glass lined tank with mechanical agitators is employed. This method is used for the preparation of wide variety of syrups. Cough syrups are commonly prepared by this process. (e.g., codeine syrup, ephedrine sulfate syrup etc.)

2. ***Solution with heat :*** This process is generally preferred as it is simple and less time consuming method, particularly if the constituents are not effected by heat and are non volatile in nature. In this process sucrose is added in the aqueous solution and heated till the sucrose is dissolved completely. Adding remaining amount of distilled water makes up volume of the solution. If the syrups containing any substances which are coagulated, it can be separated subsequently by straining. The concentration of the syrup is measured using saccharometer if the specific gravity of the solution is known. Excessive heating of syrup is not suitable because more inversion of sucrose occurs with the

increase in temperature. Syrups cannot be sterilized in autoclave without caramelization. This solution is converted in yellowish to brown color due to formation of caramel by the effect of heat on sucrose.

3. ***Addition of a medicated liquid :*** This method is put to use in those cases in which tinctures, fluid extracts or other medicated substances in liquid form are added to syrup to medicate it. In this process some time precipitation takes place due to the presence of resinous and oily substances. It is necessary to take care that medicated substance should not get precipitated in this process.

4. ***Percolation :*** In this process, purified water or an aqueous solution is allowed to pass through a bed of crystalline sucrose. A pledget of cotton is put in the neck of the percolator and purified water or aqueous solution is added in the percolator containing sucrose. The flow rate is controlled by the stopcock and maintained such that drops appear in rapid succession. If required, a small portion of liquid is re-passed through the percolator to dissolve the sugar completely in the liquid or aqueous solvent.

Preservatives

Syrup should be kept at low temperature, about 25°C is suitable for preservation. Following preservatives are used to prevent bacterial and mould growth viz. methylparaben, sodium benzoate, benzoic acid, glycerin etc.

Label and storage Syrup should be kept in well-closed containers and stored at temperature below 30 °C. Bottle should be completely filled, carefully stoppered and stored in cool dark place.

Example 01 : ***Prepare and Dispense simple syrup***

Rx

Sucrose	66.7 g
Purified water, sufficient to produce	100.0 g
or	
Rx	
Sucrose	85.0 g
Purified water, sufficient to produce	100.0 ml

Example 02 : ***Prepare and Dispense Invert syrup***

Rx

Sucrose	66.7 g
Purified water, sufficient to produce	100.0 g
Hydrochloric acid	qs
Sodium carbonate solution as neutralizing agent	

Method of Dispensing : Prepare syrup of sucrose 66.7% w/w in purified water and add hydrochloric acid slowly with continuous stirring. Neutralize the solution using sodium carbonate solution. Identify inversion of simple syrup to invert syrup by measuring optical activity of syrup.

Example 03 : ***Prepare and Dispense Lemon Syrup (100 ml)***

Rx

Lemon spirit	0.5 ml
Citric acid monohydrate	2.5 g
Invert syrup	10.0 ml
Syrup, sufficient to produce	100.0 ml
Formula for Lemon spirit (A)	

Rx

Lemon oil	100.0 ml
Ethyl alcohol (96%) sufficient to produce	100.0 ml
Formula for Invert syrup (B)	

Rx

Sucrose	*66.7 g*
Purified water, sufficient to produce	*100.0 g*
Hydrochloric acid	qs
Sodium carbonate solution as neutralizing agent	

Method of Dispensing : Cut thin slices of lemon and prepare lemon spirit by maceration process using 60 percent alcohol. Dissolve the citric acid monohydrate in simple syrup. Add freshly prepared invert syrup and lemon spirit, prepared using formula A and B, mix and add sufficient amount of syrup to produce 1000 ml. Lemon syrup has a weight per ml of about 1.33 g

Example 04 : ***Prepare and dispense Tolu Syrup (100 ml)***

Rx

Tolu balsam	1.25 g
Sucrose	66.0 g
Purified water, sufficient to produce	100.0 g

Method of Dispensing : Boil 400 ml of purified water in dish or tared vessel. Add weighed amount of tolu balsam in boiled water. Cover the vessel partially and boil the contents for 30 min. with frequently stirring. Add purified water to make the contents of the vessel about to 360 g. Cool it and filter the solution. Add sucrose in the solution and warm it on a water bath to dissolve sucrose completely. Add sufficient purified water to make 1000 g of the solution.

(b)   Elixirs

Elixirs are clear, liquid, flavored hydroalcoholic preparation intended for oral use. They contain one or more medicaments, pleasantly flavored, usually attractive color containing high proportion of alcohol or sucrose or suitable polyhydric alcohols together with suitable additives (including antimicrobial agents). The alcoholic contents in elixir vary from 5% to 40%. In general they are more stable than mixture as sufficient alcohol is added to maintain the drug in solution. Most of the elixirs become turbid when moderately diluted by aqueous fluids.

Elixirs are mainly of two types

1. *Non-medicated elixir :* They are used purely as diluting agents or solvents for drugs containing approximately 25 percent alcohol, e.g., simple elixir, Iso-alcoholic elixir or low alcohol elixir (containing 8-10% alcohol), High alcoholic elixir (containing 75-78% alcohol)

2. *Medicated elixirs :* Elixirs containing therapeutically active compounds are known as medicated elixirs. e.g., Phenobarbital elixir USP, Dexamethasone elixir USP, Chlorpheniramine Maleate elixir USP, Diphenhydramine Hydrochloride elixir USP, Piprazine Citrate elixir, Terpin Hydrate elixir etc.

The elixir is used as a vehicle for other drugs in many commercially available cough syrups viz. dextromethorphan hydrobromide, codeine phosphate, pyrilamine maleate, ammonium chloride, creosote, chloroform, and a wide variety of other drugs with expectorant and anti-tussive properties.

Some proprietary elixirs (phenethicillin and phenoxymethyl penicillin) are available in the market in granule or powder form because active ingredients are unstable in solution. They are dispersed by adding measured amount of water or at a specified point in bottle and shaken until solution is complete. The preparation is labeled so as to be stored in cool place and used within one week.

Formulation

Generally elixirs contain following ingredients.

Vehicles : About 10% to 20% of alcohol is used for keeping oils, vegetable extracts, tannin etc., in solution form. Faint opalescence from flavoring agents containing essential oils and light precipitants from vegetable extracts are not considered acceptable in elixirs. Glycerol and propylene glycol are used as solvents.

Stabilizers : In neomycin elixir, citric acid is used to adjust pH 4.0 to 5.0 to minimize the darkening that occurs on storage. Disodium edetate should be used to sequester heavy metals that catalyse decomposition of the antibiotics.

Colouring agents : Elixirs are attractive preparations containing following dyes.

Colouring agent	Color	Elixir
Amaranth	Magnetic red	Paediatric paracetamol, Paediatric streptomycin Ephedrine, Isoniazid, Neomycin, Phenobarbitone Piperazine citrate
Compound tartrazine	Saffron	
Green S, tartrazine	Green	

Flavouring agents : Sweetening agents and fruit flavors are used in many medicinal preparations e.g., Black currant syrup in chloral elixir, Concentrated raspberry juice with inverted syrup in paracetamol elixir, Lemon spirit with invert syrup in ephedrine elixir, compound orange spirits with glycerol in phenobarbital elixir.

Preservatives : In elixir, fermentation and mold growth are inhibited when it contains more than 20% of alcohol, propylene glycol or glycerol. Syrup containing saturated solution of sucrose is also inhibitory to many microorganisms because of high osmotic pressure. The commonly used preservatives are double strength chloroform, spirit, and benzoic acid and methyl ester of p-hydroxy benzoic acid.

Method of Preparation

Elixirs are prepared by dissolving the ingredients with agitation / or by admixture of two or more liquid components in the suitable solvent. Usually, the alcohol soluble substances are dissolved in alcohol and water soluble in water separately. As a rule, the aqueous solution is always added to alcoholic solution. The aqueous solution is then added to the alcoholic solution with constant stirring and make up the volume with the solvent or vehicle specified in the formulation. At this stage the product may not be clear due to the separation of some of the flavouring agents because the alcoholic strength is reduced. In such case the elixir is allowed to stand for some time to ensure the saturation of the hydroalcoholic solvent and permit the oil globules to coalesce. Talc (upto 3%) can be used to absorb the excess of oils and assist in their removal from solution. Filtration gives a bright clear product.

Container

It should be dispensed in narrow mouthed, screw capped, colorless plain bottle.

Example 01 : *Prepare and Dispense Low Alcohol Elixir*

Rx

Compound orange spirit	1.0 ml
Alcohol	10.0 ml
Glycerin	20.0 ml
Sucrose	32.0 ml
Purified water, sufficient to produce	100.0 ml

Method of Dispensing : Mix the alcohol, glycerin and 50.0 ml of purified water and add measured amount of compound orange spirit with agitation. Allow to stand for 24 hours, Filter this solvent mixture through filter papers and dissolve the weighed amount of sucrose in the filtrate by agitation or percolation and finally add the solvent mixture to make volume to100 ml.

Example 02 : ***Prepare and Dispense High Alcohol Elixir***

Rx

Compound orange spirit	: 0.40 ml
Saccharin	: 0.30 ml
Glycerin	: 20.0 ml
Alcohol, sufficient to produce	: 100.0 ml

Method of Dispensing : Dissolve the compound orange spirit and the saccharin in 70.0 ml of alcohol and add glycerin. Add sufficient amount of alcohol to produce 100.0 ml and mix properly. Filter the mixture and preserve in suitable container.

Example 03 : ***Prepare and dispense simple elixir***

Rx

Orange tincture	: 7.5 ml
Syrup	: 40.0 ml
Chloroform water, sufficient to produce	: 100.0 ml

Method of Dispensing : Mix orange tincture with the syrup and add sufficient chloroform water to produce 100.0 ml. Add 5% of purified talc and shake vigorously. Filter the elixir and preserve in a suitable container.

Example 04 : ***Prepare and dispense Paediatric Paracetamol Elixir***

Rx

Paracetamol	: 2.4 ml
Ethanol (96%)	: 10.0 ml
Propylene glycol	: 10.0 ml
Concentrated raspberry juice	: 2.5 ml
Chloroform spirit	: 2.0 ml
Invert syrup	: 27.5 ml
Amaranth solution	: 0.2 ml
Glycerin, sufficient to produce	: 100.0 ml

Method of Dispensing : Mix ethanol (96%), propylene glycol and chloroform spirit and make a mixture. Dissolve paracetamol and shake it, add other additives and sufficient amount of glycerin to produce 100 ml.

Example 05 : *Prepare and dispense Piperazine Citrate Elixir*

Rx

Piperazine citrate	18.0 ml
Chloroform spirit	0.5 ml
Glycerin	10.0 ml
Orange oil	0.025 ml
Syrup	50.0 ml
Purified water, sufficient to produce	100.0 ml

Method of Dispensing : Dissolve piperazine citrate in required amount of the purified water and add other additives to produce 100.0 ml with water.

Example 06 : *Prepare and dispense Terpin Hydrate Elixir*

Rx

Terpin hydrate	5.0 g
Orange oil	0.02 ml
Glycerin	40.0 ml
Alcohol	42.5 ml
Syrup	10.0 ml
Purified water sufficient to produce	100.0 ml

Method of Dispensing : Dissolve terpin hydrate in alcohol and add other additives. Add sufficient purified water to produce 100 ml and mix. If necessary, filter the elixir and preserve in a suitable container.

(c) Solutions

A solution is a homogeneous one-phase system consisting of two or more components. It contains two-phases i.e., solvent and solute. The solvent is the phase in which the dispersion occur and solute is that component which is dispersed as small ions or molecules in the solvent. In general, solvent part is greater than solute in the solution except a few preparation. e.g., Syrup BP, it contains 66.7% *w/w* of sucrose as solute and 33.3% of water as the solvent.

Advantages

1. Easy to swallow than solid dosage form like tablet and capsules.
2. Drug in solution form is immediately available for absorption.
3. A solution is a homogeneous system and therefore the drug remains uniformly distributed throughout the preparation.
4. Suitable for drugs that can irritate and damage the gastric mucosa, if localized in specific area. The irritation is reduced by administration in solution form.

Disadvantages

1. Inconvenient to transport and store because they are bulky.
2. Whole product is lost immediately if any breakage in the container.
3. The stability of most of substances in aqueous solution is less than solid dosage form.
4. Shelf life of solution is shorter than solid preparation.
5. Suitable media for the microbial contamination and may therefore require suitable preservatives.
6. Dose inaccuracy compared to solid dosage form.
7. Bitter unpleasant substances are not suitable for solutions and need sweetening and flavoring agent to make them more palatable.

Formulation of Solution

Following additives are generally required for the preparation of solution.

1. *Solvents :* a. Aqueous b. Non-aqueous (fixed oil, alcohol, polyhydric alcohol, dimethyl-sulphoxide, ethyl ether, liquid paraffin, etc.
2. *Buffers :* Carbonates, citrates, gluconates, lactates, phosphate, tartrate, borates, etc
3. *Colors :* water soluble dye amaranth.
4. Density modifiers
5. Flavors and perfumes
6. Taste

    (a) *Salty :* Apricot, butterscotch, liquorice, peach, vanilla

    (b) *Bitter :* Anise, chocolate, mint, wild cherry

    (c) *Sweet :* Vanilla fruits

    (d) *Sour :* Citrus fruits, raspberry

7. Preservatives
8. Antioxidants and reducing agents

Container

Narrow mouth, screw capped colorless plain bottle.

Example 01 : *Prepare and dispense Cresol with Soap Solution*

Rx

Cresol	50.0 ml
Vegetable oil	18.0 g
Potassium hydroxide	4.20 g
Purified water, sufficient to produce	100.0 ml

Method of Dispensing : Dissolve potassium hydroxide in purified water (50%), add vegetable oil and heat on a water-bath and mix thoroughly. Continue heating until a small portion dissolves in water without separation of oily drops. Add cresol and mix thoroughly with sufficient purified water.

Example 02 : *Prepare and dispense Aqueous Iodine Solution (Lugol's solution)*

Rx

Iodine	5.0 g
Potassium iodide	10.0 g
Purified water	100.0 ml

Method of Dispensing : Dissolve potassium iodide and iodine in purified water and mix thoroughly.

Example 03 : *Prepare and dispense Strong Iodine Solution*

Rx

Iodine	10.0 g
Potassium iodide	6.0 g
Purified water	10.0 ml
Ethanol, sufficient to produce	100.0 ml

Method of Dispensing : Dissolve potassium iodide and iodine in purified water and add sufficient ethanol to produce 100 ml.

Example 04 : *Prepare and dispense Weak Iodine Solution*

Rx

Iodine	2.0 g
Potassium iodide	2.5 g
Purified water	10.0 ml
Ethanol, sufficient to produce	100.0 ml

Method of Dispensing : Dissolve potassium iodide and iodine in purified water. Add sufficient ethanol to produce 100 ml.

(d) Linctuses

Linctuses are solutions of one or more medicaments, usually containing large amounts of sucrose, and sometimes glycerin as a sweetening agent, and also have a demulcent effect on the mucous membrane of the throat. The vehicle syrup has soothing effect on the soar mucous membrane of the throat. Linctuses are usually intended for use in the treatment of cough, being sipped and swallowed slowly without the addition of water. For local and prolonged action, they should be administered undiluted and sipped and swallowed slowly. The usual dose of linctuses is 5.0 ml.

Dilution of Linctuses : If a dose is prescribed which is less than or not a multiple of 5 ml, the linctus should be suitably diluted to achieve a dose-volume that is a multiple of 5.0 ml, using the specified diluent. They are diluted by syrup except codeine linctus. It is diluted by chloroform water. For this purpose chloroform water must be freshly prepared. Diluted linctuses should be used within two weeks of preparation, or any other period as may be specified. They contain following substances.

1. *Vehicles :* Syrup, tolu syrup, invert syrup, glycerin, chloroform water, sorbitol etc.

2. *Stabilizers :* Syrups

3. *Coloring agents :* Compound tartrazine solution, coal tar dyes, etc.

4. *Flavoring agents :* Tolu syrup, fruit flavored syrup, lemon syrup, blackcurrent syrup.

5. *Preservatives :* Benzoic acid, chloroform spirits, cinnamic acid, tolu syrup etc.

Example 01 : *Prepare and dispense Codeine Linctus*

   Rx

Codeine phosphate	0.3 g
Benzoic acid	2.0 ml
Compound tartrazine solution	1.0 ml
Chloroform spirit	2.0 ml
Lemon syrup	20.0 ml
Purified water	2.0 ml
Syrup, sufficient to produce	100.0 ml

Method of Dispensing : Dissolve the codeine phosphate in purified water and other additives to produce 100 ml.

Example 02 : *Prepare and dispense Simple Linctus.*

   Rx

Concentrated anise water	1.0 ml
Amaranth solution	1.5 ml
Citric acid monohydrate	2.5 g
Chloroform spirit	6.0 ml
Syrup, sufficient to produce	100.0 ml

Method of Dispensing : Separately dissolve the citric acid monohydrate in chloroform spirit and mix amaranth solution, concentrated anise water and add sufficient quantity of syrup.

Example 03 : *Prepare and dispense Paediatric Compound Tolu Linctus*

Rx

Benzaldehyde spirit	0.1 ml
Citric acid monohydrate	0.4 g
Compound tartrazine solution	1.0 ml
Glycerol	20.0 ml
Invert syrup	20.0 ml
Tolu syrup, sufficient to produce	100.0 ml

Method of Dispensing : Mix all ingredients except tolu syrup gradually one by one in a container and add tolu syrup sufficient to produce 100 ml.

II. External liquid preparations applied on the skin

(a) Lotions

Lotions are usually liquid or liquid suspensions or semi-solid preparations containing one or more medicaments, intended to be applied to the uniform skin *without rubbing*. They are lightly applied on the skin or applied on a suitable dressing and covered with waterproof substance to reduce evaporation. They may be prepared by triturating the ingredients to a smooth paste and then gradually adding the remaining liquid phase. For large quantity preparation of lotion, high-speed mixers or homogenizers produce better quality of lotions. The particles in colloidal dimension are more soothing to inflamed areas and are more effective in contact with infected surfaces. A wide variety of ingredients are employed in the preparation to produce better dispersions that show good cooling, soothing, drying or protective nature of the lotion. Following substances are used in the preparation of lotions.

1. *Bentonite :* used as a suspending agent.

2. *Methylcellulose or sodium carboxymethylcellulose :* used to hold the active ingredient in contact with the affected site.

3. *Glycerin :* keep the skin moist for considerable period of time.

4. *Alcohol :* used for accentuated action like drying, cooling etc.

5. *Miscellaneous :* benzocaine, calamine, resorcin, steroids, sulphur, zinc oxide, etc.

Lotions are generally prescribed for the following purpose – anesthetic, antiseptic, astringent, germicide, protective, antihistaminic, screening agent. Microorganisms may grow in certain lotions if no preservative is included in the preparation. Care should be taken to avoid contamination during the preparation of lotion, even if it contains preservative.

Dilution of Lotions : Care should be taken in dilution, particularly to prevent microbial contamination. The appropriate diluent should be used and heating should be avoided during mixing. Diluted lotions should be used within four weeks of their preparation.

Examples

Acriflavine Lotion	Dichloroxylenol Lotion	Salicylic acid Lotion
Boric acid Lotion	Gentian violet Lotion	Thiomersal Lotion
Calamine Lotion	Oily calamine Lotion	Zinc sulphate Lotion
Cetrimide Lotion	Phenolated Lotion	White Lotion
Dichloroxylenol Lotion	Potassium permanganate Lotion	

Labelling

Comply with the general requirements for labeling. In addition the label on the container states - 'Shake Well Before Use' and 'For External Use Only'

Example 01 : *Prepare and dispense Calamine Lotion*

Rx

Calamine	15.0 g
Zinc oxide	5.0 g
Bentonite	3.0 g
Sodium citrate	0.5 ml
Liquefied phenol	0.5 ml
Glycerin	5.0 ml
Rose water, sufficient to produce	100.0 ml

Method of Dispensing : Prepare sodium citrate solution in 70 ml rose water. Triturate calamine, zinc oxide, and bentonite with citrate solution and add other additives and make sufficient volume with rose water.

Example 02 : *Prepare and dispense Boric Acid Lotion*

Rx

Chlorinated lime	1.25 g
Boric acid	1.25 g
Purified water, sufficient to produce	100.0 ml

Method of Dispesnsing : Mix chlorinated lime and boric acid and dissolve in purified water to produce 100 ml.

Example 03 : *Prepare and dispense gentian violet lotion*

Rx

Gentian violet	1.0 g
Ethanol (95%)	10.0 ml
Purified water, sufficient to produce	100.0 ml

Method of Dispensing : Dissolve gentian violet in ethanol (95%) and add sufficient purified water to produce 100 ml.

Example 04 : *Prepare and dispense oily calamine lotion*

Rx

Calamine	5.0 g
Oleic acid	0.5 ml
Wool fat	1.0 g
Arachis oil	50.0 ml
Calcium hydroxide solution qs	100.0 ml

Method of Dispensing : Melt oleic acid, wool fat and arachis oil in a container, triturate the calamine with the mixture and transfer to a suitable container. Add calcium hydroxide solution sufficient to produce 100 ml and shake vigorously.

Containers : Narrow mouthed, fluted bottle or container distinguished from types used for orally-administered preparations.

Liniments

Liniments are solution or mixture of various substances in oil, alcoholic solution of soap or emulsions or occasionally semi-solid preparations intended for external application and should be labeled accordingly. They are applied with rubbing or massaged into the skin as counter irritating or stimulating agents to the affected area and because of this were known as embrocations.

Dental liniments, which are no longer official, are solutions of active substances and are applied onto the gums by rubbing. Liniments are usually applied *with friction* and rubbing of the skin, the oil or soap base proving for ease of application and massage. Alcoholic liniments are used generally for their rubifacient, counter irritant, mildly astringent and show penetrating effects. These types of liniments easily penetrate to the skin than those with oil base.

The oily liniments are slow in their action but are more useful when massaged. The function of liniment depends on the additives but most of liniments may function solely as protective coating on the affected area. Liniment should not be applied to the broken or bruised skin because they would be very irritating especially if alcohol is used as solvent.

They may contain following substances : (a) analgesic, (b) antimicrobial, (c) rubefacient, (d) counter irritant, (e) stimulants, and (f) soothing agents.

Although alcohol is primarily used as solvent, it enhances the penetration of the medicaments into the skin and has counter irritant or rubefacient action. Counter irritants are used to mask pain from fibrositis, sciatica, nuralgia and similar complaints by producing warmth, tingling and numbness. When rubbed onto the skin, they also cause redness and hence are called as rubefacients. Cottonseed oil and arachis oil are less irritant than alcohol and spread more easily on the skin.

Two types of vehicle are used for the preparation of liniments (i) alcohol e.g. soap liniment and aconite liniment, and (ii) oils e.g. camphor liniment and methyl salicylate liniment.

Labelling

It should comply with the general requirements for labeling. In addition the label on the container should indicate - For External Use Only, Shake Well Before Use, Not To Be Applied to Wounds or Broken Skin, Store in Cool Place, Inflammable.

Container

Narrow mouthed screw capped colored bottles can be used for dispensing liniments.

Examples 01 : *Prepare and dispense White Liniment*

Rx

Oleic acid	85.0 ml
Turpentine oil	250.0 ml
Dilute ammonia solution	45.0 ml
Ammonium chloride	12.5 g
Purified water	625.0 ml

Method of Dispensing : Mix the oleic acid with the measured quantity of turpentine oil. Mix dilute ammonia solution with 45 ml of purified water and warm it. Add warm diluted ammonia solution to the oily solution and shake to form an emulsion.

Examples 02 : *Prepare and dispense Camphor Liniment (Syn. - Camphorated oil)*

Rx

Camphor	20.0 g
Arachis oil	80.0 g

Method of Dispensing : Mix weighed amount of camphor in arachis oil in a closed vessel.

Examples 03 : *Prepare and dispense Soap Liniment*

Rx

Soft soap	1.0 g
Camphor	1.0 g
Lemon grass oil	4.0 g
Purified water	1.5 ml
Alcohol (90.0%), sufficient to produce	17.0 ml

Method of Dispensing : Dissolve the weighed quantity of soft soap, camphor and lemon grass oil in alcohol. Add purified water and remaining amount of alcohol to make up the volume and mix. Keep aside for a week and filter to remove the undissolved substance.

Example 04 : *Prepare and dispense Turpentine Liniment*

Rx

Soft soap	5.0 g
Camphor	5.0 g
Turpentine oil	65.0 ml
Purified water, sufficient to produce	100.0 ml

Method of Dispensing : Mix the soft soap with small amount of purified water (10 ml). Make solution of camphor in fresh rectified turpentine oil. Gradually add camphor solution to the soap mixture with trituration until a thick creamy emulsion is formed. Add sufficient amount of purified water to make up the volume and mix.

Example 05 : *Prepare and dispense Calamine Liniment*

Rx

Calamine	5.0 g
Wool fat	1.0 g
Oleic acid	0.5 ml
Arachis oil	50.0 ml
Calcium hydroxide solution	100.0 ml

Method of Dispensing : Melt weighed amount of wool fat, oleic acid and arachis oil. Triturate calamine with the melted oil. Add calcium hydroxide solution and shake it. Transfer it to a suitable container and shake vigorously.

Throat Paints

Paints are solutions or dispersions of one or more medicaments intended for application to the skin or, in some cases, to the mucous membrane. They may contain volatile solvent that evaporates quickly to leave a dry or resinous film of medicament. Throat paints are more viscous due to high content of glycerin. Paints are sticky and adheres to the affected site and prolong the action of the medicaments. Common examples of pastes are : 1. Brilliant green and crystal violet paint, 2. Crystal violet paint, 3. Coal tar paint, 4. Compound *mastric* paint 5. *Mandl's* paint 6. Tannic acid glycerin paints

Storage : Paints should be kept in airtight containers.

Labelling

Comply with the general requirements for labeling. In addition it should states 'For External Use Only'.

Container : Wide mouth screw capped colored bottles.

Example 01 : *Prepare and dispense Brilliant Green and Crystal Violet Paint.*

Rx

Brilliant green	0.5 g
Crystal violet	0.5 g
Ethanol (90%)	50.0 ml
Purified water, sufficient to produce	100.0 ml

Method of Dispensing : Dissolve the brilliant green and crystal violet in ethanol (90%). Add sufficient water to produce 100 ml.

Example 02 : *Prepare and dispense Crystal Violet Paint.*

Rx

Crystal violet	0.1 g
Purified water, sufficient to produce	100.0 ml

Method of Dispensing : Dissolve crystal violet in purified water. Add sufficient purified water to produce 100 ml.

Example 03 : *Prepare and dispense coal Tar Paint.*

Rx

Coal Tar	10.0 g
Acetone, sufficient to produce	100.0 ml

Method of Dispensing : Disperse the coal tar in 70 ml of acetone and allow to stand for one hour. Filter if necessary and dilute with acetone to 100 ml.

Example 04 : Prepare and dispense Iodine paint (Syn. : *Mandl's* **paint)**

In this preparation Iodine acts as antiseptic and potassium iodide dissolves the iodine, peppermint oil acts as flavoring agent and produce cooling effect, alcohol is used as a solubilizing agent for the peppermint oil. This preparation contains iodine, hence should be prepared in glass apparatus. It should not be prepared in mortar and pestle because porcelain contains pores and iodine enters in these pores. It is difficult to washout the iodine and this entangled iodine can change the color of other preparations.

Rx

Potassium iodide	2.5 g
Iodine	1.25 g
Ethanol (90%)	4.0 ml
Peppermint oil	0.4 ml
Purified water	2.5 ml
Glycerin, sufficient to produce	100.0 ml

Method of Dispensing : Dissolve potassium iodide and iodine in purified water in glass mortar and pestle with small portion of glycerin. Add peppermint oil dissolve in ethanol and mix. Add sufficient glycerin to produce 100 ml.

Collodions

Collodions are liquid preparations for external use, containing pyroxylin in a mixture of ethyl ether and ethanol. They are applied to skin by a soft brush or other suitable applicator or rod. The volatile vehicle ether and ethanol have evaporated, leave a film of pyroxylin on the skin surface. The collodions are mainly two types –

(i) *Medicated :* Official medicated collodoin, salicylic acid contains 10% *w/v* of salicylic acid in flexible collodion USP and is used as kerotolytic agent used in the treatment of corns and warts,

(ii) *Non-medicated :* for protection of small cuts and scratches,

Flexibility of collodion is made by addition of castor oil and camphor. Collodion has been used to reduce or eliminate the side effects of fluorouracil treatment of solar keratoses. In salicylic acid preparation, polyacrylic base is used as vehicle.

Pyroxylin is a nitrated cellulose obtained by treating defatted cotton with a mixture of nitric acid and sulphuric acids and its principal constituent is cellulose tetranitrate.. It is high inflammable. It is kept moist with industrial methylated spirit and stored, loosely packed in well-closed containers, protected from light.

Container : Collodions are stored in small, wide mouth, screw-capped coloured, fluted glass vial with a brush or applicator within the container or supplied separately.

Label : 'For External use Only'; 'Store in a Cool Place'; 'Highly Inflammable, keep away from naked flames'

Example

Rx

Pyroxyllin	4.0 g
Ether	75.0 ml
Ethanol	25.0 ml
To make about	100.0 ml

Procedure : Add the ethanol and ether to the pyroxylin container and closed the container. Shake the mixture occasionally until the pyroxylin is dissolved. Allow to stand for a few days while impurities settle, decant the supernatant liquid because the solution is highly inflammable. Store the preparation in well-closed container with suitable label.

External Liquid Preparations Instilled into body cavities

(a) *Douches*

A douche is an aqueous solution directed against a part or into a cavity of the body. Douches are most frequently dispensed in the form of a powder with directions for dissolving in a specified quantity of warm water. If powder or tablets are employed for this purpose, they must be completely soluble in water to produce a clear solution.

Tablets are prepared by simple process but the lubricants and diluents must be soluble in water. For preparation of tablets, boric acid is used as lubricant and sodium chloride is used as a diluent.

Tablets deteriorate on exposure to moist air and should be stored in air tight conatainers. Douches are not official preparation. Some preparations contain alum, zinc sulphate, boric acid, phenol, sodium borate. Some compendia have reported a few substances such as benzylkonium chloride to be used in various douches and compound sodium borate solution in nasal or pharyngeal douche.

Douches are mainly used as :

1. Antiseptic (e.g., chlorhexidine, chloroxylenol, lactic acid, mercuric chloride, potassium permanganate etc.)
2. Astringent (e.g., alum, tannic acid, zinc sulphate, etc.)
3. Cleaning (e.g., sodium chloride, boric acid, saponated cresol, etc)
4. Soothing action

Classification of Douches

Eye douches : It is used to remove foreign particles and discharges from the eyes use allowed to run from the inner to the outer cornea of the eye.

1. *Nasal douches :* It is used to cleanse nose by using bulb syringes.
2. *Pharyngeal douches :* It is used in infection of throat for an operation.
3. *Vaginal douches :* It is used for irrigation of the vagina by using 8-10 oz capacity bulb syringes with a large vulcanite or rubber spray tube.
4. *Rectum douches :* It is meant for irrigation of rectum using rectal syringe of the bulb type with a long narrow nozzle.

Container : It is dispensed in colored fluted bottles or single use plastic packs with rectal nozzles for enema.

Labelling : Comply with the general requirement of the label and additional information should be mentioned clearly on the label -'For external use only', 'For nasal use Only' or 'For vaginal use Only' or 'For rectal use Only'

Example 01 : Prepare and dispense Potassium Permanganate Douche

Rx

Potassium permanganate	0.1 g
Purified water, sufficient to produce	100.0 ml

Method of Dispensing : Triturate weighed amount of potassium permanganate with purified water in a pestle mortar. Allow undissolved crystals to settle and pour the supernatant into a conical flask. Filter through a clean sintered glass filter and make up the volume through filter.

Example 02 : *Prepare and dispense Astringent Douche*

Rx

Alum	0.1g
Zinc sulphate	0.5 g
Liquefied phenol	0.6 ml
Glycerin	12.5 ml
Purified water, sufficient to produce	100.0 ml

Method of Dispensing : Mixed weighed amount of alum with purified water, add zinc sulphate and dissolve and gradually add liquefied phenol and glycerin and shake.

Enemas

Enemas are aqueous or oily solutions or suspension that are employed to evacuate the bowel, to influence the general system by absorption or to affect locally the seat of disease or introduced into the rectum for cleansing, therapeutic or diagnostic purpose. Cleansing preparations are used to evacuate faeces in constipation before an operation. Enemas are usually given at body temperature in quantities of 1 to 2 pt injected slowly with a syringe. If they have to be retained in the intestine they should not be used in larger quantities than 6 fl. ounces for an adult.

Sodium chloride, sodium bicarbonate, sodium monohydrogen phosphate and sodium dihydrogen phosphate are used in enemas.

The enemas act in following ways :

1. Large volume enemas (about 0.5 to 1.0 liter) e.g., water, soap and turpentine enemas or other type of enemas stimulate peristalsis.

2. Small volume enemas (about 100 to 500 ml) like olive and arachis oil enemas act by lubricating impacted feces.

Therapeutic enemas may be used as :

1. *Anthelmintic :* Quassia enema for thread worms

2. *Sedatives :* Chloral hydrate, paraldehyde enemas.

3. *Anti-inflammatory agent :* Corticosteroids for ulcerative colitis

4. Stimulating enemas

5. *Nutritive :* When absorption by mouth is impaired, enemas are useful.

6. *X-ray examination :* Barium sulphate suspension is used for X-ray examination of the lower bowel.

Containers

Large volume enemas are administered from a douche can and should be warmed to body temperature before use. Some commercially available small volume enemas are in disposable polyethylene or polyvinyl chloride bags sealed with a rectal nozzle.

Labelling : Special labeling requirements for enemas are 1. To be warmed to body temperature before use, 2. 'Not to be taken orally', 3. 'For rectal use only'

Storage : The enema should be stored in a cool place in complete darkness and an expiry date of only two days after issue is advisable.

Example 01 : *Prepare and dispense Chloral Hydrate Enema*

Rx

Chloral hydrate	2.0 g
Mucilage of starch, sufficient to produce	100.0 ml

Method of Dispensing : Dissolve weighed quantity of chloral hydrate in mucilage of starch and add sufficient to produce 100 ml.

Example 02 : *Prepare and dispense Magnesium Sulphate Enema*

Rx

Magnesium sulphate	50.0 g
Purified water, sufficient to produce	100.0 ml

Method of Dispensing : Dissolve magnesium sulphate in purified water and shake, if required, and filter.

Example 03 : *Prepare and dispense Paraldehyde Enema*

Rx

Paraldehyde	8.0 ml
Sodium chloride	0.9 g
Purified water, sufficient to produce	100.0 ml

Method of Dispensing : Dissolve sodium chloride in purified water, filter, add paraldehyde and dissolve. Add sufficient purified water to produce 100 ml.

Example 04 : *Prepare and dispense Phosphate Enema*

Rx

Sodium acid phosphate	160 g
Sodium phosphate	60.0 g
Purified water, sufficient to produce	100.0 ml

Method of Dispensing : Mix sodium acid phosphate and sodium phosphate and powder in a pestle and mortar. Dissolve this mixture in purified water and make up volume to produce 100 ml.

Example 05 : *Prepare and dispense Soap Enema*

Rx

| Soft soap | 5.0 g |
| Purified water (lukewarm), sufficient to produce | 100.0 ml |

Method of Dispensing : Dissolve weighed amount of soft soap in warm purified water and add sufficient warm purified water to produce 100 ml.

(c) *Ear Drops*

Ear drops are liquid preparation or suspension or emulsion or solution of drug(s) in water, diluted alcohol, glycerin or polyethylene glycol intended for instillation into the ear. Aqueous solutions are not suitable because the secretions in ear are mainly fatty and aqueous solutions do not easily mix with them. Eye drops are generally safe for the ears even if there is a hole in the eardrum. The ingredients of ear drops are different depending on the purpose, 15 ml to be dispensed unless otherwise directed.

Ear drops range from liquids designed to soften ear wax, to medicines made to cure bacterial infections, to medicines against fungus. Many kinds of eye drops can be used in the ear but the opposite is *not* true. Ear drops are too harsh for the eyes.

Ear drops fall into two major practical categories

1. Those that are gentle enough to be safe in the part of ear behind the ear drum,
2. Those that are not safe for ear drum.

How to Use Ear Drops

1. Warm the ear drop bottle by holding it in your hands for a few minutes. Shake the bottle well.
2. Unscrew the cap of the bottle and draw some liquid into the dropper.
3. Either lie on your side or tilt your head over so that the ear which needs the drops is facing upwards.
4. Gently pull your earlobe upwards, away from your neck, and squeeze the correct number of drops into the ear.
5. Keep your head tilted for about five minutes so that the drops can spread into the ear.

6. Straighten your head and wipe away any extra liquid with a clean tissue.

7. Replace the cap on the bottle.

8. Store your ear drops in a cool, dark place.

9. You must use your ear drops for the full length of the treatment course, even if your ear feels better. If you stop too soon, your ear problems may return.

10. While using your ear drops, try not to get water in your ear. Be careful when washing your hair and do not go for swimming until the course is finished.

11. When you have finished your course of treatment, throw any leftover drops away, or return them to your pharmacist for disposal.

Don't mix-up! Eyes drops or ear drops? Ear drops never go in the eye, but some eye products can be used safely in the ear.

Containers

Ear drops should be supplied in containers of glass or suitable plastic which are fitted with an integral dropper or with a cap of suitable materials incorporating a suitable dropper tube and rubber or plastic teat. Alternatively, such cap assembly is supplied separately.

Labeling : Comply with the general requirements for labeling on the ear drops container. It should clearly state that the prescription is intended 'for external use only'.

Example 01 : *Prepare and dispense Aluminium Acetate Ear Drops.*

Rx

Aluminium sulphate	4.5 g
Acetate acid	5.0 ml
Tartaric acid	0.9 g
Calcium carbonate	2.0 g
Purified water	15.0 ml

Method of Dispensing : Weigh required amount of aluminium sulphate and dissolve in 10.0 ml of purified water, add acetic acid and then calcium carbonate. Add remaining amount of purified water and mix properly. Allow to stand for not less than twenty-four hours in a cool place and stir occasionally. Filter the solution after twenty-four hours. Add tartaric acid in the filtrate and mix.

Example 02 : *Prepare and dispense Sodium Bicarbonate Ear Drops.*

Rx

Sodium bicarbonate	0.75 g
Glycerin	4.5 ml
Purified water, sufficient to produce	15.0 ml

Method of Dispensing : Dissolve sodium bicarbonate in freshly boiled and cooled purified water and mix glycerin. Make up the volume with purified water to produce 15.0 ml.

Example 03 : *Prepare and dispense Hydrogen Peroxide Ear Drops.*

Rx

Hydrogen peroxide solution (6.0%)	3.75 ml
Purified water, sufficient to produce	15.0 ml

Method of Dispensing : Mix measured amount of hydrogen peroxide solution with purified water and filter the solution.

Example 04 : *Prepare and dispense Boric Acid Ear Drops*

Boric acid is produced from native borax or from the other borates by reacting with hydrochloric acid or sulphuric acid. It is colorless scales of a somewhat pearly luster or crystals but more commonly a white powder slightly unctuous to the touch. It is odorless and stable in air and volatilizes with steam. It is slightly soluble in water hence in this preparation denatured spirit is used as it enhances the solubility of boric acid in purified water. It is a very weak germicide. It is nonirritating hence suitable for application to delicate structures such as cornea of the eye.

Rx

Boric acid	0.1 g
Specially denatured spirit	3.0 ml
Purified water, sufficient to produce	15.0 ml

Method of Dispensing : Weighed quantity of boric acid is to be dissolved in denatured spirit and add purified water to make sufficient volume. Filter to remove impurities, if any and dispense in a suitable container.

Example 05 : *Prepare and dispense Chloramphenicol Ear Drops.*

Rx

Chloramphenicol	0.75 g
Propylene glycol, sufficient to produce	15.0 ml

Method of Dispensing : Dissolve Chloramphenicol in propylene glycol, shake and add remaining quantity of propylene glycol to produce sufficient volume of 15 ml.

Example 06 : *Prepare and dispense Ichthammol Ear Drops.*

Ichthammol consists of the ammonium salts of the sulphuric acids of an oily substance prepared from a bituminous schist or shale, or from other sources, together with ammonium sulphate and water. It is black viscid liquid, which has characteristic strong odor. It is miscible in water, alcohol, glycerin and with fixed oils. It is used as antiparasitic and irritant,

Rx

Ichthammol   1.5 g

Glycerin, sufficient to produce   15.0 ml

Method of Dispensing : Weighed amount of Ichthammol is mixed with glycerin and dispensed in suitable container.

(d) Nasal Drops

Nasal drops are aqueous or liquid paraffin solutions meant for instillation into the nostrils. Nasal drops often contain vasoconstrictor drugs to relieve nasal congestion. Oily solutions are not preferred since the oil may retard the ciliary action of the mucosa and may even cause lipoid pneumonia if drop of the oil enter the trachea. A vehicle for formulating nasal drops should have- (i) pH between 5.5 and 7.5, (ii) buffering capacity, (iii) tonicity equivalent to normal saline, and iv) viscosity not exceeding the normal viscosity of nasal mucosa.

Nasal drops are dispensed in 10 to 25 ml quantities in colored fluted bottles fitted with a screw cap and dropper. Commercially available products are supplied in plastic, squeeze-type containers.

(e) Nasal Sprays

Sprays are solutions of various drugs in aqueous vehicles and are applied to the mucous membrane of the nose and the throat by means of an atomizer or nebulizer. Spray devices should produce relatively coarse droplets if the therapeutic action of the medicaments is to be restricted to the upper respiratory tract. Very fine droplets penetrate into the respiratory tract. Initially the sprays were prepared by dissolving various medicaments in light liquid petrolatum. It may damage the normal ciliary activity of the nasal mucosa and, if drops of oil enter the trachea it can cause lipoid pneumonia. Because of this problem, aqueous sprays that are isotonic with nasal secretions and of approximately the same pH are preferred. Sprays contain substances such as antibiotics, antihistamines, vasoconstrictors, alcohol, solubilizers, and wetting agents.

Example 01 : *Prepare and dispense Isoprenaline Compound Spray.*

Rx

Isoprenaline	0.250 g
Papaverine hydrochloride	0.625 g
Atropine methonitrate	50.0 mg
Propylene glycol	1.25 ml
Sodium metabisulphite	25.0 mg
Purified water, sufficient to produce	25.0 ml

Method of Dispensing : Mix isoprenaline, atropine methonitrate and papaverine hydrochloride and dissolve in purified water. Dissolve sodium metabisulphite and add in the solution. Add other additives and add sufficient purified water to produce 25 ml.

Example 02 : *Prepare and dispense Compound Adrenaline and Atropine Spray.*

Rx

Adrenaline acid tartrate	0.80 g
Atropine methonitrate	0.10 g
Papaverine hydrochloride	0.80 g
Sodium metabisulphite	0.10 g
Chlorbutanol	0.50 g
Propylene glycol	5.00 ml
Purified water, sufficient to produce	100.0 ml

Method of Dispensing : Boil purified water for about 10 minutes, to remove oxygen and destroy vegetative bacteria and mould spores. Cool the water and use for the preparation of sprays. Prepare solution of adrenaline acid tartrate, atropine methonitrate and sodium metabisulphite in separate containers, respectively using small proportion of purified water. Mix three solutions and add papaverine hydrochloride in the mixture. Dissolve weighed amount of chlorbutanol in propylene glycol and mix in the mixture. Filter, if necessary and add sufficient purified water to adjust the volume 100 ml through the filter.

(f) Inhalations

The term inhalation is used commonly by the layman to describe preparations intended to be vaporized with the aid of heat, usually steam, and inhaled. Inhalations are solutions of medicaments administered by the nasal or oral respiratory route for local or systemic effect. Nebulizers are suitable for administration of inhalation solutions only if they give droplets sufficiently fine and uniform in size so that the mist reaches the bronchitis.

Another category of products also called insufflations consists of finely powdered or liquid drugs that are carried into the respiratory passages by the use of special delivery systems. Solutions may be nebulized by use of inert gases. Nebulized solutions may be breathed directly from the nebulizer or nebulizer may be attached to a plastic facemask or intermittent positive pressure breathing machines. Particle size is one of the important parameter for inhalation. The optimum particle size for penetration into the pulmonary cavity is 0.5 to 7.0 μm. Pressurized aerosols generate fine mists and hence posses basic advantages over the older nebulizers.

Example 01 : *Prepare and dispense Aqueous Inhalation.*

Rx

Eucalyptus oil	6.0 ml
Menthol	3.0 g
Light magnesium carbonate	6.50 g
Purified water, sufficient to produce	100.0 ml

Method of Dispensing : Powder weighed amount of menthol in glass mortar and pestle, add eucalyptus oil and stir until the solid has dissolved and add other additives and mix well.

Example 02 : *Prepare and dispense Benzoin Inhalation.*

Rx

Benzoin	10.0 g
Prepared storax	6.85 g
Specially denatured spirit, sufficient to produce	100.0 ml

Method of Dispensing : Benzoin and prepared storax should be macerated with 7.5 ml of specially denatured spirit for twenty four hours. Filter and add specially denatured spirit passed through filter to produce 100 ml.

Example 03 : *Prepare and dispense Menthol Inhalation.*

Rx

Menthol	1.0 g
Specially denatured spirit, sufficient to produce	50.0 ml

Method of Dispensing : Mix menthol with specially denatured spirit in mortar and pestle. Add sufficient specially denatured spirit through filter and produce 50 ml.

External Liquid Preparations Used in the Mouth

(a) Gargles

Gargles are aqueous solutions used for treating the pharynx and nasopharynx by forcing air from lungs through the gargle that is held in the throat. Gargles are generally dispensed in concentrated form. They must be diluted with water prior to use. Gargles are pleasantly flavored and medicated than mouthwashes. Many mouthwashes are used as gargles, either as such or diluted with purified warm water. Gargles generally contain following substances viz. antibiotics (e.g., benzocaine), antiseptics (e.g., borax), anti-inflammatory (e.g., clove oil), anti-fungal (e.g., phenol, thymol etc.), analgesic (e.g., potassium permanganate), astringents (e.g., benzalkonium chloride, potassium chlorate), alkalinizing agents (e.g., cresote), deodorants (e.g., sodium bicarbonate), local anesthetics (e.g., eugenol).

Container : Narrow mouthed, screw capped, colorless fluted bottles.

Example 01 : *Prepare and dispense Phenol Glycerin Gargles.*

Rx

Phenol glycerin	5.0 ml
Amaranth solution	1.0 ml
Purified water, sufficient to produce	100.0 ml

Method of Dispensing : Prepare phenol glycerin using phenol and glycerin. Mix phenol glycerin with purified water and add amaranth solution. Add sufficient purified water to produce 100 ml.

Example 02 : *Prepare and dispense Potassium Permanganate Gargles.*

Rx

Potassium permanganate	25.0 mg
Purified water, sufficient to produce	100.0 ml

Method of Dispensing : Grind weighed amount of potassium permanganate with water. Remove undissolved permanganate by filtration and add sufficient amount of purified water to produce 100 ml.

(b) Mouthwashes

A mouthwash is an aqueous solution which is most often used for its deodorant, refreshing or antiseptic effect. It may contain alcohol, glycerin, synthetic sweeteners, surface-active agent, flavoring and coloring agents. Mouthwashes generally contain following substances.

1. Antibacterial agents : alkaline phenol, hydrogen peroxide, buffered sodium perborate, thymol glycerin.

2. Astringents : zinc sulphate, zinc chloride, etc.

Container : Narrow mouthed screw capped colored fluted bottle.

Labeling : Comply with the general requirements for labeling. In addition the label on the container states - 'Not to be Swallowed in large amount', and 'Store in cool place'.

Example 01 : *Prepare and dispense Compound Sodium Chloride Mouthwash.*

Rx

Sodium bicarbonate	1.0 g
Sodium chloride	1.5 g
Concentrated peppermint emulsion	2.5 ml
Double strength chloroform water	50.0 ml
Purified water qs	100.0 ml

Method of Dispensing *:* Dissolve sodium bicarbonate and sodium chloride in purified water, add concentrated peppermint emulsion and mix. Add double strength chloroform water.

Example 01 *: Prepare and dispense Mouthwash.*

Rx

Cetylpyridinium chloride	0.10 g
Citric acid	0.10 g
Sweetener (sodium saccharin)	0.04 g
Flavor oils (peppermint, eucalyptus, and clove oils)	0.15 ml
Polyoxyethylene (20) sorbitan monostearate,	0.3 g
Ethanol	10.0 ml
Sorbitol solution	20.0 g
Purified water, sufficient to produce	100.0 ml

Method of Dispensing *:* Dissolve cetylpyridinium chloride, citric acid, and sodium saccharin in a sufficient amount of the water and add ethanol. Mix polyoxyethylene (20) sorbitan monostearate and flavor oils and add slowly hydroalcoholic solution with stirring, sorbitol and mix. Add sufficient amount of purified water to produce 100 ml.

CHAPTER 11

Suspensions

A pharmaceutical suspension may be defined as a dispersion in which finely divided solid particles are suspended in a liquid medium. Dispersed solid particles are known as internal phase and dispersion medium is known as continuous phase/external phase. Particles smaller than 0.1 to 0.2 µm are generally considered to be colloidal. A solid in liquid dispersion in which the particles are above colloidal size (upto 1000 µm) is termed as coarse suspension. In other words suspensions are heterogeneous (biphasic) system consisting of two phases. The continuous phase or external phase is generally a liquid or semisolid and the dispersed or internal phase is made up of particulate matter that is essentially insoluble in but dispersed throughout the continuous phase.

Ideal Suspension

- The suspension must remain sufficiently homogeneous for at least the period between shaking the container and removing the required dose from the container.

- The sediment produced on storage must be easily re-suspended by the use of moderate agitation/shaking.

- The suspension may be required to thicken in order to reduce the rate of settling of particles but the viscosity must not be too high that is not suitable for removing the dose from container.

- The suspended particles should be small and uniformly sized in order to give a smooth, elegant product, free from a gritty texture.

- The suspension should resist microbial attack during storage and also maintain during the shelf-life all organoleptic properties as initially.

- Topical suspension should spread easily when applied.

Advantages

- It is easy to dispense unstable or degradable drugs in solution form.

- Suspension is the only choice if the drug is not soluble in water and non-aqueous solvent is not acceptable, e.g., corticosteroids suspension.

- Suspension is most suitable for drugs having unpleasant taste and odor e.g., Chloramphenical palmitate (bitter taste).

- The insoluble solids act as a reservoir and continuously supply the drug into solution, which is absorbed over a long period e.g., Protamine zinc-Insulin.

- Drug in suspension exhibits a higher rate of bioavailability compared to the same drug of equivalent dose formulated in tablets or capsules. This is due to larger surface area and high dissolution. e.g., antacid suspension.

Disadvantages

- Sedimentation of solids occasionally gives poor form of product. It may lead to caking (formation of compact mass), which is difficult to dispense.

- Dose precision cannot be achieved unless suspensions are packed in unit dosage forms.

- Sometimes microbial contamination takes place if preservation not added in accurate proportion.

- A suspension being a bulky product, transportation cost is high.

Purpose of Suspension

- Many people have difficulty in swallowing solid dosage forms and therefore require the drug to be dispensed in a liquid. If the drug is insoluble or poorly soluble in a suitable solvent their formulation as a suspension is usually required.

- The degradation of a drug in the presence of water may also preclude its use as an aqueous solution in which case it may be possible to synthesize an insoluble derivative which can be then be formulated as suspension. eg., oxytetracyline hydrochloride is hydrolyzed rapidly in aqueous solution.

- The prolonged contact between the solid drug particles and dispersion medium can reduce the efficiency of some drugs e.g. Ampicillin. The pharmacist makes the product up to volume with water immediately before issue to the patient. Shelf-life of product is 7 days at room temperature and 14 days at refrigerator.

- Some materials are required to be present in the gastrointestinal tract in a finely divided form, their formulation as suspensions will provide the desired high surface area e.g., kaolin, magnesium carbonate, magnesium trisilicate etc. used for the adsorption of toxins or to neutralize excess acidity.

- The adsorption properties of fine powders are also used in the formulation of some inhalations. The volatile components of menthol and eucalyptus oil would be lost from solution very rapidly during use. Prolonged release suspension would contain volatile ingredients adsorbed on light magnesium carbonate.

- Tastes and odors of drugs are more noticeable if in solution than in an insoluble form e.g., paracetamol suspensions are particularly more suitable for children as compared to paracetamol elixir. Insoluble chloramphenicol palmitate is successfully formulated in the form of suspension.

- Suspension of drugs can also be formulated for topical application e.g., Calamine lotion
- Suspension can also be formulated for parenteral administration to control the rate of absorption of the drug e.g., depot, implants.
- Vaccines are often formulated as suspension for induction of immunity. They may consist of dispersions of killed micro-organisms as in Cholera vaccine, Diphtheria and Tetanus vaccines
- X-ray contrast media are also formulated in the form of suspension e.g., barium sulphate suspension for alimentary tract examination.

Classification of Suspensions

A. On the basis of Preparation

(a)   Flocculated suspensions   (b)   Deflocculated suspensions

B. On the basis of route of administration

(a)   Orally administered suspensions   (b)   Topical suspensions

(c)   Sterilized (injectable and ophthalmic) suspensions

C. On the basis of preparation

(a)   Dispersed suspensions   (b)   Open network suspension aggregates

(c)   Closed suspensions

Table 11.1 Comparison of Flocculated and Deflocculated Suspension.

S.No.	Deflocculated suspension	Flocculated suspension
1.	Particles exist in suspension form as separate entities	Particles form loose aggregates and settle down in the container
2.	Rate of sedimentation is slow, since each particles settles separately and particle size is minimal	Rate of sedimentation is high, since particles settle as a floc, which is a collection of particles
3.	A sediment is formed slowly, may take months	A sediment is formed rapidly, within minutes
4.	The sediment eventually becomes very closely packed, due to weight of upper layers of sedimenting material. Repulsive forces between particles are overcome and a hard cake is formed which is difficult to re-disperse.	The sediment is loosely packed and possesses a scaffold-like structure. Particles do not bind tightly to each other and a hard dense cake does not form. The sediment is easy to re-disperse so as to reform the original suspension
5.	The suspension has a pleasing appearance because the suspended particles remain suspended uniformly for long time. The supernatant also remains cloudy, even when settling is apparent.	The suspension is somewhat unsightly, due to rapid administration and the presence of an obvious, clear supernatant region. This can be minimized if the volume of sediment is made large.

Dispensing of Suspensions

Mainly four types of materials are used in dispensing of the suspension –

(a)   ***Suspensions containing diffusible solids :*** Insoluble lightweight powdered substances are readily mixed with water and remain suspended throughout the continuous phase after long time shaking and mixing. The uniform dispersion is based on the size distribution of the particles in continuous phase.

Examples of diffusible substances are Calcium carbonate, Magnesium trisilicate, Bismuth carbonate, Light magnesium carbonate, Kaolin, Rhubarb Powder.

Dispensing Method

Solid powder is finely divided by triturating in pestle and mortar. Make a cream of fine power with small part of vehicle and add more vehicle with stirring or slow trituration. Remove foreign particles, if visible in suspension, by muslin cloth. Mix rinsing in the mortar and pestle and add other liquid ingredients, make up the volume by adding vehicle and mix properly by shaking the final product. Store in suitable container with label having 'shake well before use' instruction and dose.

Example 1 : Dispense the suspension.

Rx

Bismuth carbonate	2.00 g
Sodium bicarbonate	1.40 g
Belladona Tincture	1.00 ml
Purified water q.s. to	60.0 ml

Example 2 : Dispense the suspension.

Rx

Light Kaolin	6.00 g
Light magnesium carbonate	1.50 g
Sodium bicarbonate	1.50 g
Peppermint water q.s. to	50.00 ml

(b)   **Suspensions containing indiffusible solids**

Indiffusible solid substances will not remain distributed throughout the vehicle for enough time to ensure uniformity of dose. The stability of suspension and uniformity of dispersed substance are enhanced by increasing the viscosity of continuous phase by adding thickening/suspending agent.

Examples of indiffusible substances include Aspirin, Chalk, Phenobarbitone, Succinylsulphathiazole, Sulphadimidine (for oral use); and Calamine, Zinc oxide, Precipitated sulphur, Hydrocortisone, Triamcinolone acetonide (for external use).

Dispensing method

Solid powders are finely divided by triturating in pestle and mortar with thickening agent. Make a cream of fine powder with 50% of vehicle and add more vehicle with stirring or triturating slowly. Remove foreign particles if visible in suspension by muslin cloth. Mix rinsing of mortar and pestle and add other liquid ingredient make up the volume by adding vehicle and mix properly by shaking the final product. Store in suitable container with label having 'shake well before use' instruction and dose.

Table 11.2 Common Suspending Agents in Dispensing Practice.

Type and name	Form in which used	Concentration	Uses	Characteristics
1. Organic Natural: Gum Tragacanth	(a) Powder (b) Mucilage 12.5% w/v (c) Compound powder 15% w/w	0.2% w/v 25% v/v 2-4% w/v	To suspend heavy indiffusible solids and resinous tinctures	Forms viscous gel in water. Mucilage is used when the vehicle is water or chloroform water. It is desirable to add a preservative.
Gum acacia	(a) Mucilage 40% w/v (b) Compound powder 20% w/v	6-12% v/v 2-4% w/v	To suspend light powders and resinous tinctures	Storage of the mucilage results in fall of pH below 4. It is rarely used for external purposes. Compound powder is used when the vehicle is other than water.
Starch (Wheat, corn, rice or potato)	a. Mucilage 2.5% w/w b. Compound powder 20% w/w	2-4% w/w 2-4% w/w	Not used orally. Makes good jellies for external use.	Good suspending agent for barium meal. Possesses good gelatinizing properties.
Sodium alginate	Mucilage 1% w/v		Used for suspending anionic substances	Viscosity is maximum after 1 hour of preparation and falls to a constant value after 24 hours.
Agar	Powder	1% w/v	Bulk laxative	In 1% concentration it produces a jelly like mass.
Gelatin	Powder	2-4% w/v	Used in pastes and external preparations .	There are two types, Pharmagel A and B. Isoletectric point of A is 7-9 and is compatible with cations. Isoelectric point of B is 5-7 and is compatible with anions.

Table 11.2 Contd...

Type and name	Form in which used	Concentration	Uses	Characteristics
Semisynthetic: Methyl cellulose	Mucilage 2% w/v in hot water	0.5-2% *w/v*	Used both for internal and external preparations .	Mucilage is clear to opalascent, It is susceptible to microbial attack; 0.001% phenyl mercuric nitrate is used to preserve it. On heating to 50^0C the mucilage gels and on cooling it becomes a sol. It is incompatible with phenol, tannic acid, chlorocresol, resorcinol and silver nitrate.
Sodium carboxymethyl cellulose	Mucilage 2% *w/v* in cold water	0.25-1% w/v	Used for oral, external and parenteral preparations .	Susceptible to pH less than 5 and more than 10 when viscosity is affected. It gets precipitated below pH 3. It is sterilizable by dry heat
II. Inorganic Bentonite	Suspension 5% *w/v* as stock suspension	1% *w/v*	Used for external preparations .	It should be sterilized before use. Bentonite is incompatible with electrolytes and positively charged particles.
III. Synthetic Carboxyvinyl polymer	Gel	0.1-0.4% *w/v*	Used for internal and external preparations , also used for gelling alcohol, glycols etc.	It possesses high viscosity between pH 6-11. The viscosity gets markedly reduced below pH 3.

Example 3 : Dispense the following suspension.

Rx

Bismuth carbonate	2.0 g
Chalk	2.0 g
Kaolin	8.0 g
Tincture catechu	4.0 ml
Purified water q.s. to	60.0 ml

Method of dispensing: Kaolin, chalk and bismuth carbonate are finely divided by trituring in pestle and mortar with tincture of catechu. Make a cream of fine powder with 50% of purified water and add more purified water with stirring or triturating slowly. Remove foreign particles if visible in suspension by muslin cloth. Mix rinsing of mortar and pestle and add other liquid ingredient make up the volume by adding vehicle and mix properly by shaking the final product. Store in suitable container with label having 'shake well before use' instruction and dose.

(c) **Suspensions containing Precipitate forming liquids**

Some liquid preparations containing resinous constituents, gums and small amounts of volatile components are precipitated on addition to water. Gum resins are oil soluble purified exudates of Myrrh, Benzoin, Galbanum, oppoponax, Tolu, Lobelia etc. The precipitated resin adheres to the side of the container and converted to non-dispersible form. To prevent this problem the pharmacist should adopt special precaution during dispensing. Two methods are commonly used for the prevention of precipitation of suspension.

A. Using Compound Tragacanth Powder

Mix finely powered substance, insoluble solid and gum intimately. Form a smooth cream with vehicle and dilute up to 50% of the final volume. Measure the precipitate forming liquid and pour in a slow stream into the center of the suspension with stirring. Avoid sticky liquid on the pestle and on the sides of the mortar. Precipitated resin particles are adsorbed by hydrocolloids over their surface conferring hydrophilic properties and preventing aggregation into clots. (Note – If electrolytes are present in the preparation, it should not be added until the resin has been protected by hydrocolloids)

B. Using Tragacanth mucilage

This method is quite easy to dispense resin-containing substances. Mix mucilage with an equal volume of vehicle in beaker and add precipitate forming liquid into the center of the mucilage with constant stirring. If any electrolyte is present, add and dilute well with vehicle.

Example 4 : Prepare and dispense Mixture of Lobelia and Stramonium.

Rx

Lobelia ethereal Tincture	8.0 ml
Tragacanth mucilage	10.0 ml
Potassium iodide	2.0 g
Stramonium Tincture	16.0 ml
Double strength Chloroform water	10.0 ml
Purified Water q.s. to	100 ml

Method of dispensing : Mix tragacanth with purified water and add Lobelia ethereal tincture and stramonium tincture with constant stirring. Add and mix potassium iodide and double strength chloroform water. Add sufficient purified water to make up the volume.

Practice Exercise

Example 1

Rx

Ammonium chloride	120 gr
Syrup of wild cherry ad	3 fluid ounces

Label : 1 tablespoonful 3 times a day

Example 2

Rx

Ephedrine hydrochloride	60 mg
Syrup of tolu ad	100 ml

One tablespoonful when the cough is severe.

Example 03

Rx

Pot citrate	5 g
Spt. ammon, aromat	15 ml
Spt. aeth, nitrosi	10 ml
Ext. glycyrrhiza liq.	30 ml
Aq. dest. ad	200 ml

One dessertspoonful 6 times a day

Example 04

Rx

Sod. Salicylate	20 gm
Sod. citrate	10 gm
Syr. crange	15 ml
Water ad	200 ml

M. ft. mist. Put 10 dose marks. One dose 3 times a day

Example 5

Rx

Codeine phos.	250 mg
Syr. Lemon	50 ml
Syr. Tolu	20 ml
Chloform water ad	150 ml

15 ml to be taken 3 times a day

Example 6

Rx

Aluminium hydroxide	20%
Magnesium oxide	10%
Water of peppermint	q.s.

M. ft. mist Mitte 4 fl.oz. One tablespoonful before meals.

Example 7

Rx

Bismuth subnitrate	8 gm
Nitric acid	18 ml
Ammonium carbonate	10 gm
Strong ammonia solution	
Purified water aa q.s.	100 ml

M.ft. mist. 5 ml three times a day

(Refer to NF XII monograph Bismuth Magma)

Example 8

Rx

Sulphathiazole	5 gm
Syrup	20 ml
Water	50 ml

M. ft. mist. Mode dicto utenda.

Example 9

Rx

Mag. Carb.	15 gm
Citric acid	27.4 gm
Syrup	60 ml
Talc	5 gm
Lemon oil	0.1 ml
Pot. Bicarb.	2.5 gm
Purified water q.s.	350 ml

M.ft. mist. To be taken as directed

Marketed Products

Generic Name	Company	Active Ingredients	Indications
Acigon	Nicholas Piramal	Each 10 ml contains Sodium alginate 440 mg, Dried aluminium hydroxide gel 160 mg, Magnesium Trisil 80 mg, Sodium bicarbonate 140 mg	Antacid
Adocid	Adoc Pharma	Each 5 ml contains Megaldrate 400 mg, semithicone 20 mg	Antacid
Diovol Forte	Wallace	Each 5 ml contains Dried aluminium hydroxide gel 300 mg, Magnesium hydroxide 250 mg, Activated dimethicone 40 mg, Deglycyrrhizinized Liquorice 400 mg	Antacid
Rcin	Lupin	Rifampicin 100 mg /5 ml	Antibiotic, Treatment of tuberculosis
Taurmox	Taurus Lab	Amoxycillin	Antibiotic, used in respiratory, genitor-urinary, skin and soft tissue infection.
Clamp	Dr. Reddy's Lab	Amoxycillin 200 mg and clavulanic acid 28.5 mg per 5 ml	Used in the treatment of respiratory and urinary tract infection
Cefspan	Glaxo-Smithkline	Cefixime 100 mg/5 ml	Infections of respiratory, urinary & biliary tract
Jucef-LB	Jollen Midicare	Cefixime 50 mg, Lactic acid bacillus 60 million spores	Infections of respiratory, urinary & biliary tract
Cefadic	Andic Lifesciences	Cefadroxil 125 mg	In the treatment of urinary tract infection caused by *E.coli*
Zedro	FDC	Cefadroxil 125 mg	In the treatment of urinary tract infection caused by *E.coli*
Zefdinir	German Remedies	Cefdinir 125 mg/5ml	Pharyngitis, tonsillitis
Roxeptin	IPCA	Roxithromycin 50 mg/5ml	Acute bronchitis, tonsillitis and genital infections

CHAPTER 12

Emulsions

Emulsions are biphasic systems consisting of two immiscible liquids, one of which (the dispersed phase) is finely subdivided and uniformly dispersed as droplets throughout the other phase is known as dispersion medium. The dispersed phase is also called as the internal phase and the dispersion medium as external phase. These immiscible liquids are made miscible by adding a third substance known as emulsifying agent. They stabilize the system by forming a thin film around the globules of the dispersed phase.

In other words an emulsion may, therefore be defined as a disperse system consisting of heterogeneous system consisting of at least one immiscible liquid dispersed in another in the form of droplets whose diameter in general exceed $0.1\mu m$. Such systems posses a minimal stability because the droplets quickly coalesce and the two liquids get separated. The stability of the emulsion is increased by adding another substance known as emulsifying agent or emulsifier. The liquid droplets, generally known as the emulsion phase or emulsion globules or dispersed phase or internal phase or the interrupted phase while the liquid in which they are dispersed is known as the continuous phase or the dispersion medium or the external phase.

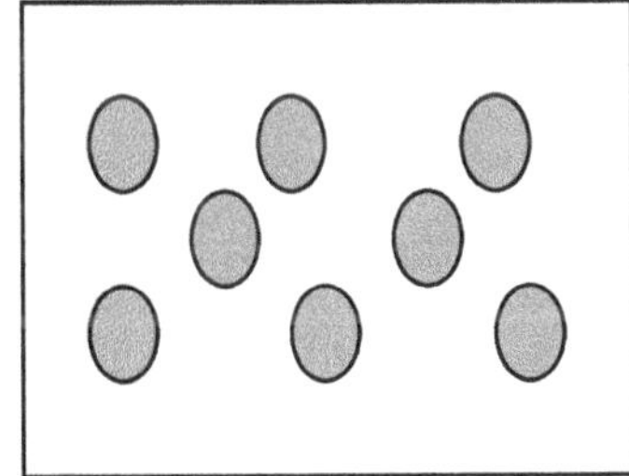
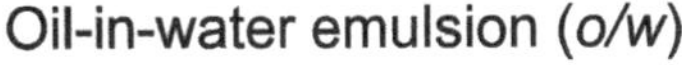

Oil-in-water emulsion (*o/w*)

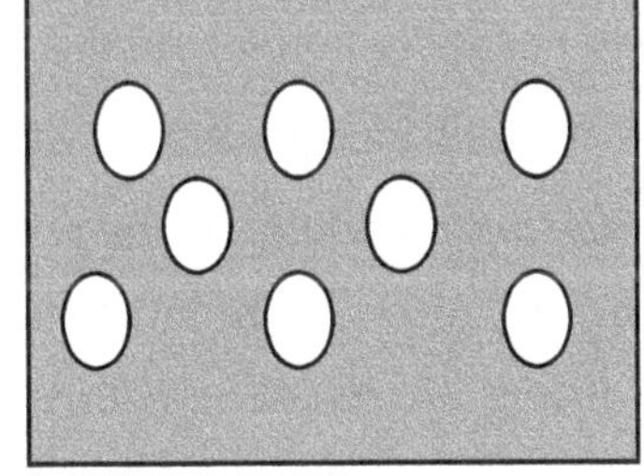

Water-in-oil emulsion (*w/o*)

Advantages

- Suitable to mask the bitter taste and odor of drug and making more palatable dosage form e.g., castor oil, cod-liver oil etc.

- Some nutrients like carbohydrates, fats and vitamins can be emulsified and can be administered to bed ridden patients as sterile intravenous emulsions.
- Used to prolong the release of the drug thereby providing sustained release action.
- Emulsions provide protection to drugs which are susceptible to oxidation or hydrolysis.
- Intravenous emulsions are useful for diagnosis and parenteral nutrition.
- Suitable to formulate externally used products like lotions, creams, liniments etc.

Purpose of Emulsion

- It increases stability of many drugs, which are unstable in aqueous solution.
- It improves the taste of objectionable medicinal agents and makes them more acceptable form.
- It improves appearance of those materials which are generally intended for topical application.
- It improves penetration and spreading ability.
- It enhances the rate and extent of absorption through alimentary canal.
- It can be used as diagnostic agent e.g., radiopaque emulsion in X-ray examination.
- It improves solubility of many drugs, which have limited solubility in aqueous phase.
- It can prolong drug action.

Emulsion Types

(a)   Water-in-oil (*w/o*) emulsion (Dispersed phase – water, Continuous phase – oil)

(b)   Oil-in water (*o/w*) emulsion (Dispersed phase – oil, Continuous phase – water)

(c)   Multiple emulsion (Water-in-oil-in-water (*w/o/w*), Oil-in water-in oil (*o/w/o*))

(d)   *Miscellaneous :* Globule size or the disperse phase size of emulsion can vary enormously but are commonly in the range of 0.25-25µm diameter.

On the basis of size emulsions are mainly of three types

(i)   *Coarse emulsion :* globule size more than 25.0 µm.

(ii)   *Fine emulsion :* globule size less than 5.0 µm.

(iii)   *Microemulsion or miceller emulsion :* globule size range of 10-75 nm, such emulsions appear transparent to the human eye in day light.

Oil-in-water (*o/w*) Emulsion

In this emulsion oil is the dispersed phase (internal phase) and aqueous is the dispersion medium (external phase). These emulsions are used mainly for internal/oral use to mask the bitter or disagreeable taste and odor of drugs. External preparations of these emulsions are used for formulating non-greasy lotions, creams and liniments. Moreover easy assimilation of oil in the body takes place as oil is present in a finely dispersed state. Cosmetic products prepared using *o/w* emulsions can easily be removed from the surface of the skin e.g., castor oil emulsion, foundation creams, vanishing creams.

Water in oil (*w/o*) emulsions

In this emulsion water is the dispersed phase (internal phase) and oil is the dispersion medium (external phase). These emulsions are mainly used for external preparations e.g., lotions and creams as the external layer of oil forms an occlusive film and prevents the evaporation of moisture from the surface of the skin. They are also effective as cleansing cream as they solubilize the oil soluble dirt from the surface e.g. Cold creams.

Multiple Emulsions

In this emulsion, oil in water (*o/w*) or water in oil emulsion (*w/o*) is dispersed in another liquid medium. Thus, oil-in-water-in-oil (*o/w/o*) emulsion consists of very small droplets of oil dispersed in the water globules of water in oil emulsion and water-in-oil-in-water (*w/o/w*) emulsion consists of droplets of water dispersed in the oily phase of oil in water emulsion. Multiple emulsions are primarily used for formulating sustained release dosage forms as the drug entrapped in the innermost layer has to pass through the other two phases before being released for absorption.

Table 12.1 Differences between *o/w* and *w/o* emulsions.

Oil in water emulsion (*o/w*)	Water in oil emulsion (*w/o*)
In this type of emulsion, water is the continuous phase (dispersion medium) and oil is the dispersed phase	While in this type of emulsion oil is the dispersion medium and water is the dispersed phase
Generally non greasy and easily removable from the skin surface	More greasy and not washable with water
This type of emulsions is generally meant for internal use as bitter taste of oils can be masked.	This type of emulsions is generally meant for external use like creams.
Externally applied emulsion e.g., vanishing cream provide cooling effect	Externally applied emulsion prevent evaporation of moisture from the surface of skin e.g., cold cream
Water soluble drugs are more quickly released from *o/w* emulsions	Oil soluble drugs are more quickly released from *w/o* emulsions
Show a positive conductivity test, as water is the external phase, which is a good conductor of electricity.	Do not give a positive conductivity test, as oil is the external phase, which is a poor conductor of electricity.

Routes of Administration of Emulsions

(a) **Oral Emulsions :** Generally *o/w* emulsions are used for oral administration of drugs or substance because oil is more readily absorbed in a fine state of subdivision through the gastro intestinal tract and secondly the preparation becomes more palatable when water forms the continuous phase. From manufacturing point of view, oil is enveloped in a thin film of emulgent, which masks the bitter and oily taste of the drug like liquid paraffin. Orally, emulsions are also used to enhance the absorption of the oil soluble drugs like vitamins A,D, E and K.

Example 1 : Liquid Paraffin Emulsion

Rx

Liquid Paraffin	50 ml
Methyl cellulose	2.0 g
Vanillin	50 mg
Chloroform	0.25 ml
Benzoic acid solution	2.0 ml
Saccharin sodium	50 mg
Purified Water q.s	100 ml

Method of Preparation : Triturate the weighed quantity of liquid paraffin and chloroform with methyl cellulose in mortar and pestle, creamy emulsion is formed. Add and mix other additives and add sufficient purified water with continuous stirring.

Uses : Laxative and acts as an emollient purgative in chronic constipation especially during pregnancy and geriatric patient.

Example 2 : Castor oil Emulsion

Rx

Castor oil	16 ml
Gum acacia	q.s
Water	80 ml

Method of Preparation : Triturate the weighed quantity of castor oil and cinnamon water with gum acacia in mortar and pestle. Add remaining quantity of cinnamon water and mix properly.

Use : Purgative

Example 3 : Cod-Liver oil Emulsion

Rx

Cod-liver oil	50 ml
Acacia powder	12.5 ml

Tragacanth powder	0.75 g
Benzaldehyde Spirit	0.25 ml
Saccharin sodium	0.01 g
Chloroform	0.25 ml
Water, to	100 ml

Method of Preparation : Mix two gums and prepare the primary emulsion by the dry gum method and add cod-liver oil. Add and mix other additives with constant stirring and make up the volume.

Uses : Source of vitamin A and D. It is used as dietary supplement in infants and children to prevent the occurance of rickets and to improve nutrition in undernourished children and patients with rickets.

(b) External Emulsions : Both types of emulsions are used for external purpose but *w/o* emulsions are more commonly used for this purpose. Emulsions find maximum use in topical preparations, both for therapeutic and cosmetic use. Therapeutically they are used as carrier for a drug. In cosmetic industry *o/w* emulsions have been used for formulation of make up foundation lotions, moisturing lotions, and hand lotions. Cold cream *w/o* is used when oily layers are desired to prevent moisture loss from the surface of skin, for barrier action and for cleansing action.

Example 1 : Antiseptic cream

Rx

Cetrimide	1g
Cetostearyl alcohol	10 g
White soft paraffin	10 g
Liquid paraffin	29 g
Purified water	50 g

Method of Preparation : Dissolve cetostearyl alcohol in the liquid paraffin with gentle heat in a beaker and in another beaker dissolve cetrimide in purified water. Add warm oily phase into aqueous phase with stirring until cold.

Uses : Antiseptic cream for the treatment of wounds, cuts and burns.

Example 2 : Cold Cream

Rx

Liquid paraffin	20 g
Hard paraffin	4.5 g
Lanette wax	3.5 g
Glycerine	4.5 g
Water	17.5 g
Propyl paraben	0.1 g

Method of preparation : Melt all oily substance in a beaker and dissolve aqueous substances in another beaker. Add aqueous solution to the mixture of oily phase with continuous and rapid stirring until it has congealed.

Uses : Skin protective and skin smoothner.

(c) *Rectal Emulsions :* Enemas are formulated as *o/w* types of emulsions for various purposes.

Emulsifying Agents

These are the substances added to an emulsion to prevent the coalescence of the globules of the dispersed phase. They are also known as emulgents or emulsifiers. These agents have both a hydrophilic and a lipophilic part in their chemical structure. All emulsifying agents concentrate at and are adsorbed onto the oil/water interface to provide a protective barrier around the dispersed droplets. In addition to this protective barrier, emulsifiers stabilize the emulsion by reducing the interfacial tension of the system. Some agents enhance stability by imparting a charge on the droplet surface thus reducing the physical contact between the droplets and decreasing the potential for coalescence.

The effectiveness of an emulsifying agent depends on the following factors viz:

- Chemical structure
- Concentration
- Solubility
- pH
- Physical properties
- Electrostatic effect

Emulsifiers act in three ways -

1. Formation of a protective barrier
2. Reduction of interfacial tension
3. Decreasing the potential for coalescence by forming an electrical double layer

Classification

I. Hydrocolloids

A. *Natural products*

(i)   *Tree exudate :* gum arabic (acacia), gum ghatti, karaya gum, tragacanth

(ii) *Sea weeds :* agar, carrageenan, alginate etc.

(iii) *Seed extracts :* locust bean, guar gum etc.

(iv) *Steroid containing substance :* beeswax, woolfat, wool alcohol

(v)   *Animal substances :* gelatin, casein etc.

(vi) *Mineral substances :* bentonite, veegum

B. Inorganic

Colloidal alumia, milk of magnesia, mag. oxide, magnesium trisilicate

C. Semisynthetic

Methyl cellulose, carboxy methyl cellulose, hydroxy methyl cellulose, micro crystalline cellulose.

D. Synthetic

Carbopol, colloidal silicone dioxide.

II. Surfactants

A. *Anionic*

(i) *Carboxylic acid :* soap, acetylates, polypeptide condensates

(ii) *Sulfuric acid esters :* sulfated monoglycerides, alkyl sulfates

(iii) *Alkyl and alkyl-aryl sulfonates :* dodecylbenzene sulfonates

(iv) *Phosphoric acid esters :* trioleyl phosphate

(v) *Substituted alkyl amides :* sarcosinates, taurates

(vi) *Hemiesters :* sulfosuccinates

B. *Cationic*

(i) *Amines :* alkoxyalkylamines,

(ii) *Quaternaries :* benzylkonium chloride

C. *Nonionic*

(i) *Polyalkoxyethers :* polyoxyethylene alkyl/aryl ethers, polyoxyethylene polyoxypropylene, block polymers.

(ii) *Polyalkoxyesters :* polyoxyethylene fatty acid esters, polyoxyethylene sorbiton acid esters

(iii) *Polyalkoxyamide fatty acid esters :* sorbitan esters, glyceryl esters, sucrose esters

(iv) *Fatty alcohols :* lauryl alcohol.

Selection of Emulsifying Agents using HLB method

In 1949 William C. Griffin developed a system to assist making systematic decisions about the amounts and types of surfactants needed in stable products. The system is called the HLB (hydrophile-lipophile balance) system and has an arbitrary scale of 1 - 18. HLB numbers are experimentally determined for the different emulsifiers in laboratory.

An emulsifier having a low HLB number indicates that the number of hydrophilic groups present in the molecule is less and it has a lipophillic character. For example, spans generally have low HLB number and they are oil soluble. Because of their oil soluble character, spans cause the oil phase to predominate and form a *w/o* emulsion.

A higher HLB number indicates that the emulsifier has a large number of hydrophilic groups on the molecule and therefore is more hydrophilic in character. Tweens have higher HLB numbers and they are also water soluble. Because of their water soluble character, tweens will cause the water phase to predominate and form an *o/w* emulsion.

HLB Range	Application
0-3	Antifoaming agents
4-6	*w/o* emulsifying agent
7-9	Wetting agents
8-18	*o/w* emulsifying agent
13-15	Detergents
10-18	Solubilizing agents

HLB values of some common emulsifying agents are given below.

Emulsifying agent	HLB Value
Oleic acid	1.0
Sorbitan tristearate	2.1
Glyceryl monostearate	3.8
Sorbitan mono-oleate (Span 80)	4.3
Sorbitan monolaurate (Span 20)	8.6
Polyethylene lauryl ether (Brij 30)	9.5
Gelatin (Pharmagel B)	9.8
Methyl Cellulose	10.5
Polyoxyethylene lauryl ether	10.8
Polyoxyethylene monostearate (Myrj 45)	11.1
Triethanolamine oleate	12.0
Polyoxyethylene Sorbitan mono-oleate (Tween 80)	15.0
Polyoxyethylene Sorbitan monolaurate (Tween 20)	16.7
Polyoxyethylene lauryl ether (Brij 35)	16.9
Sodium oleate	18.0
Potassium oleate	20.0
Sodium lauryl sulphate	40

Methods of Preparation

Preparation of emulsion depends on the scale at which it is produced. In laboratry or on small scale, mortar and pestle can be used but its efficiency is limited. To overcome these problems small electric mixers can be used although care must be exercised to avoid excessive entrapment of air. In large scale production mechanical stirrers are used to provide controlled agitation and shearing stress to produce stable emulsions. e.g.

- Kenwood mixer
- Silverson mixer
- The Q.P. emulsifiers
- Colloid mills
- Standard slurry-type dispersed mixer with vaned-rotor
- Standard paste-type dispersed mixer with clipped rotor
- Two stage homogenizer

Small Scale Preparation

(a) ***Wet gum method :*** A primary emulsion can be prepared by various methods. However it depends on the type of ingredients involved. Stable preparation of fixed oil, water and acacia (ratio in parts 4 : 2 : 1) is prepared by the following methods.

- Two parts of water and one part of acacia mixture are triturated in a mortar and pestle until a smooth mucilage is formed.
- Oil is added slowly with continuous trituration until a smooth cream of primary emulsion is formed.
- The mixture should be again triturated for another 5 minutes and then add water to make up the volume with continuous triturating.

(b) ***Dry gum method :*** A primary emulsion of fixed oil, water and acacia (ratio in parts 4: 2:1) is prepared by the following methods.

- The oil is mixed with acacia in a dry mortar and pestle until acacia powder is distributed uniformly.
- Purified water is added with rapidly trituration until a primary emulsion is formed.
- Add other additives and remaining quantity of water with continuous trituration to finish the product.

(c) ***Bottle method :*** It is a modified dry gum method. The ratio of oil, water and acacia should be 3: 2:1 or 2 :1 :1 is used for the preparation of emulsion as the low viscosity of the volatile oil requires a higher proportion of acacia.

- The oil is mixed with acacia by shaking the bottle uniformly
- Add measured quantity of water and shake until uniform emulsion is formed.

(d) *Soap method :* Soap is formed by mixing equal volumes of oil and an aqueous solution containing a sufficient amount of alkali. This method is suitable for the formation of an *o/w* or *w/o* emulsion. It is dependent on the formation of soap e.g. olive oil and lime water are mixed during the preparation of calamine lotion to form calcium oleate, an emulsifying agents.

Table 12.2 Proportions of Oil, Water and Gum required for formation of primary emulsion.

Type of Oil	Proportions of		
	Oil	Water	Gum
Fixed Oil	4	2	1
Mineral Oil	3	2	1
Volatile Oil	2	2	1

Additives

(a)   **Thickening agents :** e.g., emulsifying agent

(b)   **Antimicrobial agents**

- *Acids and acid derivatives :* benzoic acid, sorbic acid, propionic acid, dehydro-acetic acid

- *Alcohols :* chlorobutanol, phenoxy-2-ethanol

- *Aldehydes :* Formaldehyde, glutareldehyde

- *Phenolics :* phenol, cresol, chlorothymol, o-phenylphenol, p-chlorometaxylenol, methyl p-hydroxybenzoate, propyl p- hydroxybenzoate, butyl p- hydroxybenzoate

- *Quaternaries :* benzethonium chloride, benzalkonium chloride, cetyl pyridinium chloride, cetyltrimethyl ammonium bromide, chlorhexidine and salts

- *Mercurials :* phenylmercuric acetate, sodium *ethylmercurithiosalicylate*

- *Miscellaneous :* 6-acetoxy-2,4-dimethyl-m-dioxane, Imidizolidinyl urea compound

(c)   *Antioxidant :* ascorbic acid, ascorbyl palmitate, butylated hydroxyanisol, butylated hydroxytoluene, gallic acid, 4-hydroxymethyl-2,6-di-tert-butylphenol, L-tocopherol, sulfites.

(d)   *Organoleptic agent :* e.g., coloring agent, flavoring agent and sweetening agent

Evaluation of Emulsions

(a)   Organoleptic properties

(b)   Particle size or globule size analysis by microscopic method

(c)   Rate of phase separation by centrifugation

(d)   Viscosity by viscometer

(e)   Electrophoretic properties

(f)   Measurement of dielectric constant

(g)   Measurement of conductivity

(h)   Microwaves irradiation

Tests for Identification of Emulsion Type

Final preparation of both emulsions (*o/w* or *w/o*) looks the same in appearance with naked eyes, therefore certain tests are required to differentiate between them. It is also important that at least two tests should be performed to draw a final conclusion.

1. ***Dilution test :*** In this test the emulsion is diluted either with oil or water. If the emulsion is *o/w* type and it is diluted with water, it will remain stable as water is the dispersion medium but if it is diluted with oil, the emulsion will break as oil and water are not miscible with each other. Oil in water emulsion can easily be diluted with an aqueous solvent whereas water in oil emulsion can be diluted with a oily liquid (Shown in Fig. 12.1)

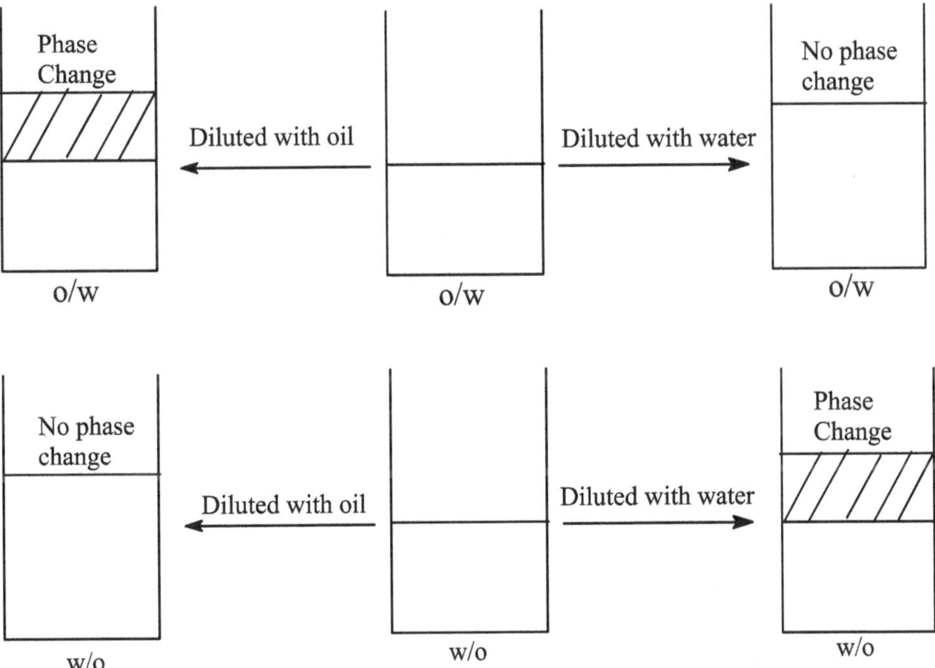

Fig. 12.1 Dilution Test for *o/w* and *w/o* type emulsion.

2. ***Conductivity Test :*** The basic principle of this test is that water is a good conductor of electricity. Therefore in case of *o/w* emulion, this test will be positive as water is the external phase. In this test, an assembly is used in which a pair of electrodes connected to an electric bulb is dipped into an emulsion. If the emulsion is o/w type, the electric bulb glows.

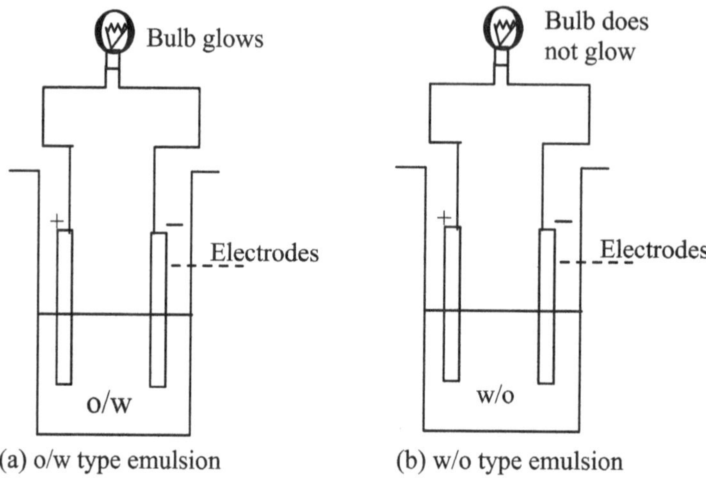

        (a) o/w type emulsion   (b) w/o type emulsion

3. ***Dye Solubility Test :*** In this test an emulsion is mixed with a water soluble dye (amaranth) and observed under the microscope. If the continuous phase appears red, it means that the emulsion is *o/w* type as water is in the external phase and the dye will dissolve in it to give color. If the scattered globules appear red and continuous phase colorless, then it is *w/o* type. Similarly if an oil soluble dye (Scarlet red C or Sudan III) is added to an emulsion and the continuous phase appears red, then it is *w/o* emulsion.

4. ***Cobalt Chloride Test :*** When a filter paper soaked in cobalt chloride solution is dipped in to an emulsion and dried, it turns from blue to pink, indicating that the emulsion is *o/w* type.

5. ***Fluorescence Test :*** If an emulsion on exposure to ultra-violet radiations shows continuous fluorescence under microscope, then it is *w/o* type and if it shows only spotty fluorescence, then it is *o/w* type.

Instability of Emulsion

A stable emulsion is one in which the globules retain their initial character like mean size and size distribution and remain uniformly distributed throughout the continuous phase. During storage of emulsions instability is endorsed by creaming, cracking, reversible aggregation and/or irreversible aggregation etc.

1. ***Cracking or coalescence :*** Coalescence is a growth process during which the emulsified particles join to form large particles. When small droplets are merged and large droplets are formed, it suggests that the emulsion will separate completely and cannot be re-

dispersed by shaking. This process is also known as cracking. Any chemical, physical or biological effects that change the nature of the interfacial film of an emulsifying agent may cause cracking. Creaming can be induced by the following methods.

- Addition of an emulsifying agent of opposite type
- Decomposition or precipitation of emulsifying agent
- Addition of a common solvent
- Addition of proper preservatives
- Incorporation of excess of disperse phase

2. *Creaming :* Under the influence of gravity suspended particles or globules tend to upward movement, known as creaming while downward movement of particles or droplets is called sedimentation. Creaming or sedimentation depends on the differences in specific gravity between the phases. If creaming take place without any aggregation, the emulsion can be reconstituted by shaking. Process of creaming is explained by Stoke's law.

$$v = \frac{d^2(\rho_1 - \rho_2)g}{18\eta}$$

where,

v = terminal or settling velocity

d = diameter of globules

ρ_1 = density of disperse phase

ρ_2 = density of continuous phase

η = viscosity of dispersion medium

g = acceleration due to gravity

Factors that influence the rate of creaming and sedimentation:

- **Globules size :** Globules of small size have less tendency to cream.
- **Viscosity :** Higher the viscosity of continuous phase, less creaming
- **Density :** Less difference in density of two phases means more stability of emulsion.
- **Temperature :** Lower temperature is more suitable for the better stability of emulsion

3. *Phase inversion :* It is known that *w/o* emulsion of benzene in water that was stabilized with sodium stearate will invert to *o/w* emulsions upon heating and reform *w/o* emulsions upon cooling. The temperature at which the inversion occurs depends on the emulsifier concentration and is called Phase Inversion Temperature (PIT). An *o/w* emulsion stabilized by a non-ionic polyoxyethylene-derived surfactant contains oil-swollen miscelles of the surfactant as well as emulsifying oil.

Containers

Emulsion should be supplied in wide mouthed bottles

Storage

Emulsion should be kept at temperature not exceeding 20°. They should not be allowed to freeze.

Labeling

Comply with general requirements for labeling, in addition the label should indicate following information : quantity of emulsifying agent, preservative, "Shake well before use", and "Keep in cool place".

Examples

Example 1 : Prepare and dispense Liquid Paraffin Emulsion

Rx

Liquid paraffin	50.0 ml
Indian gum in powder	12.5 g
Tragacanth in powder	0.5 g
Sodium benzoate	0.5 g
Vanillin	0.05 g
Glycerin	12,5 ml
Chloroform	0.25 ml
Purified water, sufficient to produce	100.0 ml

Method of Dispensing : Triturate the weighed quantity of liquid paraffin and chloroform with the Indian gum, tragacanth the vanillin in mortar and pestle and triturate until a creamy emulsion is formed. Dissolve sodium benzoate in small quantity of purified water and add other additives with continuous stirring.

Use : laxative

Example 2 : To and prepare and dispense castor oil emulsion

Rx

Castor oil	37.5 ml
Acacia in powder	10.0 g
Cinnamon water, sufficient to produce	100.0 ml

Method of Dispensing : Triturate the weighed quantity of castor oil and the cinnamon water with acacia in mortar and pestle. Add remaining quantity of cinnamon water to produce 100 ml.

Use : Laxative

Example 3 : Prepare and dispense Concentrated Peppermint Emulsion

Rx

Peppermint oil	2.0 ml
Polysorbate-20	0.10 ml
Double strength chloroform water	50.0 ml
Purified water, sufficient to make	100.0 ml

Method of Dispensing : Mix peppermint oil with the polysorbate-20 by shaking and add gradually to double strength chloroform water. Add sufficient purified water to produce 100 ml with shaking.

Use : Carminative

Table 12.3 Some Marketed Emulsion Products.

Generic Name	Company	Active Ingredients	Indications
Cremaffin	Abott. Lab.	Liquid paraffin and milk of magnesia	Stool softner
Ivelip (10%)	Baxter India Pvt. Ltd.	Intravenous fat emulsion. Not to exceed 3g/kg body weight per day	Caloric agent, Total parenteral nutrition
Restasis	Allergan India Pvt. Ltd.	Cyclosporine 0.05%	Keratoconjuctivitis
Estrasorb	Ranbaxy Research Lab.	Each g contain 2.5 mg Estradiol hemihydrate	Vasomotor symptoms in menopausal women
Diprivan	Astra Zeneca	1% Propofol Injection	General anesthesia
Lipfudin 10% Fat Emulsion	Braun India Pvt. Ltd	Intravenous fat emulsion	Total parenteral nutrition (TPN)

CHAPTER 13

Semisolid Preparation

I. Semisolid Preparations

Semisolid dosage forms include ointments, creams, pastes, suppositories and other forms of similar viscous consistency intended for external application. Semisolids may perform any one or more of the following functions

- vehicles for drugs
- emollients
- protective
- occlusive dressings on the skin.

Ointments

Ointments are semisolid preparations for application to the skin and usually contain a medicament. Ointments are used topically for several purposes, e.g., as protectants, antiseptics, emollients, antipruritics, kerotolytics, and astringents. The vehicle or base of an ointment is of prime importance if the finished product is expected to function as any one of the above categories. The consistency of ointments should be such that they may be readily applied to the skin by inunction. The medicament may be in solution, suspension or emulsified in the base. Ointment vehicles serve as protective and emollients for the skin. They usually exhibit plastic flow characteristics and hence when ointment is applied there is a definite yield value, the resistance to flow however drops as the application to the skin is continued. The present day concept of ointments is slightly different than earlier one in the sense that earlier ointments implied a semisolid preparation containing medicinal agents uniformly dispersed in a fatty base but presently ointments may be entirely free of oleaginous substances.

Ointments in the form of semisolid emulsions are also referred to as creams; and ointments and creams containing large proportions of insoluble powders are referred to as pastes.

In addition to topical ointments there are ophthalmic ointments, rectal ointments and vaginal creams depending upon the intended site of application. Thus the ointments are also applied to mucous membrane in addition to the skin.

In the case of a protective ointment, it serves to protect the skin against moisture, air, sun rays and other external factors. It is necessary that the ointment neither penetrates the human skin barriers nor facilitates the absorption of substances through this barrier.

An antiseptic ointment is used to destroy or inhibit the growth of bacteria. Frequently bacterial infections are deeply seated; a base which has the capacity to either penetrate or dissolve and release the medication effectively is therefore desired.

Ointments used for their emollient effect should be easy to apply, non-greasy and should effectively penetrate the skin.

Ideal Ointment Base

An ideal ointment base –

- should not retard wound healing,
- have a low sensitization index,
- pharmaceutically elegant,
- release the medicament efficiently at the site of application,
- have a low index of irritation,
- non-dehydrating, non-greasy and neutral in reaction,
- possess good keeping qualities,
- compatible with common medicaments,
- easily washable with water,
- have minimum number of ingredients,
- easy to compound and remain stable on storage, and
- economic and easy to transport

Ointment Bases

The earliest bases consisted of fats of animals or man and their mixtures with other substances but the modern day bases are mostly non-greasy, water-miscible and water-washable.

Classification

Although ointment bases can be classified in many ways, the simplest one based on composition is as follows.

A. Oleaginous bases.
B. Absorption bases.
C. Emulsion bases.
D. Water-soluble (hydrophilic) bases.

A. Oleaginous bases

Salient characteristics of these bases are -

* they are anhydrous,
* they are hydrophobic (do not absorb water readily),
* they are insoluble in water, and
* they are not removable by water.

These are the earliest ointment bases which consisted of vegetable and animal fats as well as petroleum hydrocarbons. A list of commonly used materials has been given here although in practice still a larger number of materials are used.

S.No.	Category	Substances
I.	Hydrocarbons	Petrolatum (white and yellow), Microcrystalline wax, Liquid paraffin, Paraffin, Ceresin, Plastibase (Jelene)
II.	Vegetable oils and animal fats	Coconut oil, Olive oil, Peanut oil, Sesame oil, Almond oil, Beeswax, Lanolin, Spermaceti wax
III.	Hydrogenated and sulphated oils	Hydrogenated castor, cottonseed, soyabean and corn oils. Hydrogenated sulphated castor oils
IV.	Alcohols, acids and esters	Cetyl alcohol, Stearyl alcohol, Oleyl alcohol, Lauryl alcohol, Myristyl alcohol, Oleic acid, Stearic acid, Palmitic acid, Myristic acid, Lauric acid, Glyceryl tristearate, Ethyl oleate, Isopropyl myristicate,Ethylene glycol, dilaurate/distearate/dioleate
V.	Sillicones	Dimethylpolysiloxanes,Methylphenylpolysiloxanes, Stearyl esters of dimethylpolysiloxanes

Oleaginous bases are expected to provide a film, which resists soap and water yet readily removable by solutions of surfactants. This can possibly be achieved by emulsifying the silicones or other hydrophobic film formers so that when the protective ointment is properly applied, an invisible protective film is left on the skin. Film forming agents are exemplified by polyvinylpyrollidone, polyvinyl alcohol and the cellulose derivatives.

B. Absorption bases

The term absorption as applied here implies the hydrophilic or water absorbing properties of the base and not the absorption of medicaments from the bases. These bases are generally anhydrous but capable of absorbing several times their own weight of water ultimately forming *w/o* type of emulsions.

Absorption bases vary in their composition and are usually mixtures of animal sterols with petrolatum. Eucerin and Aquaphor are the commercial bases consisting of combination of cholesterol and/or other suitable lanolin fraction with white petrolatum. Anhydrous absorption bases can also be formulated by the addition of lipophilic surfactants to petrolatum and anhydrous water-removable bases can be formed by the addition of hydrophilic surfactants to petrolatum. Some important formulae of absorption ointment bases are given below.

Example 01

Cholesterol	3.0
Stearyl alcohol	3.0
White wax	8.0
White petrolatum	86.0

Example 02

Wool alcohols	6.0
Hard paraffin	24.0
Yellow or white soft Paraffin Liquid	10.0
paraffin	60.0

Example 03

Cholesterol	30
Cottonseed oil	30
White petrolatum	40

Example 04

White petrolatum	41.0
Microcrystalline wax	3.0
Fluid lanolin	10.
Span 80	4.75
Tween 80	0.25
Purified water	41.0

Absorption bases were primarily developed so as to have a product to which water or an aqueous solution of medicinal substances could be easily added. These bases are usually highly compatible with the majority of drugs used topically. The limited popularity of absorption bases however is attributed to their greasiness.

C. Emulsion bases

These may be either *o/w* or *w/o* type emulsions.

(a) ***Water-in-oil type emulsion (Hydrophobic ointment)*** : The *w/o* type emulsion bases such as lanolin and cold cream are used as emollients. The aqueous phase hydrates the skin and the oily phase forms an occlusive covering which prevents loss of water by evaporation. Emulsion bases also serve as vehicle for medicaments such as sulphur, ammoniated mercury, balsam of peru, zinc oxide etc. The main drawback of *w/o* emulsion bases is their greasy and sticky nature and therefore they are less popular than *o/w* type of bases.

Earlier cold creams consisted of oil (40 to 70%), wax or spermaceti (5 to 15%), and water (20 to 35%). Thus a large proportion of water was loosely held in the water-in-oil mixture. More stable creams were later formulated employing borax which formed the sodium soap by reacting with the fatty acids present in the beeswax. Presently cold creams are also formulated by employing non-ionic surfactants alone or in combination with beeswax. When cold creams are applied, slow evaporation of the water causes a pleasant cooling sensation and hence these creams are given the name 'cold creams'. A simple formula for borax-beeswax cold cream is as follows.

Mineral oil	50.0
Beeswax	14.0
Borax	0.7
Purified water	35.3

(b) ***Oil-in-water ointment (Hydrophilic Ointment)*** *:* Oil in water type emulsion bases are used as vehicles for medicinal agents. Water being in the external phase they are easily removed with water alone from skin and linen. They are non-grease and non-sticky. Vanishing creams are often used as cosmetics.

The vanishing type of cream bases contain a large proportion of water which may be as high as 80% and this seems to account for the high release of medicaments from such bases. Vanishing creams essentially contain about 20% stearic acid (triple pressed) and a part of it is reacted with alkali to form soap *in-situ*. About 5 to 10% glycerin is also included in the formulation as humectant which can be substituted either partially or wholly by propylene glycol. The typical sheen of vanishing cream is due to stearic acid. Truly speaking, vanishing cream should be regarded as dispersion and not an emulsion. Two simple formulae for vanishing cream are given below.

<table>
<tr><td colspan="2">Example 01</td><td colspan="2">Example 02</td></tr>
<tr><td>Stearic acid</td><td>20.0</td><td>Stearic acid</td><td>15.0</td></tr>
<tr><td>Potassium hydroxide</td><td>1.4</td><td>White wax</td><td>2.0</td></tr>
<tr><td>Glycerin</td><td>10.0</td><td>White soft paraffin</td><td>8.0</td></tr>
<tr><td>Purified water</td><td>70.0</td><td>Triethanolamine</td><td>1.5</td></tr>
<tr><td></td><td></td><td>Propylene glycol</td><td>8.0</td></tr>
<tr><td></td><td></td><td>Purified water</td><td>65.5</td></tr>
</table>

D. ***Water-soluble bases*** *:* These bases are prepared from mixture of low and high molecular weight polyethylene glycols which range in their consistency from liquids to solids. Their water solubility is due to the presence of many polar groups and other linkages. They are non-volatile, unctuous, inert and possess the ability to form an emollient surface. They neither hydrolyse and deteriorate nor support mould growth.

Medicaments like benzoic and salicylic acids, phenol, tannic acid, bacitracin etc. have a solubilizing effect on bases consisting of high molecular weight polyethylene glycols. Although the diffusion of medicaments through such bases occurs readily yet the percutaneous absorption is very little. Some formulae for water-washable ointments containing polyethylene glycols are given below.

Example 01

PEG 400 monostearate	26.0
PEG 400	37.0
PEG 4000	37.0

Example 02

PEG 4000	42.5
PEG 400	37.5
1, 2, 5-Hexanetriol	20.0

Example 03

PEG 400	60
PEG 4000	40

Example 04

PEG 4000	11.2
Stearyl alcohol	20.8
Glycerin	17.0
Sodium lauryl sulphate	0.6
Purified water	50.4

Some of the water-soluble bases are also prepared by employing glyceryl monostearate (GMS), cellulose derivative, sodium alginate, bentonite, colloidal magnesium aluminium silicate, and Carbopol 934. Carbopol 934 and acid polymer disperses readily in water to yield an acid solution of low viscosity. It is physiologically inert, non-irritating and non-sensitizer. It exhibits excellent compatibility with materials frequently incorporated in ointment formulations. Some examples of ointment bases employing materials like GMS, hydrocolloids and Carbopol 934 etc. are given below.

Example 01

Calcium citrate	0.05 g
Sodium alginate	3.0 g
Methyl paraben	0.20g
Glycerin	45.0 g
Purified water to make	100 g

Example 02

Petrolatum	32.0 g
Bentonite	13.0 g
Sodium lauryl sulphate	0.5 g
Purified water	54 g
Methyl paraben	0.1 g

Example 03

Mineral oil	10
White petrolatum	30
GMS	10
Cetyl alcohol	05
Glycerin	05
Purified water	40

Example 04

Methocel 90 HC 4000	1.0 g
Carbopol 934	0.3 g
Propylene glycol	20.0 ml
Methyl paraben	0.15 g
Purified water q.s	100 ml
Sodium hydroxide q.s pH 7.0	

Each ointment base type has different physical characteristics and therapeutic uses based upon the nature of its components. The following table summarizes the composition, properties, and common uses of each of the five types of bases.

Table 13.1 Properties of ointment bases.

Properties	oleaginous bases	absorption bases	w/o emulsion bases	o/w emulsion bases	water miscible bases
Composition	oleaginous compounds	oleaginous base & *w/o* surfactant	oleaginous base & water (< 45% *w/w*) & *w/o* surfactant (HLB $\leq$8)	oleaginous base & water (> 45% *w/w*) + *o/w* surfactant (HLB $\geq$9)	Polyethylene Glycols (PEGs)
Water Content	anhydrous	anhydrous	hydrous	hydrous	anhydrous, hydrous
Affinity for Water	hydrophobic	hydrophilic	hydrophobic	hydrophilic	hydrophilic
Spreadability	difficult	difficult	moderate to easy	easy	moderate to easy
Washability	Non-washable	poorly washable	poorly washable	washable	washable
Stability	oils poor; hydrocarbons better	oils poor; hydrocarbons better	unstable, especially alkali soaps and natural colloids	unstable, especially alkali soaps and natural colloids; nonionics better	stable
Drug Incorporation Potential	solids or oils (oil solubles only)	solids, oils, and aqueous solutions (small amounts)	solids, oils, and aqueous solutions (small amounts)	solid and aqueous solutions (small amounts)	solid and aqueous solutions
Drug Release Potential	poor	poor, but > oleaginous	fair to good	fair to good	good
Occlusiveness	yes	yes	sometimes	no	no
Uses	protectants, emollients (+/-), vehicles for hydrolyzable drugs	protectants, emollients (+/-), vehicles for aqueous solutions, solids, and non-hydrolyzable drugs	emollients, cleansing creams, vehicles for solid, liquid, or non-hydrolyzable drugs	emollients, vehicles for solid, liquid, or non-hydrolyzable drugs	drug vehicles
Examples	White Petrolatum, White Ointment	Hydrophilic Petrolatum, Anhydrous Lanolin, Aquabase, Aquaphor, Polysorb	Cold Cream type, Hydrous Lanolin, Rose Water Ointment, Hydrocream, Eucerin	Hydrophilic Ointment, Dermabase, Velvachol, Unibase	PEG Ointment, Polybase

Preparation of Ointments

Ointments can be prepared either by mechanical incorporation or by fusion methods. Irrespective of the method employed for the preparation, ointments should be smooth and free from granular or gritty particles. In compounding of ointments, the following general considerations are observed.

(i)   If insoluble substances are to be incorporated in the ointment base then they should be in impalpable powder form.

(ii)   For efficient incorporation of insoluble substances they should first be levigated with a little quantity of base to form a smooth cream and then incorporated into the remainder of the base.

(iii)   Water-soluble salts are best incorporated by dissolving them in a small quantity of water and then incorporating in the base.

(iv)   Drugs soluble in ointment bases may also be incorporated by fusion (melting the highest melting point ingredient of the base and mixing the medicament into it). Remaining ingredients are then added and mixed by stirring.

A. Preparation By Mechanical Incorporation

This can be achieved by the use of (i) mortar and pestle, (ii) ointment slab and spatula, and (iii). an ointment mill. Mechanical method of incorporation is particularly advantageous when the substance to be incorporated into ointment base must be in a fine state of subdivision.

(a) *Mortar and pestle :* This method is used to a limited extent in compounding practice particularly when large quantities of liquids are to be incorporated in a base or when exceptionally large quantities of the ointments are to be prepared. Compounding a homogeneous ointment in a mortar and pestle is not as simple as compounding of a powder.

(b) *Ointment slab :* In this case both mixing and size reduction of insoluble medicaments are better than the previous method. The powder is first rubbed with a small quantity of the base to form a concentrated ointment base containing a finely divided powder uniformly distributed in it. The concentrated ointment is then gradually diluted with remaining quantity of the base by rubbing with a spatula. A small quantity (approximately 5%) of oil or oil-soluble substances can be used as a levigating agent. Large amounts of levigating agents may cause undue softening of the finished preparation. The spatula should be of stainless steel with a long, broad flexible blade. When steel spatula cannot be used for reasons of reacting with certain drugs like iodine, salicylic acid, and mercury salts etc., a hard rubber spatula or a wooden tongue depressor may be used.

(c) *Ointment mill :* Ointment mills are particularly suitable for large scale manufacture of ointments although small mills are available for laboratory scale ointment preparation. Ointments containing gritty particles are also passed through the ointment mill to ensure further uniformity and smoothness. Usually the powdered medicaments are sifted into the softened or melted base in a change can mixer, stirred into the softened or melted base in a change can mixer, stirred until congealed and then run through any ointment mill. Most popular ointment mill is the triple roller mill in which the ointment is made to pass through the narrow clearance between the rolls. This mill can be sterilized by wiping with 5% aqueous phenol solution and storage under UV light before use. There is a provision for cooling the rolls so that melted materials introduced as a liquid will emerge as an ointment.

B. Preparation by Fusion

When waxy material and hard bodies are to be incorporated in soft oleaginous materials, fusion is the best technique. It consists of subdividing the waxy components and melting together all components over a water bath starting from one having a highest melting point. Remaining components are then added in order of their decreasing melting points till all the components are added up. Thus all the components are not unduly exposed to higher temperatures. The mixture should be continuously stirred until congealed to ensure a homogeneous preparation. Powdered ingredients, if any, are then added using a small quantity of the base as a levigating agent.

Packaging and Labelling

1. Ointment jars

   (a)   Straight-sided screw cap jars of glass or plastic.

   (b)   Clear, amber or opaque glass containers

   (c)   White, opaque, plastic usually high-density polyethylene jar.

   (d)   Metal or composition plastic tops

2. Ointment tubes

   (a)   Made of tin or aluminium or plastic materials e.g., polyethylene, polypropylene.

   (b)   Ointment tube should be packed in a winged plastic board box.

   (c)   The box serves to hold and protect the ointment tube and to carry the label.

   (d)   The ointment tube is identified with an inked-on prescription number so that both tube and box are identified.

On large scale tubes are labeled in a variety of ways. Paper labels may be used. Label may be silk-screened onto plastic surfaces. Expiry dates and code lot numbers may be stamped on as a part of the tube crimping procedure.

Stability

The ointments can be dispensed in wide-mouth jars or tubes of adequate size or in collapsible tubes. While dispensing in jars, care should be exercised not to allow the contact of the ointment with the cap liner. The cap should be tightly fitted after use so as to avoid evaporation of water.

The problems of stability of ointments are mostly concerned with the initial and 'in-use' microbial contamination and its increase. Many ophthalmic ointments are found to be heavily contaminated with pathogenic micro-organisms. The main source of microbial contamination in ointments is water which supports the growth of micro-organisms.

To safeguard the stability of the packaged product the following points are borne in mind.

(i)   In general, the pharmacist or the manufacturer should follow Good Manufacturing Practice (GMP).

(ii)   Use of preservatives to protect against the contamination, deterioration or spoilage of ointment bases by bacteria and fungi.

(iii)   Use of antioxidants when there is possibility of oxidative degradation of the base.

(iv)   Use of chelating agents where the presence of traces of metallic ions is anticipated. The traces of metallic ions, if present, may catalyse oxidative degradation.

(v)   If the metallic ions are chelated their catalytic effect is nullified.

(vi)   The immediate container should not permit evaporation of water from the packaged ointments otherwise an emulsion base may lose aqueous phase and others may become dry and hard.

(vii)   The containers should ensure not only the sterility of ophthalmic ointments initially but also up to a time till whole of the preparation is consumed.

(viii)   Due to wide variations in the climatic conditions in different regions in tropical countries, maintenance of desirable consistency of an ointment is also an important consideration.

(ix)   Most of the problems related to the stability of packaged ointments can be solved by dispensing them as single application capsules although it works out to be more expensive. This is particularly recommended in case of ophthalmic ointments where sterility and absence of particles are the prime considerations.

Ophthalmic ointments

Eye ointments should be sterile and supplied in small sterile tubes with a fine nozzle for convenience in application. The tubes should be thoroughly cleaned and free from metallic and dust particles. These ointments are intended for application into the eye for the effect of a variety of medicaments on the outside and edges of the eyelids, the conjunctiva, the cornea and the iris. Most of these ointments contain petrolatum, petrolatum-mineral oil and petrolatum-anhydrous lanolin bases. Absorption and emulsion bases may irritate the eye due to the emulsifier/surfactant present in the base.

Sterility of ophthalmic ointments is a legal requirement and hence tests for sterility should always be performed on packaged products. Immediate container for ophthalmic ointment should be sealed and tamper-proof so as to ensure sterility at time of first usage.

The active ingredients should be finely divided and sterile. Petrolatum bases can be sterilized in a hot air oven at 175°C for 2 hours. The processing should be carried out under aseptic conditions employing sterile apparatus and equipment. For small scale preparations either an aseptic hood or a laminar flow unit is satisfactory. An easy method for sterilizing ointment tubes consists of keeping them immersed in 70% alcohol for 24 hours prior to use. Current trend in ophthalmic ointments is to pack them in single application capsules so as to preclude contamination during use products. Such single application ointment capsules contain a quantity sufficient for single use and have to be punctured with a sterile needle just before use and discarded afterwards.

Rectal ointments

The usual ointment bases need modification if they are to be applied rectally. Rectal ointment should be very soft in consistency and sufficiently thin; so that they can pass easily through a rectal nozzle without bursting the tube. Replacement of the 25% base with liquid paraffin usually provides desired thin and soft consistency in ointments containing soft paraffin, olive oil or arachis oil for replacing Simple Ointment, to render it suitable for rectal application. The present trend is towards the formulation of water-soluble rectal ointment bases.

General Comments on Compounding Ointment Bases

(a) Some quantity of an ointment may be lost in the compounding process between 2 and 4 grams The ointment is lost as it adheres to ointment tiles, beakers, or ointment pads, spatula etc. To compensate for this loss, make an excess of the ointment. A general rule might be to add all ingredients in 10% excess of the prescribed amount.

(b) Melt ingredients on a water bath (not more than 100°C) or special low temperature hotplate (full range is 25°C to 120°C). Most ingredients used in ointment bases will liquefy at around 70°C. These two heating devices provide adequate control over the heating and will ensure that the ingredients are not over heated.

(c) If oil and aqueous phase are being mixed together to make an ointment, it is helpful to heat the aqueous phase a few degrees higher than the oil phase prior to mixing because aqueous phase tends to cool faster than the oil phase and may cause premature solidification of some ingredients. However, use the lowest temperature possible and keep the time of heating as short as possible. This will minimize the quantity of water lost through evaporation.

(d) If a number of ingredients required melting, the ingredient with the highest melting point should be melted first. Then gradually reduce the heat to melt the ingredient with the next lowest melting point. Continue this process until all ingredients have been added.

(e) The cooling step in an ointment's preparation is an important part of the compounding process.

   - Do not cool by putting the melt in water or ice. It will change the consistency or homogeneity of the final product, making it more stiff than desired.

- If volatile ingredients such as oils, flavors, or drugs are required, add them when the product is cool to the back of the hand and apply just enough heat to evaporate the volatile substance.

- Ointments should be cooled until just a few degrees above solidification before they are poured into tubes or jars. They should be thick, viscous fluids. This will minimize layering of the ointment in the packaging container.

Example 1 : Oleagineous base

White Wax	5 %
White Petrolatum	95%

Method of Preparation : Melt the white wax on a hot plate (at 70 – 75 °C). When the wax has completely melted, add the petrolatum and allow the entire mixture to remain on the hot plate until liquified. Following liquefication, remove from heat and allow the mixture to congeal. Stir the mixture until it begins to congeal.

Example 2 : Absorption Base

Cholesterol	3%
Stearyl Alcohol	3%
White Wax	8%
White Petrolatum	86%

Method of Preparation : Melt the stearyl alcohol, white wax, and petrolatum together on a hot plate and add the cholesterol to the mixture; stir until completely dissolved. Remove the mixture from the hot plate and stir until congealed.

Example 3 : Water-in-oil emulsion base

White wax	12.0%
Cetyl Esters Wax (or Spermaceti)	12.5%
Mineral Oil	56.0%
Sodium Borate	0.5%
Water	19.0%

Method of Preparation : Melt the white wax and spermaceti on a hot plate and add the mineral oil to this mixture and bring the temperature to 70 °C. Dissolve the sodium borate in water. Heat the sodium borate solution to 70 °C. When both phases have reached the desired temperature, remove both phases from the hot plate and add the aqueous phase slowly and with constant stirring to the oil phase. Stir briskly and continuously until congealed.

Example 4 : Oil in water emulsion base

Sodium Lauryl Sulfate	1.0%
Propylene Glycol	12.0%
Stearyl Alcohol	25.0%
White Petrolatum	25.0%
Purified Water	37.0%

Method of Preparation : Melt the stearyl alcohol and white petrolatum on a hot plate at 70°C. Dissolve remaining ingredients in water and heat the solution to 70° C. Add the oleaginous phase slowly to the aqueous phase, stirring constantly. Remove from heat and stir the mixture until it congeals.

Example 5 : Water Soluble Base

Polyethylene Glycol 400	60%
Polyethylene Glycol 4000	40%

Method of Preparation : Melt the PEG 400 and PEG 4000 on a hot plate and heat the mixture to about 65°C. Remove from the hot plate and stir until congealed.

Practice Exercises

Example 01 : To prepare Emulsifying Ointment

Liquid paraffin, Emulsifying wax	2.00 g
White soft paraffin	3.00 g
	5.00 g

Method of Preparation : Melt together liquid paraffin, emulsifying wax, and white soft paraffin. Stir until cool.

Uses : Pharmaceutical aid.

Example 2 : To prepare Simple Ointment

Wool fat	0.50 g
Cetostearyl alcohol	0.50 g
Hard paraffin	0.50 g
White soft paraffin or yellow soft paraffin	8.50 g

Method of Preparation : Mix wool fat, cetostearyl alcohol, hard paraffin, and white soft paraffin or yellow soft paraffin in a container. Heat the mixture gently with stirring until homogeneous. Stir continually until cold.

Uses : Pharmaceutical aid.

Example 03 : To prepare Paraffin Ointment

White beeswax	0.20 g
Hard paraffin	0.30 g
Cetostearyl alcohol	0.50 g
White soft paraffin	9.00 g

Method of Preparation : Mix white beeswax, hard paraffin, cetostearyl alcohol, and white soft paraffin. Heat gently with stirring until homogeneous, and stir until cold.

Uses : Pharmaceutical aid and protective.

Example 4 : To prepare Wool Alcohol Ointment

Wool alcohol	0.60 g
White soft paraffin or yellow soft paraffin	1.00 g
Hard paraffin	2.40 g
Liquid paraffin	6.00 g

Method of Preparation : Melt together wool alcohol, white soft paraffin or yellow soft paraffin, hard paraffin, and liquid paraffin. Heat gentle and stir until cold.

Uses : Pharmaceutical aid, protective

Example 5 : To prepare Salicylic Acid Ointment

Salicylic acid, finely sifted	0.20 g
Wool alcohol ointment	9.80 g

Method of Preparation : Melt the wool alcohol ointment. Add gradually the salicylic acid and stir until cold.

Uses : Local anti-infective

Example 6 : To prepare Zinc Ointment

Zinc oxide, finely sifted	1.50 g
Simple ointment	8.50 g

Method of Preparation : Triturate the zinc oxide with a portion of the simple ointment until smooth. Gradually add simple ointment sufficient to produce 10 g.

Uses : Astringent, protective and antiseptic

Creams

The term cream is used in different senses. A concentrated layer separated from milk is called cream, milk of magnesia is often referred to as a cream and certain ointments are also known as creams. Many cosmetic preparations are also called creams e.g. vanishing cream, cold cream, hand cream etc. In pharmaceutical practice the term 'cream' is applied to viscous emulsions or semi-solid preparations consisting of solutions or dispersions of one or more medicaments in suitable base and intended for application to the skin or mucous membrane. They are applied to the skin for protective, beautifying, therapeutic or prophylactic purposes. Creams may contain suitable antimicrobial or preservatives unless the medicaments or basis have sufficient intrinsic bactericidal and fungicidal activity.

Creams are mainly two types

1. water-in-oil (*w/o*) 2. oil-in-water (*o/w*)

Dilution of Creams

Sometimes dilutions of proprietary creams are required. Care should be taken in diluting creams particularly to prevent microbial contamination. For dilution of creams, appropriate diluent should be used and heating should be avoided during mixing of diluent in the creams. Sometimes use of diluent may affect the stability of creams. Diluted creams should be used within two weeks of their preparation.

The stability and activity of cream may be impaired by the dilution such as :
1. Diluent without antimicrobial agent reduces the overall concentration of the preservative in the preparation.
2. Sometimes creams change from *o/w* to *w/o* by the diluent property.
3. Change of pH by dilution may cause precipitation or degradation of medicaments.
4. Choice of wrong diluent may cause poor solubility of medicament.
5. The activity of medicament may be reduced due to complex formation with the diluent.
6. It may invert the activity of emulsifying agents.

Container

Cream should be supplied in suitable containers fitted with a closure which reduces contamination of micro-organisms and evaporation of water while the product is not in use. For commercial purpose creams should be supplied in suitable collapsible tubes.

Labeling : Comply with the general requirements for labeling and should also specify i)expiry date, and ii) storage conditions

Storage : Creams should be stored at temperature not exceeding 25°C. They should not be allowed to freeze.

Example 1 : To prepare Aqueous Cream

A.

Emulsifying ointment	30.0 g
Chlorocresol	0.1g
Purified water, freshly boiled and cooled	69.9 g

B. Emulsifying ointment

Emulsifying wax	30.0 g
White soft paraffin	50.0 g
Liquid paraffin	20.0 g

Method of Preparation : Emulsifying ointment is prepared by melting all ingredients together and stirring until cold. Dissolve chlorocresol in small amount of purified water with the aid of gentle heat. Melt the emulsifying ointment and add the solution of chlorocresol while still warm.

Uses : Pharmaceutical aid

Example 2 : To prepare Buffered cream

Emulsifying ointment	30.0 g
Sodium phosphate	2.5 g
Citric acid monohydrate	0.5 g
Chlorocresol	0.1g
Purified water, freshly boiled and cooled	66.9 g

Method of Preparation : Dissolve sodium phosphate, citric acid monohydrate and chlorocresol in purified water with gently heat. Melt the emulsifying ointment with heat. Heat both solution and emulsifying ointment at the same temperature and mix with stirring gently until cold.

Uses : Pharmaceutical aid

Example 3 : To prepare Aqueous Calamine Cream

Calamine	4.0 g
Zinc oxide	3.0 g
Arachis oil	30.0 g
Emulsifying wax	6.0 g
Purified water, freshly boiled and cooled	57.0 g

Method of Preparation : By gentle heat dissolve emulsifying wax in arachis oil and add 45.0 ml of purified water at the same temperature, Stir until cool. Triturate calamine and zinc oxide with remaining quantity of purified water. Add this mixture in the cream and mix uniformly.

Uses : Astringent and protective

Example 4 : To prepare Cetrimide cream

Cetrimide	0.5 g
Cetostearyl alcohol	5.0 g
Liquid paraffin	50.0 g
Purified water, freshly boiled and cooled	100.0 g

Method of Preparation : Dissolve the cetostearyl alcohol in the liquid paraffin with the aid of gentle heat (A). At the same temperature in another beaker dissolve cetrimide in purified water (B). Add warm oily phase (A) into aqueous phase (B) with stirring until cold.

Example 5 : To prepare Cold Cream

Cetyl esters wax	12.5 g
White wax	12.0 g
Mineral oil	56.0 g
Sodium borate	0.5 g
Purified water	19.0 g

Method of Preparation : Reduce size of cetyl esters wax and white wax in small pieces. Melt them on a steam bath with the mineral oil and continue heating until the temperature of the mixture reaches 70°C (A). Dissolve the sodium borate in purified water and heat at 70°C in separate flask (B). Gradually add aqueous solution (B) to the mixture of oily phase (A) with continuous and rapid stirring until it has congealed.

Uses : Emollient and cleansing cream.

Example 6 : To prepare Vanishing cream

Stearic acid	13.0 g
Stearyl alcohol	1.0g
Cetyl alcohol	1.0g
Methylparaben	0.10 g
Propylparaben	0.05 g
Potassium hydroxide	0.90 g
Purified water, sufficient to produce	100.0 g

Method of Preparation : Melt stearic acid, stearyl alcohol, and cetyl alcohol at 75°C in a conical flask. (A). Dissolve potassium hydroxide in purified water at 75°C in another conical flask and add preservative (B). Add (A) into (B) at 75°C slowly with continuous stirring. Slowly stir the mixture until a smooth cream is formed at room temperature.

Category : Protective

Jellies

Jellies are transparent or translucent semisolids to thick viscous fluids that consist of sub microscopic particles in a somewhat plastic or rigid vehicle. They may be prepared from natural gums such as tragacanth, pectin, alginates or from synthetic derivatives of natural substances such as methylcellulose and sodium carboxymethylcellulose. Some of them are medicated or contain aromatics. Tragacanth is used in the preparation of Ephedrine Sulphate jelly. The jellies are mainly used as lubricants for surgical gloves, catheters and rectal thermometers and in haemorrhoids. They are now becoming popular for contraception purposes and contain surfactants to enhance the spermicidal properties of the jelly. Methyl salicylate and eucalyptol are commonly used aromatics which provide a desirable odour to the preparation.

Spermicidal agents commonly included in contraceptives are phenylmercuric acetate, nonylphenoxypolyethoxyethanol, methoxyppoly-ethylene glycol 550 laurate and paraformaldehydde.

Pastes

Pastes differ from ointments and creams in showing essentially dilatant flow due to the high concentration of insoluble medicament present in them. They are characterized by definite yield value and increase in the resistance to flow with increased force of application. As compared to ointments they are usually stiffer, less greasy and more absorptive. As they absorb serum secretions, pastes are used for acute lesions having a tendency to ooze.

Historically the pastes were introduced in about 1900; Unna's and Lassar's pastes are still used in practice.

The usual concentration of insoluble powders in pastes may be 20% or more and may consist of starch, zinc oxide, calcium carbonate etc. Zinc Oxide Paste USP contains as high as 50% of powdered medicament. Pastes are chiefly used as vehicles for atringent and antiseptic agents. They are not suitable for application to hairy parts like scalp because they form a densely melted mass.

Example 01 : To prepare Compound Aluminium Paste

Aluminium powder	20.0 g
Zinc oxide	40.0 g
Liquid paraffin	40.0 g

Method of Preparation : Mix the aluminium powder and zinc oxide with liquid paraffin until smooth.

Uses : Mild astringent, protective and antiseptic

Example 2 : To prepare Resorcinol and Sulphur Paste

Resorcinol, finely sifted	5.0 g
Precipitated sulphur	5.0 g
Zinc oxide, finely sifted	40.0 g
Emulsifying ointment	50.0 g

Method of Preparation : Prepare emulsifying ointment and triturate the resorcinol, precipitated sulphur and zinc oxide with a portion of the emulsifying ointment until smooth. Gradually incorporate the remaining quantity of the emulsifying ointment.

Uses : Anti-fungal, antibacterial, protective

Example 3 : To prepare Compound Zinc Paste

Zinc oxide, finely sifted	25.0 g
Starch, finely sifted	25.0 g
White soft paraffin	50.0 g

Method of Preparation : Melt white soft paraffin in a glass container. Incorporate zinc oxide and starch and stir until cold.

Uses : Protective, astringent and antiseptic

Example 4 : To prepare Zinc and Salicylic Acid Paste (**Lassar's Paste**)

Zinc oxide, finely sifted	24.0 g
Salicylic acid, finely sifted	2.0 g
Starch, finely sifted	24.0 g
White soft paraffin	50.0 g

Method of Preparation : Melt white soft paraffin in a glass container. Incorporate the zinc oxide salicylic acid, and starch stir until cold.

Example 5 : To prepare Zinc and Coal Tar Paste

Emulsifying wax	5.0 g
Zinc oxide, finely sifted	6.0 g
Coal tar	6.0 g
Starch	38.0 g
Yellow soft paraffin	45.0 g

Method of Preparation : Melt the emulsifying wax at 70 °C and add coal tar and 22.5 g of yellow soft paraffin and stir at 70 °C until completely melted. Add the remainder of the yellow soft paraffin and cool at 30 °C. Add zinc oxide and the starch with constant stirring and stir until cold.

Poultices

Poultices are viscous or paste-like preparations intended for external use only. They are applied to the skin. They may stimulate body surface or alleviate an inflamed area by supplying medicating substances in the presence of heat and moisture. Poultices must retain heat for a considerable time because they are intended to supply warmth to inflamed parts of body. They may contain following substances.

- Absorbent : e.g. kaolin
- Hygroscopic : e.g. glycerin
- Anti-rheumatic : e.g. methyl salicylate
- Bactericide : e.g. thymol, boric acid
- Flavoring agent : Peppermint oil
- Coloring agents

Container : Wide mouth screw capped colored bottle.

Example 1 : To prepare Kaolin Poultice

Heavy kaolin, finely sifted	52.7 g
Boric acid, finely sifted	4.5 g
Methyl salicylate	0.1 ml
Thymol	50.0 mg
Peppermint oil	0.05 ml
Glycerol	42.5 g

Method of Preparation : Mix the heavy kaolin and the boric acid with the glycerol. Heat the mixture at 120 °C for one hours, stirring occasionally and allow to cool (A) and dissolve thymol and methylsalicylate in separate container. (B) Mix both and add the peppermint oil and mix thoroughly.

Uses : Local anti-infective

Plasters

Plasters are solid preparations for external application of such consistency as to adhere to the skin and thereby keep a dressing in position. They are amongst the oldest class of pharmaceutical preparations. Plasters are used to afford protection or mechanical support, and to furnish an occlusive and macerating action. They also bring medicament into close contact with the surface of the skin.

Adhesive plasters consist of vinyl resin, plasticizer and other chemical additives. Such elastic-plastic adhesives are easy to apply, afford dermal protection and are easily cleaned by washing with ordinary soaps and water after soiling.

Two medicated plasters still used are Corn Plaster and Medicated Back Plaster. Back plasters contain oleoresin of capsicum as the active ingredient and are made of a heavy cotton or wool and cotton backing which provides warmth and support.

CHAPTER 14

Suppositories

Suppositories are solid or semisolid dosage forms, usually medicated, for insertion into body cavities like rectum, vagina or urethral tract. They are designed to melt, disintegrate or dissolve at the body temperature. Suppositories intended for vagina, urethra or nasal cavity are also referred to as pessaries, urethral bougies and nasal bougies, respectively. Distribution of a drug from suppositories may be either local or systemic. Pessaries are also made as compressed tablets, which disintegrate in the body fluids. They are frequently used for local effects for relief of hemorrhoids or infection in the rectum, the vagina or the urethra.

Historically suppository dosage from dates back to 2600 B.C. and were reported in the works of Hippocrates and in Papyrus Ebers, Theobroma oil and glycerinated gelatin mixtures were recommended as suppository vehicles in 1852 and 1871, respectively. Suppositories account for about 1% of all medications dispensed today.

Advantages of suppository medication

- When oral administration of a drug is not suitable as in infants or patients suffering from nausea, vomiting and gastrointestinal disturbances; suppositories serve as an alternate for drug administration.

- They have been used for a variety of conditions like hemorrhoids and local infections in vagina and rectum.

- Drugs like hypnotics, tranquillizers, antispasmodics etc., are often given as suppositories. This provides the advantage that the biotransformation of drugs in liver, pH conditions and gastrointestinal enzymes are avoided as the portal circulation is bypassed.

- Oral administration of phenylbutazone and indomethacin may cause gastric irritation hence these drugs are sometimes administered rectally.

- Suppositories have also been used for prolongation of drug action.

- Absoprtion of drugs from rectal mucosa directly into the venous circulation may bring about a faster onset of action as compared to oral administration.

- Undissociated drugs are absorbed more rapidly from gastric mucosa than the ionised ones.

- Rate of diffusion of drugs from the dosage form to the site of absorption depends upon nature of the medicament, its lipid/water solubility, physical state of the colon and the amount and nature of the solids and lipids present in the colon.

- In general, presence of surfactants may increase the rate of diffusion unless complexation takes place. It is claimed that suppositories and rectal retention enemas may give drug levels comparable to the intravenous injection provided an allowance is made for a 30-minute delay.

Classification

Suppositories are classified as -

1. ***Rectal suppositories :*** Rectal suppositories for adults are tapered at one or both ends and usually weigh about 2.0 g each. Infant suppositories usually weigh about one-half that of adult suppositories. Sedatives, tranquilizers, and analgesics are administered by rectal suppositories. They are used as hemorrhoid remedies dispensed over-the-counter. An adult suppository of 2.0 g weight is based on use of cocoa butter as the base. If other bases are employed in place of cocoa butter, weight may be increased or decreased.

2. ***Vaginal suppositories (Pessaries) :*** These are usually globular, or oviform and weigh about 4.0 to 8.0 g each. Vaginal medications are available in various physical forms like cream, liquids, and gels for the management of vaginal disorders. These suppositories are also known as pessaries.

3. ***Urethral suppositories (Bougies) :*** These are cylindrical dosage form, diameter 5.0 mm, and length 50 mm for female and 125 mm for male. Weight for urethral male suppository is 4.0 g while for female weight is 2.0 g. It is not popular dosage form and is rarely encountered. These are also known as urethral bougies.

4. ***Nasal bougies :*** These are similar to urethral bougies slightly thinner, not more than 8 mm in size and weigh about 1.2 g. In dispensing practice nasal bougies are prepared from gelato-glycerin base.

5. ***Ear cones :*** These are rarely used and whenever required they are prepared from cocoa butter.

Suppository Bases

Ideal suppository base

It should possess the following properties-

1. It should melt at body temperature or dissolve or disintegrate in body fluids.
2. Higher melting point bases may be necessary for eutectic mixtures. Addition of balsams to suppositories is intended for use in tropical climates.
3. It should be inert, non-irritating and non-sensitizing.
4. It should release the medicament readily.
5. It should be compatible with a broad variety of drugs.

6.   It should be stable on storage and transportation

7.   It should have wetting and emulsifying properties.

8.   It should be able to incorporate a high percentage of water in it i.e., a high water number.

9.   It should shrink sufficiently on cooling to release itself from mold and should be moldable by pouring or by cold compression.

10. Fatty bases should have acid value below 0.2, saponification value in between 200 to 245, iodine value less than 7 and a small range between the melting and solidification points.

Classification of Suppositories Bases

Suppository bases can be broadly divided into following categories-

A. Oleaginous bases. B. Aqueous bases. C. Emulsifying bases.

A. Oleaginous bases : Theobroma oil or cocoa butter was introduced as base in 1852 and has been one of the most widely used bases. It satisfies most of the criteria of an ideal suppository base but it melts at 32 $^{\circ}$C i.e., below the body temperature. Overheating alters its physical characteristics and it has a tendency to adhere to the mold when solidified. It may exist in 4 crystalline states.

α Form : This form is obtained by suddenly cooling the melted mass to 0 $^{\circ}$C. Its melting point is 24 $^{\circ}$C.

β Form : This form is obtained when cocoa butter is melted at 35 to 36 $^{\circ}$C and slowly cooled. It melts at 18 to 23 $^{\circ}$C.

β'Form : It reverts back to β form and melts at 34 to 35 $^{\circ}$C.

γ Form : It is obtained by pouring a cool (20 $^{\circ}$C) cocoa butter into a container before it is solidified and cooled at deep freeze temperature. It melts at 18 $^{\circ}$C.

All the four forms are unstable and are converted to stable form over a period of several days. Thus extreme care should be exercised while melting and cooling cocoa butter. As a general rule, the minimal use of heat during the melting process is recommended.

Cocoa butter can take up to 20 to 30g of water per 100 g. The incorporation of emulsifiers such as Tween 61 (5 to 10%) increases the water absorption capacity of cocoa butter.

Drugs like volatile oils, cresol, phenol and chloral hydrate lower the melting point of cocoa butter considerably and hence some wax and spermaceti can be used to correct such a problem.

To overcome drawbacks of cocoa butter, hydrogenated palm kernel and soyabean oils have been suggested. Palm kernel oil is particularly suggested for use in tropical countries. Completely or partially hydrogenated cottonseed oil such as `Cotoflakes' and `Cotomar' together with hexanediol has also been suggested.

Edible hydrogenated vegetable oil in combination with some waxes has been worked out in India. Pharmacopoeia of India recommends Kokum fat as a major constituent of the official suppository bases.

B. Aqueous bases

(i) ***Glycero – gelatin :*** It is a mixture of glycerin and water made into a stiff jelly by the addition of gelatin. The proportion of gelatin can be varied according to the intended use of the preparation.

Gelato-glycerin bases dissolve in the body fluids liberating contained medicaments. Gelato-glycerin Mass BP contains 14% gelatin, 70% glycerin and water. USP formula contains 20% gelatin together with 70% of glycerin. For dispensing purposes, good quality powdered gelatin should be used. In order to control the consistency, glycerin can be partially or wholly substituted by propylene glycol and polyethylene glycols. The incompatibility of some medicaments can be avoided by the use of either Pharmagel A (cationic) or Pharmagel B (anionic). Glycerin suppositories being liable to mould growth, preservatives should be added.

(ii) *Soap glycerin :* In this case, soap is employed instead of glycerin for hardening. Sodium stearate can incorporate up to 95% of glycerin. Sodium stearate (soap) is produced *in situ* by interaction of sodium carbonate with stearic acid. Soap glycerin suppositories are however hygroscopic.

(iii) *PEG bases :* Different mixtures of polyethylene glycols are marketed under the trade names of Postonals, Carbo waxes and Macrogols. Some important PEG bases used in the preparation of suppositories are as follows.

I		III	
PEG 1000	96	PEG 1540	70
PEG 4000	4	PEG 6000	30
II		IV	
PEG 1000	75	PEG 1540	30
PEG 4000	25	PEG 6000	50

Base I is a low melting, rapidly disintegrating base and requires refrigeration during summer. Base II is much more stable, harder and gives a slower release. Base III is particularly suitable for those drugs having a melting point lowering effect on the base. Base IV contains water and facilitates incorporation of water-soluble and PEG insoluble substances.

Most of the drugs commonly administered in suppository form are compatible with these bases. Polyethylene glycols are however incompatible with phenols and reduce the antiseptic effects of quaternary ammonium compounds.

C. Emulsifying bases : Massa Esterinum, Witepsol and Massupol are the trade names under which the emulsifying bases are marketed. Massa Esterinum is a mixture of the mono-, di- and tri-glycerides of the fatty acids having the formula $C_{11}H_{23}COOH$ to $C_{17}H_{35}COOH$. Witepsol bases consist of hydrogenated triglycerides of lauric acid with added monoglycerides. These are available in 9 grades. Massupol consists of glyceryl esters namely of lauric acid and addition of very small quantity of glyceryl monostearate.

All these bases are free from the drawbacks of cocoa butter and don't require any mold lubricant.

Water-dispersible bases essentially consist of surfactants. They melt at body temperature. Some formulae of dispersible bases containing surfactants are outlined below.

I		II		III	
Glyceryl monostearate	10	Glyceryl monostearate	15	Twenn 60	40
Tween 61	90	Tween 61	85	Tween 61	60

Preparation of Suppositories

1. *Hand Mould Suppositories :* This is the oldest and simplest method of preparing suppositories. A skilled person is required for the preparation of suppositories.

   General process for preparation of suppositories is as follows :

   (a) Mix measured quantity of medicinal substances with sufficient quantity of theobroma oil.

   (b) Triturate and, if required, soften with diluted alcohol and rub until a smooth paste is formed.

   (c) Add remaining quantity of theobroma oil and add wool fat for consistency.

   (d) When the mass becomes plastic by vigorous kneading of the pestle quickly remove from the mortar with a spatula.

   (e) Transfer with spatula to a piece of filter paper and keep in hands during the kneading and rolling procedure.

   (f) Roll the mass by quick rotating movements of the hands and immediately place on a pill tile.

   (g) Rolling the mass on the tile with a flat board forms a cylindrical suppository.

   (h) Cut in pieces by spatula.

   (i) Give the shape by rolling one end on the tile with a spatula.

   (j) Pack in butter paper or in proper container and store in cool place.

2. **Compression mould suppositories (Cold compression)**

   (a) Mix theobroma oil and drug.

   (b) Mixture is forced into a mould under pressure, using a wheel-operated press.

   (c) Mould is removed, opened and replaced.

   (d) On large-scale cold-compression machines are hydraulically operated by water-jacketed cooling and screw fed.

3. Fusion or melt mould suppositories

(a)   Drug is dispersed or dissolved in a melted suppository base.

(b)   Pour the mixture into suppository moulds and allow cooling in ice bath.

(c)   Finished suppositories are removed by opening the mould.

(d)   Various types and sizes of moulds are available for preparation of suppositories. Moulds are made of aluminum alloys, brass or plastic and are available with from six to several hundred cavities.

4. Automatic mould Machine

All filling, ejection, and mould cleaning operations are fully automatic. The output of a typical rotary machine ranges from 3500 to 6000 suppositories per hour. The suppository mould is lubricated by brushing or spraying and then filled to a slight excess. Excess material is removed after the mass gets solidified and collected for re-use. All heating and cooling systems are fully automatic.

Suppositories are usually formulated on weight basis. The medicament replaces the portion of base having same density as that of theobroma oil. If the drug substance is heavier, it will replace a proportionally smaller amount of theobroma oil.

Example 1

Prepare six suppositories containing 0.1 g tannic acid in each suppository.

Density of tannic acid is 1.6 as compared with cocoa butter.

Weight of blank suppositories = 2.0 g

Cocoa butter replaced by drug = 0.1/1.6 = 0.062 g

Cocoa butter required for one suppository = 2.000 − 0.062 = 1.938 g

Actual weight of one suppository = 1.938 + 0.10 = 2.038 g

Weight of cocoa butter for 8 suppositories (take excess weigh of 2 suppositories as required) = 1.938 × 8 = 15.504 g

Weight of tannic acid for 8 suppositories (take excess weigh of 2 suppositories as required) = 0.10 × 8 = 0.80 g

Total weight of all suppositories = 15.504 + 0.80 = 16.304 g

Example 2

Prepare 0.1 g tannic acid 6 suppositories using polyethylene glycol as base. Density factor of cocoa butter is 1.6 and density factor of polyethylene glycol is 1.25.

Weight of polyethylene glycol suppository = 1.75

Cocoa butter replaced by drug = (0.1/1.6) × 1.25 = 0.078 g

Polyethylene glycol required for one suppository = 1.750 − 0.078 = 1.672 g

Actual weight of one suppository = 1.672 + 0.10 = 1.772 g

Weight of polyethylene glycol for 8 suppositories (take excess weigh of 2 suppositories as required) = $1.672 \times 8 = 13.376$ g

Weight of tannic acid for 8 suppositories (take excess weigh of 2 suppositories as required) = $0.10 \times 8 = 0.80$ g

Total weight = $13.376 + 0.80 = 14.176$ g

Displacement Value of Medicaments

The quantity of medicament that displaces one part of cocoa butter is called displacement value. The volume of particular suppository mould is uniform but fill weight will vary according to the density of medicaments as compared with cocoa butter with which the mould was calibrated.

Determination of Displacement value

Weight of six suppositories of theobroma oil or any other base = a g

Weight of six suppositories containing, say 40 percent of drug(s) = b g

Calculate weight of theobroma oil = $60 / 100 \times b = c$ g

Calculate drug(s) = $40/100 \times b = d$ g

$(a - c)$ g = the weight of theobroma oil displaced by d g of drug substances

Displacement value of the medicament = $d / (a - c)$

Displacement Values (DV) of Solid Medicaments

Medicament	DV	Medicament	DV	Medicament	DV
Alum	2.0	Hydrocortisone	1.5	Phenol	1.0
Aminophyllin	1.5	Ichthamol	1.0	Quinine HCl	1.0
Bismuth oxynitrate	5.0	Iodoform	4.0	Resorcinol	1.5
Bismuth subgallate	2.5	Lead acetate	3.0	Salol	1.5
Boric acid	1.5	Lead Iodide	5.0	Silver Proteinate	1.5
Chloral hydrate	1.5	Mercury ointment	1.5	Tannic acid	1.0
Cinchocaine	1.5	Morphine HCl	1.5	Zinc oxide	5.0
Cocaine HCl	1.5	Opium	1.5	Zinc sulphate	2.0
Hydrocortisone	1.5	Peptone	1.5		

Packaging and Storage

Suppositories are packaged in partitioned boxes or in tightly closed screw-capped glass container or wrapped individually in aluminium foil. In large scale production suppositories are wrapped individually or separately in foil packs. Candy wrapping is the more familiar aluminium foil or PVC polyethylene strip. Low melting point suppositories should be store in cool place and theobroma oil suppositories should be stored in refrigeration.

Mould Lubricant

Mould lubricants are used to remove theobroma suppositories without damaging their surfaces unless a lubricant is used. Lubrication is essential for glycero-gelatin bases because of their sticky nature. Following lubricants may be used for the preparation of theobroma oil suppositories.

Soft soap	10.0 g
Glycerin	10.0 g
Ethanol, (90%)	50.0 ml

Lubricant must be compatible with medicament or adjuncts. In industry silicone fluid is used as lubricant. Mould is lubricated using a pad of gauze or muslin or with a small fairly stiff brush. Cotton wool is not used because some fibers adhere to the mould. Excess of lubricant can be removed by inverting the mould on a clean white tile.

Example 1 : Prepare and dispense Compound Bismuth Subgallate Suppositories.

Rx

Bismuth subgallate	200.0 mg
Resorcinol	60.0 mg
Zinc oxide	120.0 mg
Castor oil	60.0 mg

Theobroma oil, sufficient to fill a mould

Method of Dispensing : Melt theobroma oil and add other additives and mix uniformly. Properly lubricate the suppository mould and pour the hot base in the moulds and cool immediately in ice bath. Excess of substance is scrapped off and re-used in next lot. Open the mould and remove the suppository carefully. Pack in butter paper and store in a well-closed container.

Uses : Astringent and antacid

Example 2 : Prepare and dispense Glycerol Suppositories.

Rx

Gelatin	14.0 g
Glycerol	70.0 g
Purified water, sufficient to produce	100.0 g

Method of Dispensing : Soak gelatin in purified water for about five minutes or until thoroughly softened. Drain well and add glycerin and heat on water bath. Evaporate excess quantity until the mixture weighs 100 g. Pour the products into suitable moulds.

Uses : Rectal evacuant.

Example 3 : Prepare and dispense Glycerin Suppositories

Rx

Glycerin	91.0 g
Sodium stearate	9.00 g
Purified water	5.00 g

Method of Dispensing : Heat the weighed amount of glycerin in a suitable container to about 120°C. Sodium stearate is dissolved in the heated glycerin with stirring. Add purified water and mix. Pour the hot mixture in the suitable mould.

Uses : Local application

Example 4 : Prepare and dispense Glycerinated Gelatin Suppositories.

Rx

Drug and purified water	10.0 g
Gelatin	20.0 g
Glycerin	70.0 g

Method of Dispensing : Dissolve the drug in purified water and moisten the gelatin. Heat the glycerin and add gelatin and drug solution. Mix uniformly and pour this mixture in a mould.

Uses : Antimicrobial.

Example 5 : Prepare and dispense Tannic Acid Suppositories.

Rx

| Tannic acid | 0.2 g |

Theobroma oil, sufficient to produce qs

Method of Dispensing : Add lubricant in the mould and remove the excess of lubricant by draining and cool the lubricated mould over ice. Theobroma oil is heated in a porcelain dish over a water bath and avoid over heating. Remove dish from the water bath as soon as the mass is molten. Weighed amount of tannic acid is powdered and added in the molten theobroma oil. Mix the tannic acid by spatula (sometimes molten theobroma oil divided in two parts) and pour the mixture into the holes in the moulds. Place the mould on ice and remove excess mass carefully by sharp knife. When the suppositories have completely set hard, open the mould and remove the suppositories by slight pressure on the broad ends. Remove any lubricant on final product, by rolling on the filter papers.

Uses : Astringent.

Practice Exercises

1. Rx

Sulphur	10%
Benzoic acid	1.5%
Pertrolatum q.s. ad	30.0
Ft. ung.	

2. Rx

Tannic acid	20 %
Distilled water	40 %
Ointment of wool alcohols	40%

    Label : Astringent ointment.

3. Rx

    Supply 50g. of hydrophilic petrolatum USP.

    (The official formula includes cholesteroal 3g. stearyl alcohol 3g.

    white beeswax 8g and white soft paraffin 86g).

4. Rx

Iodine	4 g
Pot. Iodide	4 g
Glycerin	12 g
Wool fat	4 g
Yellow beeswax	4 g
Yellow soft paraffin	72 g
Supply 40 g.	

    Label : Apply to the affected parts as directed.

5. Rx

Sorbitan monooleate	6 %
Beeswax	3 %
Soft paraffin	36%
Liquid paraffin	15 %
Purified water	40 %

    Label : The oily cream base.

6. Rx

Zinc oxide	10 g
Glycerin	10 g
Bentonite	10 g
Distilled water to	100g

Label : The paste.

7. Rx

| Zinc oxide | 4 gr |
| Gelato-glycerin BPC | q.s. |

Make a 30 gr suppository. Send such 20.

8. Rx

| Chloral hydrate | 200 mg |
| Oil of Theobroma | q.s. |

Make a 1g suppository. Send such 12.

Label : The suppositories. Use one at night.

CHAPTER 15

Ophthalmic Preparations

Medication meant for the eye may be a liquid in the form of solution or suspension, or a semisolid in the form of an ointment or a cream. These preparations require special techniques, processes and theoretical considerations for compounding. Several factors have to be taken into account e.g., rendering the solution isotonic, adjusting it to proper pH and buffering if necessary, incorporating stabilizing agents, increasing the viscosity, adding preservatives etc. Further, all preparations for the eye have to be sterile. This requires considerable skill and caution on the part of the pharmacist.

Ophthalmic preparations are sterile products, essentially free from foreign particles, suitably formulated and packaged in suitable container for either topical application to the eyelids or instillation into the cul-de-sac between the eyeball and eyelids.

Following categories of drugs are used in and as ophthalmic preparations.

1. Anti-inflammatory agent
2. Anti-microbial drugs e.g., beta adrenergic blocking agent, cycloplegics, miotics, mydriatics and vasoconstrictors.
3. Anti-microbial drugs e.g., antibiotics, antiseptics, antivirals, fungicides and sulfonamides
4. Local anaesthetic
5. Others e.g., chelating agents, hyper osmolar agents, diagnostic products, lubricant ointments, artificial tears, eye washes, artificial eye solution and contact lens solution.

Drug from the ophthalmic preparation may be required to penetrate through the cornea or exert only local action. Drug absorption and permeability in the eye depends on the solubility of the drug in water. The extent of absorption is also dependent upon the quantity of the drug present and its concentration in the medication in the dosage form. Addition of buffers may be of assistance in stabilizing some of the preparations and adjustment of pH as well as in the absorption of the drug. This area however, concerns more the manufacturing pharmacist and has limited application in dispensing of extemporaneously prepared solutions for the eye. Some of the drugs are inherently irritating to the eye and initiate secretion of tears thus washing off the drug from the site of absorption and action.

Isotonic Solutions

Solutions meant for the eye should be isotonic with the tear secretion to prevent irritation due to difference in the tonicity. If the concentration of the drug is not sufficient to yield an isotonic solution, addition of requisite amount of an inert substance compatible with drug is essential. The pharmacist is required to select the substance and calculate its quantity necessary to render the solution isotonic. A given solution, from tonicity considerations, may be either isotonic or paratonic in relation to the tear secretion. If the quantity of the drug(s) prescribed is just sufficient to produce, on appropriate dilution, the same tonicity as the tear secretion, no substance should be added. Such a solution is isotonic by itself. Some prescriptions direct that an isotonic solution of a drug be dispensed without stating the concentration of the drug in solution. In such cases a pharmacist may calculate the quantity of the drug required to dispense the volume of the solution but in case that concentration is too high, he may have to refer either to the physician or use the quantity normally prescribed in the conditions for which the prescription is meant. However, it is not infrequent that a pharmacist receives paratonic prescriptions. Such prescriptions may be of two types-hypertonic or hypotonic in relation to the tear secretion. Hypertonic solutions contain more quantity than required to have the same tonicity as the tear secretion. It is not possible to render a hypertonic solution isotonic unless the quantity of the medicament is reduced to tonicity level. Reducing the quantity of the medication amounts to altering the prescription. The pharmacist may have to consult the physician in such circumstances. However, a pharmacist adjusts the tonicity of the hypotonic solutions by adding appropriate quantity of soluble substances. The required quantities of such additive substances may be calculated by any one of the methods. In practice, by experience pharmacist prepares tables of the medication in different concentrations and the concentration of the adjusting substance for the drug for all generally prescribed solutions. Whereas it is desirable to make solutions isotonic with the tear secretion, it may be remembered that paratonic solutions within the range of 0.7 to 1.5% of sodium chloride or its equivalent in relation to other substances are easily tolerated by the eye.

Adjustment of pH, Stabilization and Preservation

Tonicity of a solution and pH appear to be independent but there is some bearing of one over the other. Drugs in solutions may ionize and dissociate at alkaline pH. Solutions having a pH value between 6.5 to 7.5 are very well tolerated by the eye. However, solutions having a pH as low as 4 and as high as 10 are known to be prescribed and instilled without extraordinary pain and irritation. Pain and irritation in the eye due to acidic drug solutions are immediately felt on instilling the solution and this results into tear secretion which is slightly alkaline. The alkaline tear fluid gradually neutralizes the acidity resulting in the reduction of irritation and pain. The degree of the tear secretion depends on the extent of acidic nature and the volume of the solution instilled. Buffer solutions are included in the eye solutions sometimes which serve many a purpose maximizing therapeutic activity of the medicament, bringing about stability of the solution, reducing pain etc. Lot of investigations has been recently carried out with regard to the choice of buffers to be included in eye drops and eye washes. However, this area relates more to the manufacturer than the practicing pharmacist as he faces lesser problems of stabilizing than the manufactured products. Sodium EDTA (Sodium ethylene diamine tetraacetate) in a concentration of 0.1% acts as a good preservative of eye solutions as it performs antibacterial action as well. Very often it is used in conjunction with boric acid. Salts of the alkaloid-pilocarpine are more stable in presence of phosphate buffer. Sodium borate is another substance employed for preservation of eye solutions.

Viscosity of the Eye Medication

For providing prolonged contact of the medication to the eye and reducing the possibility of being washed away, it may be desirable in certain cases to increase the viscosity of the preparation. However, it is imperative that the agent used to increase the viscosity should possess the properties of compatibility, inertness, clarity and refractive index, Polyethylene glycol, methyl cellulose, polyvinyl alcohol and polyvinylpyrollidone are the main additives employed for this purpose. Since sterility is an essential requirement for eye preparations, the additives employed ought to be sterilizable by the commonly used methods of sterilization. If heat is to be used for sterilization, the additive should not undergo any physical or chemical change in itself or bring about any coagulation or precipitation of the medication. Enhanced therapeutic action from a preparation with increased viscosity or reduction in the concentration of the drug in the presence of viscosity increasing agents is a subject which is receiving great attention of the investigators. However, this aspect has greater and deeper implications in ophthalmic formulations designed and manufactured by the industry.

Sterility aspects of Eye Preparations, aseptic Processing and choice of Preservatives

Preparations for the eye, till about 1953, were not required to be sterile which was a serious shortcoming in ophthalmic medication. However, in the present time sterility of eye medication has been prescribed officially by the Pharmacopoeias. This applied both to the manufactured preparations as well as to the dispensed preparations. In extemporaneous dispensing of prescriptions to sterilize a preparation may be time consuming and sometimes impractical. Thus medication for the eye is generally dispensed in manufacturer's sealed containers. It is essential, however, that a pharmacist though not very often required to compound and sterilize eye medication, must be familiar with every aspect of these preparations and their preservation. Facilities for dispensing such preparations must exist in the Pharmacy and a pharmacist must receive adequate training in the techniques associated with the compounding, sterilizing and filling the containers aseptically. Generally, a manufacturer's original package is a small sealed sterile container. A dropper may be an integral part of the closure device or may be supplied duly packed in the carton for instilling the solution in the eye. Once a sealed container is opened and the medication used, it becomes increasingly contaminated following each usage and therefore the supply is in a small container. Larger packages are also manufactured for clinics and hospitals where a large number of patients call for the treatment. However, in such institutions, a separate sterile dropper is used for each patient. In view of the unavoidable contamination, inclusion of chemical preservatives is essential in ophthalmic preparations. Common preservatives are listed below.

Table 15.1 Common Preservatives for Ophthalmic Preparations.

Preservative	Concentration
Phenol	0.25-0.50%
p-chlorometaxylenol	0.03%
Phenylethyl alcohol	0.5%
Phenoxyethanol	0.3%
Chlorobutanol	0.5%
Nitromersal	1 in 2,500
Thiomersal	1 in 500
Phenylmercuric nitrate	1 in 1,00,000 to1 in 25,000
Polymyxin B sulphate	1000 units/ml
Benzalkonium chloride	1 in 1,00,000 to 1 in 10,000

Preparations for the eye can be sterilized by any method depending upon the nature of the drug and its stability under the conditions of sterilization. It is presumed that a pharmacist is familiar with the principles, methods and techniques of sterilization and the equipment to be used. The most common method for sterilizing aqueous liquid preparations is with the help of steam under pressure (autoclaving). For a pharmacy a pressure cooker is good enough and sterilization can be brought about within half an hour at 121^0C and 15 lb per square inch pressure which is attainable in a pressure cooker. Thermolabile medication can be sterilized under aseptic condition by filtering the solution through bacteria-proof filters. It is desirable to have a few varieties of filters and candles available in the pharmacy for this purpose.

A modern pharmacy is expected to have an aseptic room to carry out aseptic operations. even small pharmacies must be equipped with a glass hood for aseptic work. Aseptic work is a specialized technique and a pharmacist is expected to master it during the period of his training so as to handle aseptic problems with confidence. A brief outline of the sources of likely contamination and aseptic operation is given below.

Two classes of pharmaceutical preparations are required to be sterile - injectables and preparations for the eye. The purpose of employing aseptic process is to eliminate the possibility of contamination with micro-organisms during preparation, packaging and testing of the medication. If the medicament is packed and sealed in such a container, which after sterlization, dose not permit contamination; there is no necessity of aseptic technique. In other words, the heat treatment at the end of the process and the sealed container safeguard the sterility of the product till the container is opened. But in cases there such terminal heat treatment is not possible; one has to resort to aseptic processing. Example of this type include thermo-labile drugs in solution and suspension form, thermo-labile drugs in powder form meant for dusting or for dilution just before use and thermo-labile substances to be mixed with the base as in case of eye ointments. In addition to the above requirements for preparation and packaging, aseptic handling is essential is testing the medication for sterility.

Aseptic technique precludes the possibility of contamination, which should ensure an aseptic operation. The biggest source of contamination is air. Although atmospheric air does not provide any nutrition to the micro-organisms and thus does not promote their growth, yet it acts as an effective agency for carrying micro-organisms in it. It carries in itself several substances on which micro organisms get conveniently deposited e.g. dust, droplets, and droplet nuclei. The air that one breathes can hold a considerable number of micro organisms. Other agencies that cause heavy contamination include hands, clothes, hair of the workers in the area, the working area and the equipment used.

From the above it is apparent that aseptic processing requires aseptic working condition and a good training in functioning of the pharmacist in a manner that will lead to minimal contamination. Working conditions embody the aseptic laboratory, its furniture, services and equipment needed therein. Functioning of the pharmacist requires a consciousness to the possibility of contamination and conducting oneself in a suitable manner.

Design of an Aseptic Laboratory

As long as a laboratory meets certain essential requirements, it is suitable for aseptic work. These requirements are given below.

The Aseptic Room

All openings except the openings for entry need perfect sealing and horizontal surfaces including windows should be eliminated. These surfaces may allow retention of dust and may create problems. The structure should be tight enough to prevent infiltration of uncontrolled air. All exposed surfaces should be smooth and impervious, easily cleanable and in no way prone to settling of dust upon them. The surfacing material should not be susceptible to hold dust, flaking or chalking under normal operative procedures. Uncoated smooth surfaces e.g. stainless steel, aluminium and chromium plating, plastic laminates and plastic films make satisfactory surfaces. Cement concrete is a very undesirable surface.

Air-conditioned Atmosphere

In view of the sealed structure, preventing any source of entry of air, air conditioning is essential. Since no special requirement of temperature and humidity are prescribed, conventional air conditioning may be suitable enough. It is however preferable to have the humidity on the lower side to avoid contamination by the perspiration of the workers. Air cleaning part of the air conditioning system is a critical factor as the nature of the atmospheric air may differ considerably from time to time. Cooling and heating coils, humidity control apparatus, reheat coils; blowers etc. are the equipment that should be of standard specifications. However, the fans selected should be such that can provide high pressure. The room has to be constantly maintained under positive pressure to prevent inlet of air from entry point whenever it is opened. Dust, temperature and humidity control are interdependent functions. Dust control is impossible without confining the area. Confined space is unlivable without air-conditioning. If temperature and humidity are controlled by air conditioning, dust control measures are automatically taken care of.

Cleaning of Air

Cleaning of air is the key factor of the aseptic processing. The usual approach is a combination of the conventional cleaners e.g. regular filters or electronic air cleaners located within the system and some kind of super-interception or an ultra cleaner located down stream from all coils, blowers etc. Bactericidal equipment is incorporated in the assembly for providing sterile air in addition to be devices stated above. The air in the aseptic area should be free from fibers, dust and microbes. This can be conveniently achieved by the use of High Efficiency Particulate Air (HEPA) filters which can remove particles up to 0.3 μm with an efficiency of 99.7% or more. HEPA filters made use of in Laminar Air Flow in which air moves with uniform velocity along parallel lines with minimum of eddies. The air flow can be either horizontal or vertical and 100 ± 10 ft/min. is considered to be the minimum effective air velocity. Such laminar flow stations and work benches are commercially available and should find immense use in compounding and dispensing practice.

Air Distribution

Materials of construction for the air distribution system should be made of non-rusting and non-flaking materials (e.g. ducts, air outlets etc.). Duct insulation, if needed, should be applied on the outer side and only on the ducts that are located out of the clean area. Joints and other fittings, if any, should be sealed to prevent leakage and contamination. Air distribution is also employed for 'washing' the workers off dust who enter the sterile area. These are called air showers which are strictly blasts or air directed on the person to remove dust.

Controls

Conventional controls are used in the system for regulating humidity and temperature. Sometimes greater pressure may have to be maintained in critical areas and for this purpose additional controls may have to be installed. Interlocks may be required between the sterile area and the entrance or passing doors. In a highly elaborate system, alarm circuits are introduced to warn against the malfunctioning or inadvertent misuse of the air locks.

Instruments

Highly sophisticated instrumentation has to be installed which constantly or intermittently monitors and samples the clean atmosphere for analyzing its cleanliness. These devices immediately indicate the contamination, if any.

Furniture

Seating, work tables, racks etc. are essential requirements of furniture inside he clean area and have to be specially designed and built to meet certain rigid specifications. Adjusting mechanisms on the chairs should either not exist or ought to be sealed. These may be potential dust setting surfaces. Conventional upholstering of the chairs is completely out of question. Dust catching surfaces should be minimum and all parts should be readily cleanable and resistant to the action of the cleaning agents. Worker comfort is a very important factor in a confined area. The requirements of the job in a sterile room keep the workers chained to the work over long periods of time continuously without leisure and with minimum exits from the room and thus warrants high degree of comfort for carrying out the critical operations. Special jigs, fixtures and tools are developed for specific purposes but many operations need dust-free hoods-miniature aseptic rooms located on the working bench. Even when the aseptic hoods or chambers are located in dust free rooms, they may have to be provided with supply of pressurized air in each one of them. The air may be either super cleaned or an inert gas. Further these hoods have to be independently illuminated.

There are many several important factors to consider when called upon compounding a sterile ophthalmic preparation. Eyes are very sensitive to heat, light, drugs and chemicals. In many cases, the drugs involved have a narrow therapeutic range and even small errors when introduced have the potential to cause irreversible damage to the eye or loss of the eye sight. The following considerations are recommended whenever preparing such a product.

1. Ensure concentration is within the acceptable range or not before dispensing of the product.

2. Sterility of the final product is a must, strictly handled in aseptic area.

3. The pH of the final product must be within an acceptable range.

4. Stability of the final product must be known, as well as the recommended storage requirements.

5. Suitable knowledge of potential diluents or vehicles is required in order to ensure proper tonicity, viscosity, or dissolution of the final product.

6. Proper documentation of each step is an important consideration to reduce error.

7. If the preparation of a product requires the breaking of an ampoule or the reconstitution of a powder, it is recommended that the final product be made in sterile water for injection and free from particulate matter.

8. The preparation of intra-occular products requires the use of preservative-free ingredients. Many preservatives have been found to be toxic to the inner ocular tissues.

9. Finally, before dispensing the finished product, always indicate the storage requirements, concentrations of ingredients, and the expected expiration date.

Ophthalmic Products

    (a) Eye drops

    (b) Eye ointments

    (c) Eye suspension

    (d) Eye lotions

    (e) Contact lens solutions

Eye Drops

Eye drops are sterile aqueous or oily solutions or suspension of one or more medicaments intended for instillation into the conjunctival sac for diagnostic or therapeutic purposes. Oily eye drops are less used but may nevertheless occasionally be requested. They are usually prepared with sterile castor oil and alkaloids incorporated in a vehicle suitable to be used in the form of the base (e.g., pilocarpine eye drops contains pilocarpine dissolved in sterile castor oil). Certain eye drops may be supplied in a drug, sterile form to be reconstituted in an appropriate sterile liquid immediately before use. In such cases the label should state clearly on the container 'Powder for Eye Drops' and should include direction for the use of eye drops.

Aqueous eye drops contain suitable antimicrobial preservatives at appropriate concentrations because it is intended for use on more than one occasion. The antimicrobial preservatives should be compatible with the other ingredients of the preparations and should remain effective throughout the shelf-life of the eye drops.

Formulation

Eye drops may contain the following ingredients:

1.   *Medicaments :* anti-microbial agents, local anaesthetic, diagnostic agents, miotics, mydriatic, sulfonamides etc.

2.   *Vehicle :* sterile distilled water, sterile castor oil etc.

3.   *Viscosity :* polyethylene glycol, polyvinyl alcohol, polyvinylpyrrolidone, hydroxypropyl methylcellulose, methylcellulose, carboxymethylcellulose and hydroxyethyl cellulose.

4.   *Surfactant :* Benzthonium chloride, polysorbate-20 etc.

5.   *Hydrogen ion concentration :* The greatest comfort for the patient is expected to be found at the normal pH approximately 7.4, of lachrymal fluid but usually adequate in the pH range of 6 to 8. Most of the active ingredients used in ophthalmic solution are salts of weak acids and have low buffer capacity e.g. sodium acid phosphate solution, sodium phosphate solution, sodium chloride solution etc.

6.   *Buffers :* Monobasic sodium phosphate solution, dibasic sodium phosphate solution and sodium chloride solution.

7.   *Tonicity modifiers :* sodium chloride and boric acid.

8.   *Antioxidant :* Solution metabisulphite(0.1%) and sodium thiosulphite (0.1%)

9.   *Chelating agent :* Disodium edetate

10. *Antimicrobial :* Benzylkonium chloride, chlorahedine acetate, chlorbutol, thromersal, phenylethyl alcohol, PMN and PMA.

11. *Clarity :* All solutions for the use in the eye should be clear and free from foreign particles.

12. *Sterilization :* Ophthalmic solution are required to be sterile when prepared and great care must be exercised subsequently to prevent contamination to use. The microbe must frequently found as a contaminant is *Pseudomonas aeruginosa* and the solution most

often found contaminated is of sodium fluerescein. It is very dangerous and opportunistic organism that grows well on most culture media and produces both toxin and anti-bacterial products. This Gram (-)ve bacillus also grows readily in ophthalmic solutions which may become the source of extremely serious infections of the cornea. The common methods of sterilization are moist heat under pressure (autoclave), bacterial filtration (pore size 0.22 µm) and use of chemicals.

Containers

1. ***Single dose containers :*** It is minimum unit and consists of a disposable, pliable, tube-like applicator made from polypropylene by ultrasonic sealing. It has a nozzle protected by a cap. It is generally enclosed in a heat-sealed envelope.

2. ***Multiple application containers :*** The traditional container for eye drops is a glass bottle carrying in the cap a dropper fitted with a teat. e.g.,

3. Amber colored container to provide protection from light

4. Hexagonal in cross-section and vertically ribbed on three adjacent faces, the ribs indicate that the contents must not be taken orally.

5. Made from neutral or treated soda glass.

6. Screw capped bottle with separate droppers.

Labelling

Comply with the general requirements for labelling, following information is mentioned on the label clearly.

1. Name and concentration of medicaments.

2. Name and concentration of antimicrobial agent.

3. Date after which the product is not intended to be used.

4. Discard the contents at a specified time after opening (about one month).

5. If any discomfort or irritation discontinue use of the eye drop.

6. 'For External use Only'.

How To Use Eye Drops

1. Wash hands with soap

2. Pull lower eyelid down with one hand gently

3. If dropper is separate, squeeze rubber bulb once while dropper is in bottle to bring liquid into dropper.

4. Holding dropper above eye, drop medicine inside lower lid while looking up.

5. Do not touch dropper to eye or fingers.

6. Lift lower lid and try to keep eye open.

7. Do not blink for at least 30 seconds.

8. If dropper is separate, replace on bottle and tighten the cap.

9. Keep the dropper tip always down.

10. Never rinse the dropper.

11. Never use drops that have changed color

12. Open one bottle at a time if you have more than one.

13. If you are using more than one kind of drop at the same time, wait several minutes before using the other drop

14. After instillation of drops, do not close eyes tightly and try not to blink more often than usual.

Eye Ointments

Ophthalmic ointments are ointments meant for application to the eye. It can be used to obtain the effect of a variety of medicaments on the outside and edges of the eyelids, the conjunctiva, the cornea and the iris. It contains sterilized ingredients packed under rigid aseptic conditions and meets the requirements of the official sterility tests. Ophthalmic ointments must contain a suitable substance or mixture of substances to prevent growth of or to destroy, microorganisms accidentally introduced when the container is opened during use. The medicinal agent is added to the ointment base either as a solution or as a micronized powder.

The finished ointment must be free from large particles. Most ophthalmic ointments are prepared with a base of white petroleum and mineral oil often with anhydrous lanolin.

Container

1. Ointments are packed in collapsible metal or plastic tubes or in single dose containers

2. Plastic tubes are used for some proprietary formulations of eye ointments

3. Certain proprietary formulations of eye ointments are available in single dose containers, elongated, flexible gelatin capsule with one end constructed and are opened by cutting off the constructed end with sterile scissors.

Labeling

The label on the tube or outer sealed envelop should state that the contents are sterile provided that the container has not been opened. Other information should be similar as discussed for eye drops.

Eye Lotions

Eye lotions are sterile aqueous solutions for first aid purposes over a maximum period of twenty four hours without bactericide. In another words, eye lotions are aqueous solutions for intermittent domiciliary administration for up to seven days having bactericide. Eye lotions are usually applied with an eye bath, for first aid purposes only hence it has limited use nowadays but may be prescribed e.g., sodium bicarbonate eye lotion is used for the emergency treatment of acid burns of the eye and is popular as **Factory eye drops No.2.** Sodium chloride is an isotonic solution which is occasionally used for irrigating the eye.

Containers

Eye lotions are dispensed in colored fluted bottle closed with a screw-cap. It is important to ensure that the liner of the screw cap is not covered by cork as it may be a source of microbial contamination. Rubber or plastics liners are suitable and the screw cap may be either of metal or plastics. Uncolored or non-fluted bottles may be used if a suitable colored, fluted bottle is not available.

Labeling

Following information is stated on the eye lotion label

1.   'For External use only'.
2.   Discard any lotion remaining after use when the seal is first broken.
3.   Eye lotions which are issued for domiciliary purposes should be labeled to indicate-
4.   Not to be used more than 24 h. (without bactericide)
5.   Not to be used more than 7 days (with bactericide)

Practical Exercises

Exercise 1 : To prepare and dispense solution for eye drops.

Eye drops must be freshly prepared aseptically and dispensed in previously sterilized containers. A suitable fungistatic should be used in preparations liable to support the growth of moulds. For oily eye drops the oily vehicle, which has been previously sterilized by heating at 160°C for one hour must be used.

Eye drops should be made approximately isotonic with lachrymal secretion by the addition of sodium chloride or other suitable substance. Care should be taken to avoid contamination during use.

Rx

Methyl hydroxybenzoate	22.0 mg
Propyl hydroxybenzoate	11.4 mg
Purified water, sufficient to produce	100.0 ml

Method of Dispensing : Dissolve methyl hydroxybenzoate and propyl hydroxybenzoate in boiling water under aseptic condition. Add freshly boiled and cooled purified water to produce the required volume.

Exercise 2 : To prepare and dispense Zinc sulphate eye drops.

Rx

Zinc sulphate	12.5 mg
Sodium chloride	40.0 mg
Solution for eye drops, q.s. to	5.0 ml

Method of Dispensing : Dissolve weighed amount of zinc sulphate in purified water with aseptic precautions. Dissolve phenylmercuric acetate in small amount of purified water and mix the solution.

Use : Astringent

Exercise 3 : To prepare and dispense atropine sulphate eye drops.

Rx

Atropine sulphate	50.0 mg
Sodium chloride	37.5 mg
Solution for eye drops, q.s. to	5.0 ml

Method of Dispensing : Dissolve sodium chloride in solution of eye drop, add atropine sulphate and dissolve it by shaking and sterilize the product by autoclaving.

Uses : For acute inflammation of the anterior tract. The half-life in the eye is long, and effects may lasts for 7 to 12 days after topical application to the eye.

Exercise 4 : To prepare and dispense Fluorescein eye drops.

Rx

Fluorescein sodium	100.0 mg
Sodium chloride	16.0 mg
Purified water, q.s. to	5.0 ml

Method of Dispensing : Dissolve sodium chloride in purified water and add fluorescein sodium and dissolve it. Sterilize by autoclaving.

Uses : Diagnostic aid and to the conjunctiva.

Exercise 5 : To prepare and dispense Framycetin eye drops

Rx

Framycetin sulphate	25.0 mg
Sodium chloride	37.5 mg
Solution for eye drops, q.s. to	5.0 ml

Method of Dispensing : Dissolve sodium chloride in solution of eye drop and prepare a solution and add Framycetin sulphate and dissolve it by shaking. Sterile by autoclaving.

Uses : Anti-microbial

Exercise 6 : To prepare and dispense Physostigmine eye drops.

Rx

Physostigmine salicylate	25.0 mg
Sodium chloride	40.0 mg
Sodium metabisulphate	2.0 mg
Solution for eye drops, q.s. to	5.0 ml

Method of Dispensing : Dissolve sodium chloride in small volume of solution for eye drops, add physostigmine salicylate and dissolve sodium metabisulphate in solution for eye drops. Sterile the product.

Uses : Anticholinesterases

Exercise 7 : To prepare and dispense Pilocarpine eye drops.

Rx

Pilocarpine nitrate	50.0 mg
Sodium chloride	34.0 mg
Solution for eye drops	5.0 ml

Method of Dispensing : Dissolve sodium chloride in solution of eye drops, add pilocarpine nitrate and dissolve it by shaking. Sterilize by autoclaving.

Uses : glaucoma

Exercise 8 : To prepare and dispense Silver nitrate eye drops.

Rx

Silver nitrate	25.0 mg
Sodium chloride	65.0 mg
Solution for eye drop	5.0 ml

Method of Dispensing : Dissolve sodium chloride in solution of eye drop and prepare a solution. Add Silver nitrate and dissolve it by shaking. Sterilize by autoclaving.

Uses : Antiseptic, disinfectant, caustic and astringent

Exercise 9 : To prepare and dispense Sodium chloride eye lotion

Rx

Sodium chloride	0.9 g.
Purified water, sufficient to produce	100.0 ml

Method of Dispensing : Dissolve the sodium chloride in the purified water. Clarify by filtration and transfer the solution in a well-closed container. Sterilize by autoclaving

Uses : Pharmaceutical aid

Exercise 10 : To prepare and dispense Simple eye ointment.

Eye ointments must be free from large particles and should be prepared with aseptic precautions. For the preparation of simple eye ointment, it is often necessary to vary the proportion of the different ingredients of the bases to maintain a suitable consistency under different climatic conditions. Liquid paraffin, white soft paraffin and hard paraffin may be adjusted for this purpose. However, the proportions of the active medicaments must not be altered.

Rx

Wool fat	10.0 g
Yellow soft paraffin	80.0 g
Liquid paraffin, sufficient to produce	100.0 g

Method of Dispensing : Melt together weighed amount of wool fat and yellow soft paraffin in a container. Add liquid paraffin to make up weight 100 g. Filter the hot mixture through coarse filter paper placed in a heated funnel. Filtrate is sterilized by dry heat at 150°C for sufficient time to ensure that the whole is maintained at this temperature for one hour. Allow to cool at room temperature without opening the container.

Use : Pharmaceutical aid.

Exercise 11 : To prepare and dispense Chloramphenicol eye ointment.

Rx

Chloramphenicol	0.1 g
Simple eye ointment	10.0 g

Method of Dispensing : Triturate chloramphenicol with simple eye ointment aseptically. Add sufficient quantity of sterile simple eye ointment.

Uses : Antimicrobial.

CHAPTER 16

Parenterals

The term parenteral is derived from greek word *para* meaning beside and *enteron* meaning the intestine. Thus parenteral administration should include the administration of drugs by any route other than intestine. In pharmaceutical practice however parenteral products are considered to be those sterile drugs, solutions, suspensions or emulsions that are administered by hypodermic injection either in the form in which they are supplied or after the addition of suitable solvent or suspending agent etc.

Terminology

Ampoule : An all-glass hermetically sealed container for a parenteral or other sterile product.

Aseptic : It means **without sepsis,** a condition in which every reasonable means has been used to destroy and/or eliminate viable microorganisms but this condition is not achieved absolutely.

Clean : It is a relative term describing freedom from contamination. When used with parenteral medications 'clean' normally designates highly efficient cleanliness level.

Large volume parenteral (LVP) : A liquid intended for infusion and hermetically sealed in a container of greater than 100 ml volume.

Small volume parenteral (SVP) : A parenteral preparation hermetically sealed in a container of 100 ml or less volume.

Multiple-dose vial : A container usually of glass, having a relatively large opening closed by means of a rubber stopper which permits the insertion of a sharp needle and withdrawing a part of its contents.

Nosocomial : It is infection associated with a hospital.

Pyrogen : It is lipid associated with a polysaccharide or polypeptide of microbial origin and produces fever.

Injections are sterile products intended for administration of drugs by injection under or through one or more layers of skin or mucous membrane. The parenteral routes of drug administration are indicated for one or more of following reasons :

Less amount of drug is required because the drug reaches the site of action in adequate concentration.

It controls some pharmacological parameters such as time of drug onset, serum peak level, tissue concentration and rate of elimination of drug from the body.

Useful when other routes are not available for administration of drug.

It also provides a local effect when it is desirable to minimize or avoid systemic toxic effects or reactions.

It is helpful in administration of drugs to unconscious, non-cooperative or uncontrolled patients.

It exhibits biological effect that can not be achieved through oral administration because of non-absorbance of drug from the alimentary canal.

It controls correction of fluid and electrolyte imbalance rapidly.

It minimizes side effect of drug in the body.

Advantages

As compared to other dosage forms, parenteral administration offers some selective advantages.

- It provides a direct route for achieving the drug effect within the body.
- Modification of the formulation can however slow down the onset and prolong the action. This may also be achieved by the change in the route of injection.
- An immediate physiological response is usually provided by an intravenous injection of an aqueous solution.
- Free from hepatic first pass effect
- Low drug concentration
- Low toxicity as compared to solid dosage form
- Most suitable route for those drugs which are degraded or erratically or unreliably absorbed when administered orally
- Most suitable if the patient is unconscious, difficult to swallow drug etc.
- No chance of missing dose.

Disadvantages

The main disadvantages of parenteral products are :

- Requirement of aseptic technique in production, compounding and handling of product
- Requirement of trained personnel for administration
- Real or psychological pain associated with the injection
- Highly risky if any mistake at happens any point
- High cost as compared to solid dosage form

Types of Injections

- Solutions ready for injection
- Dry, soluble products ready to be combined with a solvent for injection.
- Suspensions ready for injection
- Dry insoluble products ready to be combined with a vehicle just prior to use.
- Emulsion

Routes of Administration

Route	Description
I. Primary route	
Intramuscular	Directly into the body of a relaxed muscle.
Intravenous	Directly into a vein.
Subcutaneous	Into the loose connective and adipose tissue beneath the skin.
II. Secondary route	
1. Intra-arterial	Into an artery which leads directly to the target organ.
2. Intra abdominal	Directly into the peritoneal cavity via needle or in-dwelling catheter or directly into an abdominal organ such as the kidney or bladder.
3. Intra-articular	Into synovial sacs of various accessible joints.
4. Intracardiac	Directly into chambers of the heart.
5. Intracisternal	Directly into the cisternal space surrounding the base of the brain.
6. Interadermal	Into the dermis located just beneath and adjacent to the epidermis.
7. Intralesional	Directly into or around a lesion, usually located in or on the skin or soft tissues to achieve a therapeutic effect.
8. Intraocular	Four types of intraocular injections are utilized
a. Anterior chamber	Directly into the anterior chamber of the eye.
b. Interavitreal	Directly into the vitreous cavity of the eye.
c. Retrobulbar	Around the posterior segment of the globe.
d. Subconjunctival	Injection is given beneath the conjunctiva.
9. Intrapleural	Usually single injection into the pleural cavity.
10. Intrathecal	Directly into lumbar sac located at the caudal end of spinal cord.
11. Intrauterine	Injection via a needle inserted percutaneously into pregnant uterus.
12. Intraventricular	Directly into the lateral ventricular of the brain.
13. Hypodermoclysis	Subcutaneous route of administration for infusion of large volume.

General Requirements

General requirements of parenteral products are (i) sterility (ii) freedom from physical and chemical contaminants, (iii) freedom from microbial products such as toxins, pyrogens etc. (iv) isotonicity and (v) matching of specific gravity with the body fluid(s). The general requirements of parenteral products lead to a difficult problem of selection of the vehicle, additives, stabilizers, buffers, preservatives, containers and closures, a reliable method of sterilization and measures to check the sterility, physical and chemical contamination, pyrogenicity etc., for the product. However, as a rule, one should always endeavor to use minimum number of essential additives in smallest possible quantities.

1. *Vehicle :* Water for injection (WFI) is the vehicle of first choice. It should be free from ions and pyrogens. Medicaments like barbiturates and sulphonamides need water free from carbon dioxide. Oxygen-sensitive drugs call for oxygen-free water. Water of suitable quality must be prepared by distillation or reverse osmosis. It can also be rendered free from ions by passing through an ion-exchanger. Sterile Water for Injection (SWFI) is water for injection sterilized and suitably packaged in single dose containers not exceeding 100 ml capacity and contains no bacteriostatic agent.

   Bacteriostatic Water for Injection (BWFI) is sterile water for injection containing one or more suitable bacteriostatic agents. Boiling of water makes it free from atmospheric gases and such water should be stored suitably so that the re-absorption of oxygen and carbon dioxide is not possible.

   In addition to water, some cosolvents are sometimes used to replace a portion of water in certain formulations. Thus cosolvents may be used either to increase the stability of the drug or to reduce its hydrolytic degradation. Commonly used water-miscible co-solvents include ethyl alcohol, glycerin, propylene glycol, polyethylene glycol and dimethylacetamide. Limited solubility and poor stability of some drugs either in water or in aqueous solvents may necessitate the use of non-aqueous hydrophobic solvents like fixed oils. Such vehicles must meet the requirements of degree of saturation, saponification value, iodine number, free fatty acids and unsaponifiable matter. Most commonly used oils include peanut, sesame, corn and cottonseed. Non-aqueous vehicles should be disposable by the body and should be non-irritant to the tissues. Mineral oils are rarely used as vehicles for parenteral preparations as these are not metabolisable. Primary considerations involved in the selection of a vehicle are solubility, stability and safety.

2. *Additives :* Apart from the vehicle, parenteral products contain many solutes as stabilizers of additive substances. All the solutes employed in the preparation of parenterals should be of highest purity. In addition, solutes should be free from microbial contamination and pyrogens. They should be free from microbial contamination and pyrogens. They should also conform to the solubility characteristics as desired by the physical form for the compound and should be free from gross dirt.

   (a) *Stabilizers :* Stabilizers ensure the stability of the drug compound in the preparation. Drugs in the form of their solutions are more liable to degradation through oxidation and hydrolysis and hence the stability of parenteral products against such degradation should be ensured. Oxidative degradation can be minimized by the use of antioxidants and when this course is not feasible, the products may be sealed in an inert atmosphere of nitrogen or carbon dioxide. Hydrolytic degradation can be minimized by adjustment of pH or by replacing water with other vehicles, partially or wholly. Some degradations are catalyzed by stray metallic ions and such a problem can be overcome by the use of sequestering or chelating agents like EDTA.

(b) ***Buffering agents :*** Formulations must maintain the intended pH. Changes in the pH of a product may occur during storage because of degradative reactions taking place in the product, interaction of the product with the components of the containers and loss or dissolution of gases and vapors. Such problems are avoided by the use of buffering agents to suppress the changes in pH. Commonly used buffering systems include acetates, citrates, phosphates etc.

(c) ***Antioxidants :*** Antioxidants are needed in the parenteral products containing oxygen-sensitive drugs so as to avoid oxidative degradation. Sodium bisulphite (0.1%) is the most commonly used antioxidant. Other antioxidants include acetone, sodium formaldehyde sulphoxylate and thiourea. Activity of certain antioxidants may be enhanced by the sodium salt of EDTA because it can chelate the metallic ions which otherwise catalyze the oxidative degradation reactions.

(d) ***Antimicrobial agents :*** These agents are to be essentially included in multiple-dose packagings to prevent multiplication of any accidentally introduced microbes in the products during the withdrawal of doses. Such agents should always be used with full recognition of their potential toxicity. Frequently used antimicrobial agents include phenol or cresol (0.5%), cholorocresol (0.2%), phenylmercuric nitrate (0.002%), chlorobutanol (0.5%), benzethionioum chloride and benzalkonium chloride (0.001%).

(e) ***Tonicity Contributors :*** Some parenteral solutions are required to be isotonic with blood serum or other body fluids. The overall tonicity of a solution can be calculated by computing the molecular concentration of the solute or by determining the freezing point of the solution. Tonicity of a solution is a function of the quality and quantity of sum total of the solutes present. If necessary, the tonicity of a solution may be increased by the addition of calculated amounts of substances like sodium chloride, borax etc. The materials used for tonicity adjustment must be compatible with other ingredients of the solution.

(f) ***Wetting, Suspending & Emulsifying agents :*** Wetting agents are used in injectable suspensions to maintain the particle size and to counteract caking. Commonly used wetting agents include tween-80, sorbitan trioleate, Pluronic F-68 etc. Commonly used suspending agents in parenteral suspensions are sodium CMC, methylcellulose, acacia, gelatin, polyvinylpyrrolidone etc. Sodium citrate may be included to prevent flocculation of suspended particles. Lecithin is the most commonly employed emulsifying agent for parenteral emulsions.

3. ***Containers and closures :*** Any container for parenteral product should maintain the integrity of the product as a sterile, pyrogen-free, high purity preparation till it is used. It should also be attractive, allow the withdrawal of the contents and be strong enough to withstand processing and shipping; and finally it should not interact with the product.

Glass seems to be the material of choice for containers for parenteral products. Glass containers may either be sealed or closed with rubber stoppers. Containers of Type-I glass are best for aqueous preparations. Siliconization i.e. the application of a thin film of silicone to coat the inside surface of the vials and ampoules, has been employed to prevent interaction of the product with the glass surface. The process also minimizes adsorption of active ingredients from homogeneous solutions, prevents adsorption of solids from suspensions and prevents aggregation at the glass surface in colloidal preparations.

Plastics used in the packaging of parenteral products are based on polyethylene or polypropylene. Plastic containers are much less used as compared to glass but the former are becoming increasingly popular for intravenous fluids. Only polypropylene containers can withstand sterilization by autoclaving. Many plastics contain additives like plasticizers, antioxidants, antistatic agents and lubricants. These additives may leach out from the plastic into the product. Most plastics selectively permit passage of chemical molecules and are permeable to gases. Plastics are extensively used for containers of administration sets particularly disposable type.

As compared to glass, plastics are light weight, less fragile and easy to handle but most of them are not as clear as glass.

Rubber is the material of choice for closures for multi-dose vials, intravenous fluids bottles, plugs for disposable syringes and bulbs for ophthalmic pipettes. Rubber closures permit the introduction of a needle from a hypodermic syringe into a multi-dose vial and provide for resealing of the vial after the needle is withdrawn. Rubber closure is held in place by an aluminium band. Such closures are composed of several ingredients, basic structural unit being a linear unsaturated hydrocarbon, isoprene. All or part of the natural polymer is sometimes replaced by a variety of synthetic rubber polymers. In addition, a vulcanizing agent usually sulphur; an accelerator e.g., 2-mercaptobenzothiazole; an activator, usually zinc oxide; fillers such as carbon black or limestone; antioxidants and lubricants etc., may also be present in rubber closures. These substances may be leached into the product or may cause chemical interaction. Lacquer or plastic coating applied to the surface of the rubber closures in contact with the product may partially reduce leaching and also permeation. Another most commonly encountered problem with rubber closures is that of **coring** i.e., the generation of rubber particles cut from the closures when needles are inserted; the particles are known as cores. Selection of the proper gauge needle and its proper use may minimize the problem of coring.

Adjustment of Tonicity and Specific Gravity

When red blood cells are introduced into water or sodium chloride solution containing less than 0.9% of the solute, they swell and often burst due to the diffusion of water into the cells and the fact that the cell wall is not strong enough to resist the pressure. This phenomenon is called haemolysis. Parenteral products are made isotonic with the body fluids otherwise they may penetrate the red blood cells and cause haemolysis. Additives present in parenteral solutions contribute to the overall hemolytic character of the solution. If the solutions are hypotonic, the osmotic pressure of the solutions can be increased by the addition of either sodium chloride or dextrose. Compounds which contribute to the isotonicity of a product also reduce pain at the site of injection in areas with nerve endings. A 1.8% solution of urea has the same osmotic pressure as 0.9% sodium chloride solution but the urea solution produces haemolysis. Hence a product should not be considered isotonic until it has been tested in the biological system.

Administration of hypertonic solutions into the blood stream may cause crenulation of cells which may return to normal with equalization of osmotic pressure. In such cases a slow injection into a vein, in which circulation is rapid, is indicated as the solution is thereby rapidly diluted and swept away.

Parenteral products are sometimes required to possess specific gravity matching with that of the body fluids and hence such adjustments may also be called for. The intraspinal injections should have predetermined specific gravity as compared to body fluid into which it is to be injected. This is of particular importance in spinal anesthesia. In case the upper part of the patient's body is raised by slopping the operating table, the solution of lower specific gravity than the spinal fluid will tend to rise on injection and that of higher specific gravity will tend to sink. For operation on the lower part of the body where the patient is titled head downwards the opposite effects will occur. Hence a careful choice must be made of the specific gravity of the solution and the position of the patient. The average specific gravity of spinal fluid at 37°C may be taken as 1.0059. The specific gravity of injection solution with respect to that of spinal fluid is expressed as isobaric (i.e. of equal) hypobaric (i.e. lower) and hyperbaric (i.e. higher). A 1 in 5000 solution of cinchocaine hydrochloride in 0.5% saline is a hypobaric solution having a specific gravity of 1,0036 at 37°C. A 1 in 200 solution of cinchocaine hydrochloride in 6% dextrose gives a hyperbaric solution having specific gravity of 1.02.

Precautions for Aseptic Work

The prime object of aseptic work is to keep the products being processed free from microbial contamination. The following precautions should always be observed in aseptic work.

- Whenever possible, a non-touch technique should be used.
- Air disturbance should be minimum.
- Interruption should be minimum.
- There should be a program for maintenance of the area and the personnel.
- Only trained personnel should perform aseptic work.
- Frequent tests should be performed in the aseptic area to monitor the level of contamination.

- Whenever contamination is detected, the sources should be identified and dealt with accordingly.
- After the aseptic work is over, the product should be removed to quarantine and aseptic area should be thoroughly cleaned, disinfected and kept ready for next operation.

Filling, sealing and sterilization

Mixing, clarification, filling, sealing and sterilization are the common techniques involved in the preparation of parenteral products.

Filling

Solutions sterilized by filtration are to be filled under aseptic conditions. The containers and closures must be properly cleaned, sterilized and made available for use at this point in the process. Filling consists of transferring a quantity of the product measured with precision and accuracy from a bulk container to a unit container. The transferring device should not contribute any contamination and the product at this stage should be adequately protected so that it does not pick up any particulate or microbial contamination from the environment. Modern day automatic high speed filling machines can fill up to 300 or more containers per minute. As a safeguard against the entry of particulate matter in a product during filling, a final filter is often inserted in the system between the filter and the delivery tube.

Sealing

Sealing of the filled container should be done as soon as possible to prevent the contents from being contaminated. Sealing represents the final aseptic procedure. Ampoules are sealed by melting a portion of the glass neck with a fine jet of flame. For rapid sealing, a high temperature gas-oxygen flame is most suitable. A variety of automated sealing devices are available today. For making 'pull-seals', the neck of the ampoule is heated below the tip leaving most of the tip for grasping with forceps or other mechanical devices. The ampoule is constantly rotated in the flame from a single burner to soften the glass and then the tip is grasped firmly and pulled quickly away from the body of the ampoule which still continues to rotate. A small capillary tube is formed which is closed by twisting. Although pull-sealing is slow yet the seals are more perfect than tip sealing.

Vials and bottles are sealed by closing the opening with a rubber closure which is held in position by means of aluminium caps. An intact aluminium cap is the proof that the closure has not been removed. Single layered aluminium caps may be applied by means of a hand crimper while double or triple layered caps are crimped by means of heavy duty mechanical crimpers.

Sterilization

Sterilization is process of complete destruction or removal of all forms of life. Except in case of thermolabile substances, parenteral products are commonly sterilized after filling and sealing in the final containers and the process is called terminal sterilization.

Injections are sterilized by following methods :

- Moist heat sterilization

- Dry heat sterilization

- Filtration through bacteria proof filters

- Using aseptic techniques

Thermolabile preparations should be sterilized by non-thermal methods. Thermo-labile solutions are mostly sterilized by filtration through bacteria proof filters. Other thermo-labile preparations like colloids, oleaginous solutions, suspensions and emulsions may require a process of sterilizing each component separately and the product is processed under aseptic conditions. Sterilization by radiation is another non-thermal method. Dry solids such as penicillin, streptomycin, polyvitamins and certain hormones can be effectively sterilized by ionized radiations. Gaseous sterilization is no good when a glass container or other impervious barrier prevents the gas from permeation to the material.

Dry heat sterilization is also of limited application because the materials being sterilized by this method should not be adversely affected by the elevated temperatures.

Most useful sterilization method is autoclaving which employs steam under pressure. It is probably the most effective method for sterilization of aqueous liquids or substances that can be reached or penetrated by steam. This method is ineffective under anhydrous conditions like a sealed ampoule containing dry solid or anhydrous oil. To prevent subsequent contamination after sterilization, the materials subjected to autoclaving must be wrapped or covered but this is not necessary in case of parenterals. Solutions as they are already sealed. The effectiveness of sterilization method should be verified from time to time. Biological indicators are a useful tool for ascertaining the effectiveness of this method.

Aseptic Technique

Aseptic technique is defined as procedures that will minimize the chance of contamination with micro-organisms. Contaminants may be brought into the aseptic area by equipment, supplies, or people, so it is important to control these factors during preparation. A number of simple guidelines should be followed:

- Before using the laminar air flow hood the operator should wash his hands with a suitable antimicrobial / detergent at the beginning of their work and when re-entering the aseptic preparation area.

- Gown, gloves or mask if needed thereof should be sterilised.

- Activities unrelated to product preparation should be kept to a minimum.

- Eating or drinking, or the storage of food, or personal items should not be allowed in the aseptic area.

- One person should working in the hood at a time.

- All items that will be used during preparation should be checked for defects and expiry dates prior to use.

- All non-sterile item surfaces should be disinfected prior to being placed into the hood.

- All items necessary for the preparation should be placed into the hood prior to commencing the procedure.

- Direct contact between a sterile product and any non-sterile product should be avoided.

- All non-sterile surface areas should be swabbed with alcohol (70% isopropyl) and left for 30 seconds.

- Ampoules and vials should be opened and contents aspirated using appropriate techniques to avoid particulate contamination.

- Reconstituted powders should be mixed carefully according to manufacturer's recommendations to ensure complete dissolution of the drug.

- Needle entry into vials with rubber stoppers should be done at a 45^0 angle to minimize rubber core particulates.

- All finished products should be carefully inspected after preparation for visible precipitation.

- Each prepared sterile product should be assigned an expiry date based upon available data.

Small Volume Parenterals (SVPs) : Small volume of parenterals include ampoules of 1 ml, 2 ml, 3 ml, 5, ml up to 20 ml and vials of 1 ml, 2 ml, up to 30 ml. They are administered by various routes such as intramuscular, intravenous, subcutaneous, intraspinal, intracisternal, intrathecal etc.

Large Volume Parenterals (LVPs) : LVPs contain 100 ml and more of injectable solution. They are generally administered by intravenous route. Two types of solutions are available in the market.

Electrolytes : sodium chloride and potassium chloride solutions, etc

Non-electrolytes : Dextrose and mannitol solutions, etc

Powder Parenterals : Dry powders are available in the market. They are soluble in water for injection or in another sterile solvent just prior to use. They are available in the form of vials containing rubber closure and sealed with aluminium file. Following antibiotics are available in the form of dry powder e.g. penicillin, ampicillin, chloramphenicol, amoxycillin, sterptomycin, etc.

Table 16.1 Container Materials.

Material	Water vapor permeation	Gas permeation	Reaction with product	Physical properties
I. Thermoplastic				
Polymers				
1. Polyethylene				
a. Low density	High	Low	Low	Translucent, flexible
b. High density	Low	Low	Low	Translucent, semi-rigid
2. Polypropylene	Moderate	Low	Low	Translucent, semi-rigid
3.Polyvinyl chloride				
a. Flexible	High	Low	Moderate	Transparent, flexible
b. Rigid	High	Low	Low	Transparent, rigid
4. Polycarbonate	High	Low	Low	Transparent, rigid
5. Polyamide	High	Low	High	Translucent, rigid, tough
6. Polystyrene	High	High	Moderate	Transparent, rigid
7. Teflon	Low	Low	Nil	Translucent, rigid, tough temperature resistant
II Glass				
1. Soda-lime	None	None	High	Optically clear, rigid
2. Borosilicate	None	None	Low	Optically clear, rigid
II.Rubber				
1. Butyl	Low	Moderate	Moderate	Opaque, flexible
2. Natural	Moderate	Moderate	High	Opaque, flexible
3. Neoprene	Moderate	Moderate	High	Opaque, flexible
4. Polyisoprene	Moderate	Moderate	Moderate	Opaque, flexible
5. Silicone	Very high	Very high	Low	Translucent, flexible

Volume of Injection

Each single dose container contains slightly excess amount that can not be withdrawn. The excess volumes usually permitted are shown in the following Table 16.2.

Table 16.2

Volume specified (ml)	Excess volume permissible (mobile liquid) (ml)	Excess volume permissible (viscous liquid) (ml)
0.5	0.10	0.12
1.0	0.10	0.15
2.0	0.15	0.25
5.0	0.30	0.50
10.0	0.50	0.70
20.0	0.60	0.90
50.0 or more	about 2%	about 3%

Cleaning and Sterilization of Vials

- Vials are cleaned and sterilized before filling. Following procedure is used for cleaning and sterilization of vials.
- Soak the vial with detergent solution overnight to remove any sticking particles, grease, etc.
- Wash with tap water three to four times till soap solution is completely removed.
- Remove surface alkalinity using 1.0% hydrochloric acid solution.
- Again wash the vial using tap water till free from alkalinity.
- Rinse with de-ionized water and finally with distilled water.
- Cleaned vials are sterilized by dry heat sterilization at 200°C for 4 hours.
- Cool sterilized vials at room temperature under the closed condition prior to filling the vials.
- Cleaning and Sterilization of Rubber closures
- Rubber closures are boiled with 1.0% solution of liquid detergent for 30 minutes.
- Wash with tap water till free from detergent.
- Boil for 30 min. using 1.0% solution of hydrochloric acid.
- Wash to make them free from acid.
- Boil the acid washed rubber closures with 1.0% sodium carbonate solution and wash till free alkali.
- Treat rubber stoppers with double strength bacteriostatic solution.
- Wash three to four times using pyrogen free water.
- Sterilize by autoclave at 115°C for 30 minutes.

Exercise 1 : To prepare Water for Injection (WFI)

WFI can not be prepared by simple distillation method because in that case the pyrogens may enter mechanically into the condenser and ultimately into the receiver. Injection of distilled water may cause rise in body temperature due to the presence of pyrogens. Water, which increases body temperature, is known as apyrogenic.

It can also cause chills, pains in back and legs. Pyrogens are metabolite end products of bacteria. They are non-filterable, thermo-stable, and non-volatile in nature. The pH of water for injection should be as near as possible to pH 7.0.

It should also be free from carbon dioxide because slight acidity of WFI is sufficient to precipitate the alkaloidal salts like phenobarbitone and sulphonamides. Water for injection should be free from dissolved air. It is necessary to prevent sensitive medicament from oxidation.

Method of Preparation : Distilled **portable** water from a neutral glass or metal still fitted with an efficient device from preventing the entrapment of droplets. The first portion of distillate should be rejected and remaining amount of water should be collected in suitable container and immediately sterilized by heating in an autoclave or by filtration without addition of a bacteriostatic.

Exercise 2 : To prepare Ascorbic acid injection

Rx

Ascorbic acid	1.03 g
Sodium bicarbonate	2.47 g
Propyleneglycol	2.50 g
Sodium hydrosulphite	0.25 g
Disodium edetate	0.05 g
WFI, qs	50.0 ml

Method of Preparation : Dissolve ascorbic acid slowly under constant stirring and nitrogen bubbling and add sodium bicarbonate with slow stirring. Separately prepare solution of sodium hydrosulphite in small proportion of WFI and add in the solution, add solution of disodium edetate and mix uniformly. The pH is adjusted to 5.5 to 6.5 using sodium hydroxide solution or ascorbic acid solution. Make up the volume and mix with water for injection. Sterilize by passing through sterilized 0.22 μm membrane filter into sterilized filling vessel. Aseptically fill 5.3 ml in sterilized 5 ml amber colour ampoules.

Exercise 3 : To prepare Dextrose Injection

Dextrose Injection is a sterile solution of anhydrous dextrose or an equivalent quantity of dextrose monohydrate for parenteral administration. If the concentration of the solution is not reported, a 5% *w/v* solution should be prepared because it is isotonic with blood serum. Dextrose decomposes on heating. The rate of decomposition depends on sterilization temperature, duration of sterilization and presence of other substances. Decomposition of dextrose is reduced by adjusting the pH between 3.5 to 6.5 with hydrochloric acid; heating time should be minimum and over heating should be avoided. It should be cooled as quickly as possible after sterilization of the solution. Solution should not adhere to the neck of ampoules because it gets charred during the process of sealing. Injection should not be used if it contains a precipitate or any suspended particle.

Rx

| Dextrose | 5.0 g |
| WFI | 100.0 ml |

Method of Preparation : Dissolve the weighed quantity of dextrose in WFI and add sufficient WFI to produce 100 ml. The ampoules are sealed and sterilized immediately by autoclaving.

Exercise 4 : To prepare Sodium Chloride Injection

Rx

| Sodium chloride | 0.9 g |
| WFI, qs | 100.0 ml |

Method of Preparation : Dissolve sodium chloride in sufficient quantity of WFI and add sufficient WFI to produce 100 ml. Fill the solution into the ampoules and seal them. Sterilize by autoclaving as quickly as possible. Sterilization can also be done by filtration.

Exercise 5 : To prepare Calcium Gluconate Injection

Rx

Calcium gluconate	.0 g
Calcium D-saccharate	1.75 g
WFI, qs	100.0 ml

Method of Preparation : Dissolve calcium gluconate in WFI and add calcium D-saccharate in solution. Adjust the pH between 6.0 to 8.2 using 10% solution of sodium hydroxide. Filter through 0.45 µm membrane filter. Sterilize by autoclave at 121°C for 30 minutes.

Exercise 6 : To prepare Chloramphenicol Injection

Rx

Chloramphenicol	12.5 g
Lignocaine hydrochloride	0.514 g
Lignocain base	0.405 g
Chlorocresol	1.0 g
Distilled water	12.0 ml
Propylene glycol	100.0 ml

Method of Preparation : Add chloramphenicol in hot propylene glycol and stir till dissolved, add lignocaine base and dissolve with continuous stirring. Dissolve chlorocresol and lignocaine hydrochloride separately in distilled water and add in the solution and stir well. Add sufficient propylene glycol to produce sufficient volume up to 100 ml. Adjust pH of the solution between 6.5 to 6.8. Filter the solution by vacuum filtration using Whatman filter paper No.1 and then pass through G-3 sintered glass funnel. Aseptically fill 10.5 ml of solution in dry sterile 10 ml amber color vials with washed sterile butyl grey plugs and seal.

Exercise 7 : To prepare Cyanocobalamin Injection

Rx

Cyanocobalamin	0.12 g
Sodium chloride	0.75 g
Sodium dihydrogen phosphate	0.30 g
Benzyl alcohol	1.0 ml
WFI, qs	100.0 ml

Method of Preparation : Dissolve cynocobalmin in WFI and add benzyl alcohol and mix. Add sodium chloride, and sodium dihydrogen phosphate separately in WFI. Add the solution to the mixture of vitamins. Adjust pH between 4.0 to 5.5. Fill aseptically in 10 ml amber color vials.

Exercise 8 : To prepare Dextrose with Sodium Chloride Solution

Rx

Dextrose5.0%

Sodium chloride0.9%

Activated charcoal5.0%

WFI, qs100.0 ml

Method of Preparation : Dissolve excess amount of dextrose in WFI and add activated charcoal and other additives, filter and sterilize by autoclaving.

Exercise 9 : To prepare Compound Sodium Chloride Injection

Rx

Sodium chloride	0.86 g
Potassium chloride	0.030 g
Calcium chloride hydrated	0.033 g
WFI, qs	100.0 ml

Method of Preparation : Dissolve sodium chloride, potassium chloride, calcium chloride hydrated in WFI and add sufficient WFI to produce 100 ml. Filter the solution and immediately sterilize by autoclave. It can be sterilized by filtration.

Exercise 10 : To prepare Sodium Citrate Anticoagulant Injection

Rx

Sodium citrate	4.0 g
WFI qs	100.0 ml

Method of Preparation : Dissolve the sodium citrate in 90 ml of water for injection. Filter and add sufficient water for injection to produce 100 ml, immediately sterilize by heating in an autoclave or by filtration.

CHAPTER 17

Incompatibility

Incompatibility signifies the problems arising when two or more ingredients prescribed, result into undesirable changes in the appearance, safety or therapeutic purpose of the product. Interaction of a drug with another drug, or of a drug with additives or adjuvants, dosage errors, omissions etc., also fall under incompatibility. Incompatibility may occur in compounding and dispensing of prescriptions so also at any stage during formulation, manufacturing, packaging, storage or administration of drugs. Contrary to expectations, the importance of incompatibility has increased in modern pharmaceutical practice mainly due to the introduction of large number of newer and more complex drugs as well as the indiscriminate use of combination therapy. In present day dispensing practice since the pharmacist invariably reviews each and every prescription, he should be in a position to detect and overcome the incompatibilities. This calls for the ingenuity of a pharmacist who is knowledgeable in pharmacy, pharmacology and chemistry. The problem of incompatibility is to be solved mainly through two angles firstly the detection or prediction of possible occurrence, and secondly, the correction which comprises of preventing or minimizing the incompatibility.

Incompatibility may be classified as physical, chemical and therapeutic.

I. Physical Incompatibility

Physical incompatibility is mostly due to insolubility. However, liquefaction and physical complexation are not uncommon. Such incompatibilities are easier to predict, detect and correct by applying proper technique, mixing, selection of additives etc. Physical incompatibilities are commonly manifested by non-uniform, unsightly or unpalatable products. Physical incompatibilities may be classified as follows:

A. *Insolubility :* Insolubility or immiscibility results in non-homogeneous product when two or more substances are combined. Separation of two phases when oil and water are shaken together (i.e. emulsion) is the classical example of such incompatibility but it is corrected by the use of an emulsifying agent whereby a uniform dispersion of one phase into the other is obtained. Gums are insoluble in alcohol and resins are insoluble in water. Insoluble substances like phenacetin, salol, precipitated sulphur etc. in mixtures require the use of a thickening agent. Use of another solvent or a cosolvent usually resolves the problem of insolubility.

Example 1

Rx

Terpin hydrate			3.0 g
Simple Syrup	q.s.	ad	120.0 ml
M. Ft. Sol.			

In this preparation terpin hydrate is not soluble in syrup and hence half of the vehicle may be replaced by alcohol or isoalcoholic elixir. Alternate remedy would be to use any suspending agent (acacia, tragacanth or methocel) and dispense the product with a `shake well' label.

Example 2

Rx

Phenobarbital	250.0 mg
Elixir Phenobarbital q.s. ad	30.0 ml
M. Ft. Sol.	
Sig : Teaspoonful at bedtime	

In this preparation phenobarbital is in excess and hence all of it is not soluble in the elixir. 10 ml of the elixir should be replaced by alcohol and 40 mg more of phenobarbital added to compensate the loss in phenobarbital (10 ml of the elixir).

Sometimes the prescriber may intend for reasons of stability or for therapeutic efficacy that insoluble compound be suspended rather than solubilized. Thus it is recommended that the intention of the prescriber should be held supreme.

Example 3

Rx

Aspirin			gr V
Cherry syrup	q.s.	ad oz i.	
D.T.D. $\neq$ 24			

Here a suspension is prepared because of better stability of aspirin in suspension than in a solution.

Example 4.

Rx

Zinc sulphate	4.0
Sulphurated potash	4.0
Rose water q.s ad	60.0

Again a suspension is intended because the active ingredients are the insoluble polysulphides formed by the reaction of the two compounds employed. A suitable suspending agent is to be included.

B. *Precipitation :* A drug in solution may be precipitated upon addition of a solvent in which it is insoluble. Thus resins are precipitated from alcoholic solution on addition of water. Mucilaginous and albuminous substances may be precipitated from aqueous solution on addition of alcohol.

Precipitation from a saturated solution is often referred to as salting out.

- Camphor and volatile oils may get salted out of aromatic waters when salts of metals are dissolved in the liquid.

- Addition of electrolytes to colloidal solutions often results into precipitation.

- Addition of tragacanth is responsible for precipitation of boric acid from a saturated solution.

C. *Separation of immiscible liquids :* A prescription containing ethyl nitrite spirit and substantial amount of potassium citrate will separate out and a layer of spirit will float.

Example 5

Rx

Chloral hydrate	15.00 g
Sodium bromide	11.25 g
Elixir aromatic q.s. ad	60.00 ml

Soluble bromide is responsible for separating an immiscible layer consisting of chloral alcoholate, chloral and alcohol. In order to obtain a clear solution the alcoholic strength of the prescription should be above 50% or below 10%. A simple remedy would therefore be to dilute it with water to bring alcohol concentration to below 10% and inform the physician.

D. *Liquefaction of Solid :* Liquefaction of dry solid materials may result from eutexia, release of water of hydration or absorption of water. Many drugs containing a phenol, aldehyde, or ketone group possess this tendency. Phenol, menthol, thymol and salol when mixed with one another, form eutectic mixtures. Liquefaction occurring at room temperature due to depression in melting point of a solid in contact with certain other components is known as eutexia. Eutectic forming ingredients may be dispensed separately or if a pasty mass has already resulted, the eutectic may be absorbed on sufficient inert diluent such as kaolin, talc, starch, magnesium carbonate, light magnesium carbonate, light magnesium oxide; and suitably dispensed.

Example 6

Rx

Menthol	5.0
Camphor	5.0
Ammonium chloride	30.0
Magnesium carbonate, light	60.0

Make insufflation, send 4 oz.

Menthol, Camphor and ammonium chloride can be diluted separately with light magnesium carbonate and then mixed with gentle trituration in ascending order of weights.

Example 7

Rx

Aminopyrine	0.3 g
Codeine sulphate	15.0 mg
Belladonna extract	10.0 mg
Acetyl salicylic acid	0.2 g

M.ft. Caps. ≠1. DTD ≠ 12.

Aminopyrine and acetyl salicylic acid form eutectic mixture. The resultant wetting of belladonna extract is further responsible for intensification of its green colour. 65 mg of light magnesium oxide per capsule should be included as diluent. One half of the quantity of the diluent is mixed with aminopyrine and the other half with acetyl salicylic acid and both are combined with gentle trituration. The remaining ingredients are then incorporated as usual.

E. ***Physical complexation :*** Preparations containing carbowax and phenols, salicylic acid or tannic acid are known to show loss in elegance and acceptability due to physical complexation. Their complexation is attributed to hydrogen bonding between the hydroxyl groups of the active ingredient and the ether oxygen of the polyether chain. Complexation of benzoic acid, salicylic acid, sulphonamides and barbiturates with urea is also reported.

Example 8

Rx

Phenol		1.0 g
Polyethylene glycol 400		10.0 ml
Zinc oxide		15.0 g
Purified Water q.s.	ad	100.0 ml

M.ft. lotion.

Unsatisfactory suspension is produced due to complexation of phenol and PEG, and phenol is inactivated. PEG may be substituted by bentonite magma. Physical complexation may not be physically evident and hence prediction may be difficult. But it may result in therapeutic incompatibility.

F. ***Miscellaneous :*** Drugs insoluble in water are not uniformly distributed in the bulk of the preparation and these results in non-uniform dose delivery. The problem is solved by (i) increasing the viscosity of the vehicle, and (ii) using suspending agents. In fact the suspending agents also act by enhancing the viscosity of the vehicle thus minimizing the settling of the solids. Suspending agents which are commonly used include acacia, tragacanth, methylcellulose derivatives; clays like bentonite; glycerin and syrups.

II. Chemical Incompatibility

This term signifies the chemical changes which occur due to the interaction of the prescribed substances leading to the formation of a harmful or dangerous product. Chemical incompatibilities often occur due to oxidation-reduction, hydrolysis or combination reactions. A chemical incompatibility, which is visualized rapidly by effervescence, precipitation or colour change, is called **immediate** incompatibility. An incompatibility without immediate and visible physical change is known as **delayed** incompatibility and may or may not result in loss of therapeutic activity.

Unintentional incompatibility may be **tolerated** i.e. interaction is minimized but composition of the prescription is not altered; or **adjusted** i.e. interaction is prevented by addition or substitution of constituents without affecting the medicinal action of the preparation. It is recommended that the pharmacist must consult or notify the prescriber about the suggested modification in the prescription while overcoming the incompatibility. However, this should be done in such a manner as not to raise any doubt in the mind of the patient.

Chemical incompatibilities may be classified as follows:

A. ***Oxidation-reduction*** : Oxidation refers to the loss of electrons and reduction to the gain of electrons. Prescription mixtures are usually oxidized on exposure to air, higher storage temperatures, light, over dilution, incorrect pH adjustment or in presence of catalysis. Use of antioxidants such as ascorbic acid, sodium sulphite or sodium metabisulphite is often helpful. Trace metal ion catalysis may be counteracted by complexing agents such as disodium edetate and sodium calcium edetate. Auto-oxidation in fats and oils, phenolic substances, aldehydes and vitamins is controlled by agents such as propyl gallate, thymol, butylated hydroxyanisole (BHA), butylated hydroxytoluene (BHT), and hydroquinone etc. Silver, mercury and gold salts may be reduced by light to the metallic form although such reactions are rare in prescriptions.

Example 9

Rx

Sodium salicylate	8.0 g
Sodium bicarbonate	16.0 g
Peppermint water q.s. ad	180.0 ml
M.ft. sol.	

The solution darkens on standing due to alkali catalysed oxidation of salicylate to quinoid form. Sodium bisulphite (0.1%) may be used as antoxidant to prevent the development of colour.

Example 10

Rx

Potassium chlorate	4.0 g
Syrup ferric iodide	15.0 ml
Purified Water q.s. ad	180.0 ml

The probable reaction is $KClO_3 + 3FeI_2 = 3 FeOI + KCl + 3I$

Ferric oxide is oxidized with potassium chlorate. This mixture remains quite clear when fresh but on standing for some time, crystals of iodine are deposited. For solving this problem, the two reacting substances must be dispensed separately.

Example 11

Rx

Mild mercurous chloride	gr XVIII
Potassium bromide	gr XXX
Sucrose	gr XXIV

M. Ft. powders = 12

The incompatibility occurs in the presence of moisture. Mercurous chloride reacts with potassium bromide, resulting in simultaneous oxidation and reduction of the mercurous salt to mercuric bromide and free mercury. The prescription should not be dispensed.

B. *Acid-base reactions* : Such reactions result into precipitation, gas formation, colour development or colour change.

Precipitation

Except for the alkali metals, soluble inorganic salts react with hydroxides to yield water-insoluble compounds. Soluble salts of phenols, carboxylic acids and barbituric acids also yield free acid in the presence of relatively strong acids. Similarly, soluble salts of amine drugs liberate free base in the presence of relatively strong bases. Correction of acid-base incompatibilities requires thorough knowledge relating to acid-base strengths and solubilities of the acidic and basic forms of the particular compounds in question.

Example 12

Rx

Cocaine HCl	0.3 g
Boric acid	0.3 g
Sodium borate aa	1.2 g
Purified water q.s. ad	60.0 ml

Sodium borate imparts alkalinity and the water-insoluble cocaine base is precipitated. Elimination of sodium borate would solve the problem.

Evolution of gas : Gas may be evolved due to a chemical reaction between ingredients. Evolution of carbon dioxide resulting from the reaction of carbonates and acids in aqueous media, and decomposition of syrups of p-amino salicylic acid, are common examples. Boric acid in the presence of glycerin forms glyceroboric acid that reacts with bicarbonates and gas is evolved.

Example 13

Rx

Sodium bicarbonate		1.50
Borax		1.50
Phenol		0.75
Glycerin		25.00
Purified Water q.s. ad		100.00

Make a spray.

The substances should be mixed with water in an open vessel until effervescence ceases.

Change in or Development of Colour : Most of the dyes employed in pharmaceutical practice and their colour are influenced by their ionization depending on pH of the solution. Laxative phenolphethalein is colourless in acid solution but red in alkaline mixtures. Gentian violet is a basic purple compound but on addition of acid, the compound changes the colour through green to yellow. Such incompatibilities are corrected by the addition of a buffer or change of the vehicle to prevent formation of free acid or base from the salt.

C. ***Hydrolysis :*** Many substances hydrolyse in water and their reaction may be facilitated by heat catalysts, hydrogen ions and hydroxyl ions. Esters, amides and metals like Zn and Fe etc., are common examples. Soluble salts of barbituric acid derivatives and sulphonamides hydrolyze in water and yield insoluble free acids. Phenyl salicylate hydrolyses in basic media to salicylic acid and phenol. Addition of any of the species formed as a result of hydrolysis is a common method employed to prevent or reverse the ionic hydrolysis. Examples of drug substances which may undergo hydrolytic decomposition include procaine, sulphonamides, chlorothiazide, barbituric acid derivatives, aspirin, some alkaloids, and penicillin. Similarly gelatin, sucrose, sodium acetate, flavouring oils and chlorobutanol; some of the common ingredients in prescriptions; are also liable to decomposition by hydrolysis.

Example 14

Rx

Sodium salicylate	8.0 g
Phenobarbital sodium	5.4 g
Vitamin B complex elixir	240 ml

The alkalinity of salts causes decomposition by hydrolysis of the B vitamins of the acidic vitamin B complex elixir and precipitation of the acids of the sodium salts. To overcome the problem the salts should be dispensed separately.

Example 15

Rx

Penicillin G sodium	1,000,000 u
Syrup of cherry q.s. ad	30 ml
M.ft. sol.	

Penicillin salt is hydrolyzed in acidic medium and penicillin is precipitated as free acid. Rate of hydrolysis can be slowed down by employing a neutral vehicle.

D. *Explosive combinations :* Oxidizing agents are chemically reactive with reducing agents and some of these combinations may be potentially explosive.

Example 16

Rx

Potassium chlorate	0.6 g
Tannic acid	0.3 g
Sucrose aa	0.3 g
Make a powder. DTD $\neq$ 20	

Ingredients of this prescription can be compounded with minimum rubbing. Tumbling the powders on a sheet of paper is also satisfactory. Alternately, each ingredient powdered individually, can be dispensed separately with adequate directions to the user. Explosion may take place if the ingredients are mixed by simple trituration in a pestle and mortar.

E. *Racemization :* It is the conversion of an optically active form of a drug substance to an optically inactive form without a change in chemical constitution but is usually associated with a reduction in pharmacological activity. Examples of substances undergoing racemization are adrenaline, ephedrine, norephedrine etc. In alkaline solution but not in acid solutions, l-hyoscyamine may undergo racemization to form atropine.

F. *Other changes :* Other types of chemical incompatibility may occur as a result of cementation (due to formation of hydrates e.g., plaster of Paris, polymerization, or conversion to new crystal habits), development of heat or lowering in temperature, polymerization, double decomposition, substitution, addition etc.

III   Therapeutic Incompatibility

When the response to one or more drugs in the patient is of a nature or intensity different from that intended, it is known as therapeutic incompatibility. It is within the realm of the physician and mainly concerned with prescribing errors and post-administration effect. Some of the adverse drug reactions may be considered as examples of therapeutic incompatibilities. Drug interactions have been dealt with in a separate chapter in this book. Common types of therapeutic incompatibilities are due to:

A. *Dosage errors :* Dispensing of an overdose of a prescription constitutes the most serious type of dosage errors. Any experienced pharmacist should be able to detect such an error while checking the prescription.

Example 17

Rx

Atropine sulphate	0.006
Phenobarbital	0.015
Aspirin	0.300

M.ft. cap. 1. Disp.≠12.

Sig : One capsule t.i.d.

The quantity of atropine sulphate for a single capsule is more than the recommended maximum dose. The physician should be contacted.

B. ***Wrong dose or dosage form :*** As many drugs have confusingly similar names, there is always a possibility of dispensing the wrong drug e.g., prednisone and prednisolone, protamine and protamide, digoxin and digitoxin. Similarly many dugs are available in different dosage forms and hence if the dosage form is not mentioned clearly on the prescription, the pharmacist must seek clarification from the prescriber. It is highly desirable that the pharmacist should be aware of the potential hazard of such errors.

C. ***Contraindicated drugs :*** Certain drugs may be contraindicated in a particular disease or when a particular patient is allergic to it. Thus corticosteroids are contraindicated in patients having an active peptic ulcer. Morphine, barbiturates, and related drugs may be dangerous in severe asthma. Vasoconstrictors should not be given to any hypertensive patient.

Example 18

Rx

Sulphadiazine	0.25 g
Sulphamerazine	0.25 g
Ammonium chloride	0.5 g

M.cap. DTD ≠ 36.

Sig : 2 caps. q 4h for cough.

Ammonium chloride being a urinary acidifier, would cause deposition of sulphonamide crystals in the kidney. It being a contraindicated combination, the physician should be contacted.

E. ***Synergistic or antagonistic drugs :*** Prescribing of synergistic or antagonistic drugs may be either deliberate or by mistake. The activity of penicillin derivatives may be prolonged by the use of probenecid and hence this combination is advantageous therapeutically as well as economically. Prescribing an amphetamine with a babiturate is apparently antagonistic combination but has been accepted in modern therapeutic practice to help in weight control. Some other antagonistic combinations would result in prescribing stimulants with sedatives, cholinergic drug with anticholinergic drug, purgatives with antidiarrhoeals etc. Concurrent use of an antacid with tetracycline will lead to decreased absorption of the antibiotic.

In conclusion it must be emphasized that although incompatibility continues to pose a serious problem in drug therapy, an experienced pharmacist should be able to detect and reasonably correct the same through his professional knowledge, skill and common sense. Drug interactions also lead to incompatibility.

CHAPTER 18

Community Pharmacy

The drugs are vital to the health of individuals and hence the drugs are classified as "essential commodity" under the Essential Commodities Act, 1955. The manufacture, sale and distribution etc., of drugs warrant the specialized knowledge, skill and experience. The Drugs and Cosmetics Act, 1940 and Rules 1945 have been passed with the objective of regulating the import, manufacture, distribution and sale of drugs and cosmetics. Cosmetics are although a luxury item, they may contain some ingredients, the constant use of which might prove to be harmful and hence need control. The Act regulates the manufacture and sale of drugs and cosmetics through licensing so that these are manufactured, distributed and sold only by qualified persons. To have a check on such operations, the Central and State Drugs Control authorities are established. Prior to the enactment of this Act, any drug or cosmetic could be imported into India and hence a drug banned in the country of origin could be easily imported and sold in India. Now no such misbranded, adulterated or spurious drugs or drugs not of standard quality, can be imported into India. The Act and Rules have been amended from time to time, the major amendment was made in 1982.

Health is a word very known to all but it also carries a lot of complications and difficulties. According to the World Health Organization (WHO) health is a state of complete physical, mental and social well-being and not simply absence of any illness. To make the above definition of health practical we have to depend upon a "health care team". A health care team is the group of community who contribute to a common health goal and common objectives determined by community needs. India with the greatest cultural diversity, health though an important issue is being neglected due to many hindrances. The condition is more worsened due to inappropriate drug use problems. It is in the hands of the pharmacist particularly the community pharmacist, to take up the challenge for providing better health care and better outcomes reasonably.

Community pharmacy may be defined as that area of Pharmacy Practice or Profession in which medicines and other related products are sold or provided (dispensed) directly to the public from a retail counter intended primarily for medicines. He dispenses medicines with a prescription and in certain cases without a prescription where applicable "over the counter" (OTC). Although community pharmacist is of key importance in providing better healthcare the patient. In India, Pharmacist has no any recognition in the healthcare system as compare to other well-established countries. For making for peaceful and well aware about the drug and disease, the need of the hour is to make community pharmacist a key towards better health care. The community pharmacist can take part in health promotion campaigns, locally and nationally, on a wide range of drug related and health related topics.

According to the drug and cosmetic Act, the premises for the retail sale of drugs may be described as:

1. Drug Store where the licencees do not engage the services of a qualified person or

2. Chemists and Druggists where licencees employ the services of a 'qualified person' but do not maintain a 'Pharmacy' for compounding against prescriptions, or

3. Pharmacy, Pharmacist, Dispensing Chemist, or Pharmaceutical Chemist, where the licencees employ the services of a 'qualified person' and maintain a Pharmacy for compounding against prescriptions.

Organisation and structure of retail and wholesale drug store

All types of business mainly includes:

   (a) Manufacturer

   (b) Wholesaler

   (c) Retailer

and it also includes marketing representative, transportation, warehousing, banking, insurance, storage etc. The main aim of any business is to give more satisfaction and quality to customers. Mainly four types of business organizations i.e.,

   (a) The Sole Trader (Proprietorship)

   (b) The General Partnership (Private Ltd.)

   (c) The Joint Stock Company (Public Ltd.)

   (d) Corporation – (i) Co-operation (ii) Public corporation

(a) The Sole Trader (Proprietorship)

This is the simplest form of business organisation in which one man show and controlled by one person. Example: retail drug store.

Advantages :

   (a) Less man power required

   (b) Ease to start the business

   (c) Capital of business can be increased or decreased

(d) Direct contact with customer, convenient to give more customer satisfaction

(e) The business includes both manufacturing and selling activities being concerned with both the producer and the trader who purchases.

The main purpose of any business is to earn the profits and send the product from manufacturer to consumers.

Types of Drug Store and Design

Based on their layout design, drug stores may be categorized as :

1. *Traditional Drug Stores:* These types of drug stores are designed in such a manner that the entire area of Drug store is exposed to customers. Such a design has pleasing and professional appearance and is convenient for both workers and customers. It provides opportunity for maximum sales but there are good chances of theft in such design.

2. *Personal Service Drug Stores :* In this type of design, the whole of the area is not exposed to the customer but the customer is required to interact with the drug store personnel at the service counter. During the purchasing process the customer demands an article and the personnel provide the articles. This service and design facilitates maximum interaction between drug store employee and the customers. The success of the drug store depends upon the convenience and friendly service of the personnel at the service counter.

3. *Prescription Oriented Drug Store:* These types of drug stores provide a comfortable waiting area where the customers are expected to wait while his prescription is proceeding. In this type of design health related items, drugs and prescription accessories are displayed in the vicinity while orthopedic and surgical appliances are kept in a separate room. Cosmetics and gifts are arranged in a suitable area in the store.

4. *Pharmaceutical Centre :* These types of centre sell medicines, convenience articles, orthopedic and surgical appliances. The store has sufficient floor space and is properly decorated.

5. *Super Drug store :* Such types of drug stores have a huge floor area ranging from 5,000 to 10000 with a square design. The customers have access to all-most-all the area in the drug store and can inspect, handle and select articles themselves. The design is on self service pattern except for the prescription department where self service is not possible.

Site Selection

The site selection is one of the most important success parts of any business. Number of factors are required to consider during the site selection. Following factors are considered for the selection of proper site for drug store.

1. *Hospital/Nursing Homes :* Near by hospital, drug store location is quite good because maximum patients are moving toward the hospital for treatment and also multi-facilities are available near to the hospitals.

2. ***Prescriptions :*** Every one is knows that the business of drug store is depending on the prescription written by physicians. One of the best locations is having the good and more physicians.

3. ***Drug Store market :*** It was found that in good cities one is the common place known as "Daba Bazar". This is one of the most suitable location for drug store if potential is very high and dedication for business. It is true if more retail drug stores at one place, people always stop to purchase drugs because they think availability of all types medicines are only in this place.

4. ***Flow of Traffic:*** The best way is to select left hand side or right hand side of road where suitable parking place is available. Identify the purchasing power of particular side and select the location accordingly. In the way of people's office site is good location for drug store. One way traffic should be avoided, location near traffic signals have to face the parking problems.

5. ***Near by Amenities :*** Enough parking, toilets, small play ground etc., are always advisable particularly when you are selecting the location in the market.

6. ***Near by Common Requirements (Hotel, School, Cinema, Play Ground etc.) :*** Near all these point from morning to evening all people are going because of any reason. These points are found most suitable for drug store business.

7. ***Business Locality :*** Number of people coming to such locality is very high and if the shop is made with modern and high-tech, many people can purchase the drugs simultaneously but required more investment for establishment of the business.

8. ***Residential Area:*** Such type of location is always advisable because you may start your business in minimum investment and customers are well known, while going for evening walk people can prefer to purchase medicine.

9. ***New Establishment:*** Now-a-days in cities number of new site as residential are developing very fast because in the city land cost is very high. It is an ideal location to serve the needs of customers initially, by providing all types of services.

10. ***Special Service/Products:*** Number of times some shops are well known for their category of drugs e.g. only Ayurvedic drugs or homeopathic drugs, veterinary drugs. For special purpose medicine people are always preferred such places for marketing.

11. ***Customer Services :*** Identifying customer in particular location will tell you which products will be sold more. In rich areas cosmetics and OTC products and in slum areas cheep products sell is very high.

12. ***Shopping centres :*** In modern time, shopping molls are very popular and the good gentry are preferred to purchase goods as well other things under the one roof. This is very costly but at the same time it is most suitable site for drug store.

Layout Design

Mainly three factors are responsible for success of drug store/wholesale store.

1. Location
2. Professional management
3. Strong financial support

Other factors are also playing important role in the success of drug store such as – design, placement of article, display, supporting staff, advertisement etc.

Common Design of Drug Stores

It is very difficult to classify the design of drug store because it is depend on the size of drug store and organization according to product as well as approach customers. Some common designs are given here.

(a) *I shape counter :* Very common, need less space, most suitable for small drug store.

(b) *L Shape counter :* Very common, need more space as compare to I shape for semi drug store.

(c) *T shape counter :* Not very common but most suitable if delivery place is different.

(d) *U shape counter :* Very common but need big space, most suitable in big drug store.

(e) *F shape counter :* In big cities and also in shopping moll, have separate cash counter with modern technology, very useful and also minimize the theft.

(f) *E Shape counter :* not very common but most common in shopping moll where purchasing, delivery and payment counter all are not at common place.

Main purpose of a good layout design

It is found that the owners are investing a huge amount in interior and designing of drug store as compare to old system of business. The main of aim of a good layout design to achieve the following objectives:

(a) To draw more attention of customers toward the drug store.

(b) To provide maximum facilities to customers so that purchasing is increased from each customer entering inside the store.

(c) Full on display including new products for kids growth and ladies requirements.

(d) All schemes and professional leaflet for introducing new common product (not required prescription)

(e) Some other specific objectives includes:
   - Fixed cost of articles
   - Availability of professional image
   - Provide customers satisfaction and convenience

- Provide sufficient parking place near to store
- Properly attending of the customer up to the satisfaction
- Proper utilization of space
- Provide hygienic place and drinking water facility

Characteristic of good layout design of Drug Store

A good drug stores layout design should have the following characteristic:

(i)   There should provide sufficient and properly ventilated space inside the store and comfortable to customers.

(ii)   There should have air conditioner/cooler in side the drug store.

(iii)   There should be proper labeling and partitioning of aluminum patrician and lighted properly.

(iv)   There should be soft light (not irritating) in side of the store.

(v)   The wall and roof should be painted properly using light colour because of pleasant nature of light colours.

(vi)   Sufficient number of wooden or steel racks should be arranged for storage of drugs.

(vii)   Maintain dust free environment using glass paneling and proper transparent gate with door closure.

(viii) Use proper stainless steel stool or stair to pick the material stored upper part of shelves at height inside the store.

(ix)   Sufficient waiting space should be provided for the customers if required arrange comfortable chairs.

(x)   Delivery counter /Cash Counter should be made from wood /glass and at properly maintained with decorative material and also instructions if any.

(xi)   Use suitable carry bags (paper/poly materials) with instruction slip helpful to patient.

(xii)   Maintain the computerized billing system.

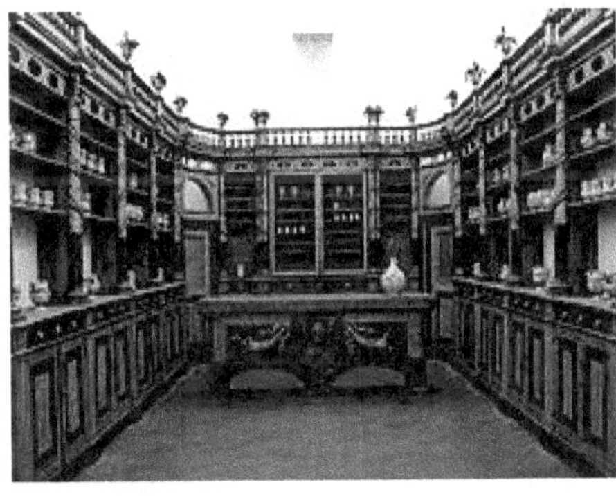

Fig. 18.1 Old Pharmacy

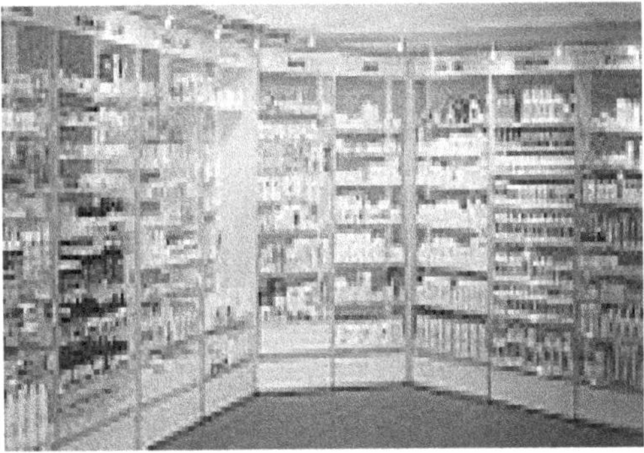

Fig. 18.2 Latest Pharmacy

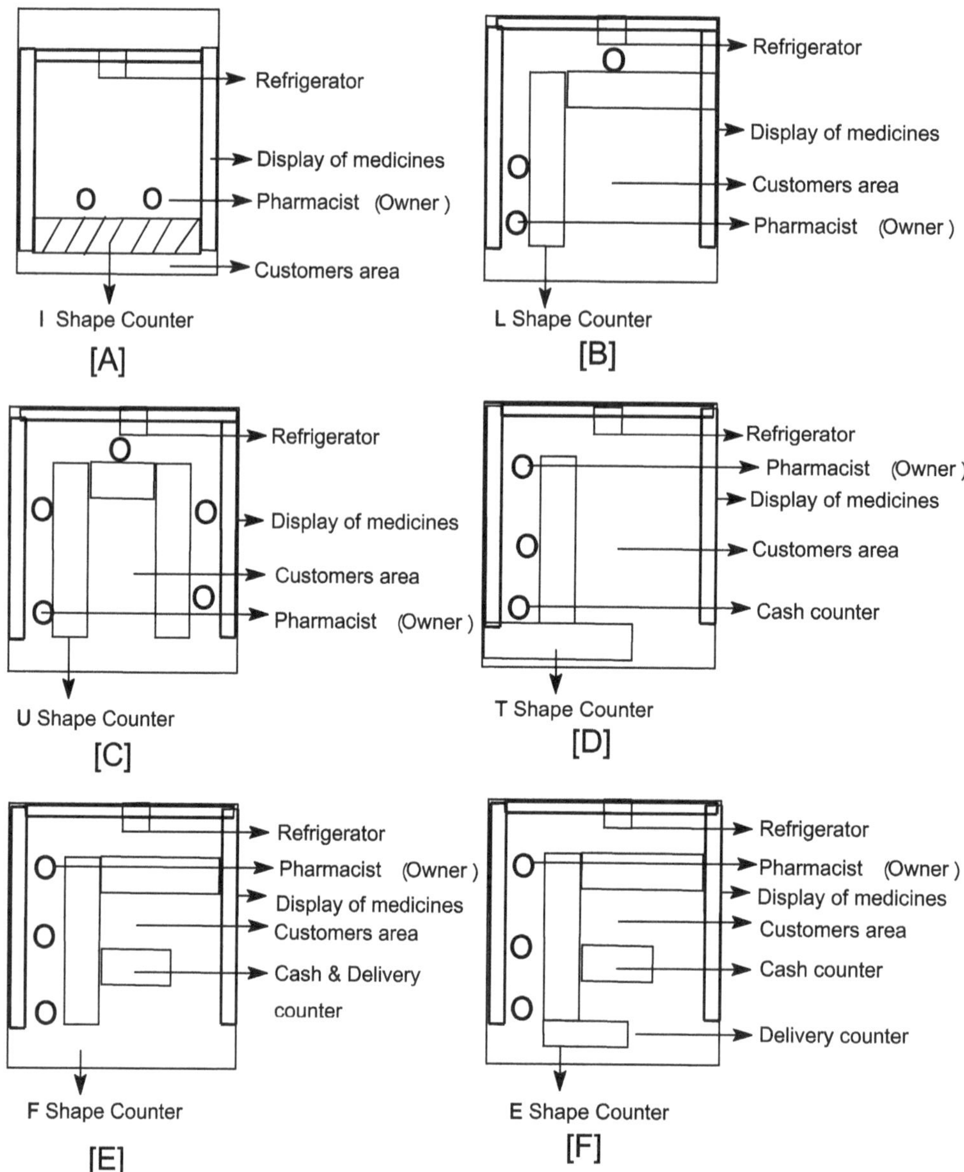

Figures A to F : Common design of Drug Stores.

Legal Requirements for Establishment of Drug Stores

Under the Sale of Goods Act, the term 'sale' is defined as 'a contract for sale of goods is a contract whereby the seller transfers or agrees to transfer the property in goods to the buyer for a price'. The drugs reach the consumers from the manufacturers by retail through shopkeepers. Manufacturers generally sell their goods to the stockiest who in turn sell the same to the shopkeepers. This transaction between the stockiest and the shopkeepers is the wholesale. Under the Drugs (Prices Control) Order, 1987 'wholesaler' means a dealer or his agent, or a stockiest appointed by a manufacturer or an importer for the sale of his drugs to a retailer; and a retailer means a dealer carrying on the retail business of sale of drugs to customers.

Sale of drugs being a specialized job, different from the sale of common goods, the Drugs and Cosmetics Act, 1940 and the Rules there under provide for a licence for the purpose. If drugs are sold or stocked for sale at more than one place, separate licence should be taken in respect of each such place. However, this is not applicable to itinerant (travelling from place to place) vendors. For the purposes of issuing licences, the State Government is empowered to appoint Licensing Authority (LA) for specified areas. A LA may, with the written approval of the State Government, delegate the powers to sign licences and other specified powers to any person under his control.

Sale of Drugs

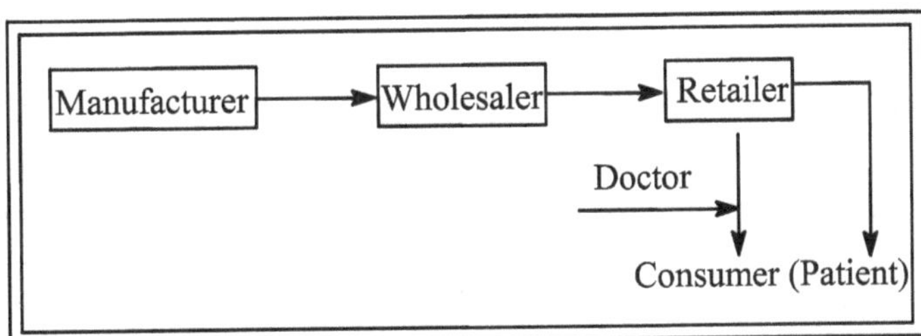

Wholesaler of Drugs

Nobody can be permitted to store drugs under the Act, without licence, for sale. Since risk to life and health is avoided by tightening up the dealer with expenses, the storage, even though for short spells and on adhoc basis and without intent to sell at that place but as part of the sales business, comes within the scope of 'storage for sale'. To loosen the law on its joints is to play with life and therefore, anti-humanist and it is a punishable offence. Even physician sample drugs 'not to be sold in the market'. A person possessing expired date medicines and physician's free samples is liable for conviction if he sells those items to anybody.

For the purposes of issuing sale licences, the drugs are divided into the following categories:

(a) Drugs other than those specified in Schedule C, C_1 and X

(b) Drugs specified in Schedule C and C_1 but excluding X; and

(c) Drugs specified in Schedule X.

The Rules also provide for the wholesale and retail sale of these drugs.

The wholesale and distribution of drugs specified in Schedule C and CI and other than those specified in Schedule C, CI and X is also permitted by motor vehicles provided a licence is taken. All the three categories of drugs can also be sold on retail. Restricted licences for the sale of drugs other than those specified in Schedule C and C_1 excluding X are also issued to the itinerant vendors and other dealers who do not engage the services of a *qualified person*.

Area required

Minimum area of 10-16 sq. meters is required for running wholesale drug store. The Licensing Authority must be satisfied that the premises in respect of which the licence is to be granted are adequately equipped with proper accommodation for preserving the properties of drugs to which licence applies and it is in charge of a person competent to supervise and control the sale, distribution and preservation of drugs. For the storage of thermolabiles substances some antibiotics, vaccines, sera, vitamins etc., are required to store in refrigerator temperature 2-8 ^{0}C. All requirements should be maintained as specified in Schedule N to the Drugs and Cosmetics Act.

Qualification

Person who is interested to start a wholesale drug store should be a registered pharmacist or who has passed the matriculation examination or its equivalent with 4 years experience in dispensing of drugs.

Renewal of Licence

An original licence or a renewed licence to sell drugs remains valid unto 31st December of the year following the year in which it is granted or renewed, unless suspended or cancelled earlier. The licence shall be deemed to have expired if application for its renewal is not made within six months after the expiry. In the event of any change in the constitution of a licenced firm, the licencee should inform the LA. Licences of such firms remain valid for a maximum period of 3 months from the date of change unless in the meantime a fresh licence has been obtained. It is no doubt true that under rule 59(3) of the Rules framed under the Drugs and Cosmetics Act a licence can be renewed even after its expiry. This does not, however, mean that a person whose licence has expired can go on selling medicines without a licence or without getting it renewed.

A licence or its renewal may be refused if the applicant is not considered to be a fit person, by the LA, for the grant of a licence because of his conviction for an offence under the Act or Rules, or the previous cancellation or suspension of any licence granted thereunder.

1. **Drugs other than those specified in Schedule C, C1 and X**

    The licence issued in Form 20B is subject to the following conditions in addition to the general conditions discussed earlier.

    1. The licence should be displayed in a prominent place open to the public.
    2. The licencee should comply with the provisions of the Drugs and Cosmetics Act, 1940 and the Rules thereunder in force.
    3. Drugs should be purchased only from a duly licenced dealer or manufacturer.
    4. Sale can be made to a person holding requisite licence to sell or distribute the drugs.

    However this shall not apply to the sale of any drugs to:
    (a) An office or authority purchasing on behalf of Government, or
    (b) a hospital, medical, educational or research institution or a RMP for the purpose of supply to his patients, or

(c) a manufacturer of beverages, confectionary biscuits and other non-medical products, where such drugs are required for processing their products.

2. Other than Schedule C and C_1 drugs from a Motor Vehicle

The licence issued in Form 20BB is subject to the following conditions in addition to the general conditions discussed earlier.

1. The licence should be displayed in a prominent part of the vehicle.
2. As for drugs other than those specified in Schedule C, C_1] and X.
3. The licencee should inform the LA in writing in the event of any change in the ownership of the vehicle specified in the licence within 7 days of such change.

3. Schedule X drugs

The licence issued in the Form 20G is subject to the following conditions in addition to the general conditions discussed earlier:

1. The licence should be displayed in a prominent part of the premises open to the public,
2. the licencee should comply with the provisions of the Drugs and Cosmetics Act, 1940 and the Rules thereunder, and
3. drugs should be purchased from a duly licenced dealer or manufacturer,
4. the licencee should forward to the LA copies of the invoices of sale made to the retail dealers,
5. sale can be made to a person holding requisite licence to sell or distribute drugs specified in Schedule X. This however does not apply to the sale of any drug to:
   (a) An officer or authority purchasing on behalf of government, *or*
   (b) a hospital, medical, educational or research institution, nursing home, RMP for the purpose of supply to its/his patients or manufacturers holding a licence to manufacture drugs containing the drugs specified in Schedule X.

4. Drugs specified in Schedule C and C_1 excluding those specified in Schedule X

The licence issued in the Form 21B is subject to the following conditions in addition to the general conditions discussed earlier:

1. The licence should be displayed in a prominent part of the premises open to the public.
2. The licencee should observe precautions prescribed for stocking or sale of drugs.
3. For the sale of each additional category of drugs the permission should be obtained from the licensing authority.
4. No sale of any drug should be made for the purpose of resale to a person not holding the requisite licence to sell or distribute the drugs. Provided that this shall not apply to the sale of any drug to:
   (a) An officer or authority purchasing on behalf of Government; *or*
   (b) *a* hospital, medical, educational or research institution or a RMP for the purpose of supply to his patients; *or*

    (c) *a* manufacturer of hydrogenated vegetable oils, beverages, confectionary and other non-medicinal products, where such drugs are required for processing their products.

5. The licencee should inform the LA in writing in the event of any change in the constitution of the firm operating under the licence.

5. Drugs specified in Schedule C and Cl from Motor Vehicle

The licence issued in the Form 21BB is subject to the following conditions in addition to the general conditions discussed earlier:

1. The licence should be displayed in a prominent place on the vehicle.

2. Precautions prescribed by the LA for the storage of drugs should be observed.

3. For the sale of additional categories of drugs not included in the licence, the licencee should take permission from the LA.

4. Drugs should be purchased from a duly licenced manufacturer.

5. Wholesale or resale can be made to a person holding the requisite licence to sell or distribute the drugs. Provided that this does not apply to the sale of any drug to:

    (a) An officer or authority purchasing on behalf of Government, *or*

    (b) *a* hospital, medical, educational or research institution or a RMP for the purpose of his patients, *or*

    (c) a manufacturer of hydrogenated vegetable oils, beverages, confectionery and other non-medicinal products,

6. The licencee should inform the LA in writing in the event of any change in the constitution of the firm operating under the licence.

7. The licencee should inform the LA in writing in the event of any change in the ownership of the vehicle specified in the licence within 7 days of such change.

Retail Sale of Drugs

The sale of drugs is different from the sale of other goods/articles in the market. For sale of medicines, required a qualified person and licence issued by Licencing Authority for specified schedule and time period. Before opening of a drug store, there is certain legal documentation and licence is compulsory.

Area required

Minimum area of 106 sq. meters is required for running retail sale of drug store. The Licensing Authority must be satisfied that the premises in respect of which the licence is to be granted are adequately equipped with proper accommodation for preserving the properties of drugs to which licence applies and it is in charge of a person competent to supervise and control the sale, distribution and preservation of drugs. For the storage of thermolabiles substances such as antibiotics, vaccines, sera, vitamins etc. are required to store in refrigerator temperature 2-8 ^{0}C.

Qualification

Person who is interested to start a retail drug store should a registered pharmacist himself or engage the registered pharmacist. The qualification of registered pharmacist is diploma or degree in pharmacy passed by PCI approved institute or universities. Registered pharmacist means a person whose name is for the time being in the register of the State in which he is for the time being residing or carrying on his profession or business of pharmacy.

Types of Licence for retail sale

For retail sale two types of licences are issued

A. General licences

General licences are granted to persons who have premises for the business and who engage the services of a *'Qualified Person'* to supervise the sale of drugs and do the compounding and dispensing.

Licences for retail sale of drugs other than those specified in Schedule C, C1 and X are issued in Form 20, for drugs specified in Schedule C, C1 excluding those specified in Schedule X in Form 21 and for Schedule X drugs in Form 20F.

Conditions

1. The licence should be displayed in a prominent place in a part of the premises open to the public.
2. The licencee should comply with the provisions of Drugs and Cosmetics Act and Rules thereunder in force.
3. Any change in the qualified staff in charge should be reported by the licencee to the LA within one month.
4. Drugs should be purchased only from a duly licenced dealer or manufacturer.
5. Any change in the constitution of the licenced firm should be informed to the LA within three months and in the meantime a fresh licence should be obtained in the name of the firm with the changed constitution.
6. Precautions prescribed by the LA for the storage of Schedule C and C1 drugs should be observed.
7. For the sale of additional categories of drugs listed in Schedule C and C1 excluding X, the licencee must take prior permission of the licensing authority.

B. Restricted licences

The licences for the restricted sale of drugs other that those specified in Schedule C, C1 and X and those specified in Schedule C and C1 but not in Schedule X are issued in Form 20A and 21A, respectively.

Restricted licences can be given to:

1. Dealers or persons in respect of drugs whose sale does not require the supervision of a qualified person,

2. itinerant vendors in exceptional cases, for bonafide travelling agents of firms dealing in drugs, or

3. to a vendor who purchases drugs from a licenced dealer for distribution in sparsely populated areas where other channels of distribution of drugs are not available.

Restricted licences may also be issued to a travelling agent of a firm for the special purpose of distribution to the medical practitioners or dealers, for supply of biological and other special products specified in Schedule C.

Travelling agents of licenced manufacturers, agents of such manufacturers and of importers of drugs need not take licences for the free distribution of samples of medicines to any member of medical profession, hospitals, dispensaries and the medical or research institutions.

Conditions for restricted licence:

1. The licencee must have adequate premises equipped with facilities for the proper storage of drugs to which the licence applies provided that this condition does not apply to vendors.

2. The licence should be displayed in a prominent place in a part of the premises open to the public or should be kept on the person of vendor who shall produce the same on demand by an Inspector or other officer authorized by the State Government in this behalf.

3. The licencee should comply with the provisions of the Drugs and Cosmetics Act and Rules thereunder in force.

4. Drugs should be purchased only from a duly licenced dealer or manufacturer.

5. The licencee can deal only in such drugs as can be sold without the supervision of a '*qualified person*'.

6. If the licencee be a vendor having no fixed place of business, he should buy drugs only from such dealers as may be specified in his licence.

7. Drugs should be sold in their original containers.

Before granting the restricted licence, the LA may take into consideration the number of licences granted in a locality during last three years and the occupation, trade or business of the applicant.

Renewal of Licence

An original licence or a renewed licence to sell drugs remains valid up to 31st December of the year following the year in which it is granted or renewed, unless suspended or cancelled earlier. The licence shall be deemed to have expired if application for its renewal is not made within six months after the expiry.

Dispensing and compounding of drugs

For the purposes of this Act and Rules, "*Pharmacy*" means and includes every store or shop or other place:

(i) where drugs are dispensed *i.e.* measured, weighed or made up and supplied; or

(ii) where drugs are prepared; or

(iii) where prescriptions are compounded; or

(iv) which by sign, symbol or indication gives the impression that the operations mentioned or

(v) which has upon it or displayed within it or affixed to or used in connection with it a sign bearing the word or words 'Pharmacy', 'Pharmacist', 'Dispensing Chemist', or 'Pharmaceutical Chemist', *or*

(vi) which is advertised in these terms.

In granting licence for a *pharmacy* the licensing authority may have regard to:

(i) average number of licences granted during the period of 3 years immediately preceding; *and*

(ii) the occupation, trade or business ordinarily carried out by such applicant during the preceding 3 years.

Supply of any drug other than those specified in Schedule X on a prescription of a RMP should be recorded at the time of supply in a prescription register maintained for the purpose and the serial number of the entry in register should be entered on the prescription. Following particulars should be entered in the register:

1. Serial number of the entry
2. The date of supply
3. Name and address of the prescriber
4. Name and address of the patient/owner of the animal if the drug is supplied for the veterinary use
5. Name and quantity of the drug
6. In case of Schedule H and X drugs the name of manufacturer, its batch number and expiry date, if any
7. Signature of the registered pharmacist under whose supervision the medicine was made or supplied.

If the drugs are not compounded in the premises and supplied in the original container, then particulars specified in (1) to (6) above may be entered in a cash or credit memo book.

In the case of refill prescriptions it shall be sufficient if the new entry in the register included a serial number, the date of supply, the quantity supplied and a reference to the entry when the drug was dispensed on the previous occasion.

It is not necessary to record the particulars in the register or cash or credit memo in respect of:

1. Drugs supplied against prescriptions under the Employee's State Insurance Scheme if all the particulars are given on the prescription, and
2. Any drug other than those specified in Schedule C and H if it is supplied in the original container.

Supply of Schedule C and C₁ Drugs

Retail supply of such drugs except on a prescription of a RMP should be recorded at the time of supply either *(i)* in a register maintained for this purpose in which the following particulars should be entered:

1. Serial number of the entry
2. The date of supply
3. The name and address of the purchaser
4. The name and quantity of the drug
5. Name of the manufacturer, batch number and date of expiry
6. Signature of person under whose supervision the drug was sold; *or*

   In a cash or credit memo book serially numbered containing all the particulars specified in items (1) to (6) above.

Carbon copies of the cash or credit memo retained by the licencee should be maintained in a legible manner. The option to maintain a register or a cash or credit memo book should be made in writing to the LA.

Supply of Schedule H and X Drugs

Substances specified in Schedule H or X should not be sold by retail except on the prescription of a RMPs and in case of substances specified in Schedule X, prescriptions should be in duplicate, one copy of which shall be retained by the licencee for a period of 2 years.

A prescription for Schedule H or X drug should:

(i)   be in writing and signed by the prescriber and dated by him, *and*

(ii) specify the name and address of the owner of the animal if the drug is meant for veterinary use; *and*

(iii) indicate the total amount of medicine to be supplied and the dose to be given.

The supply of drugs specified in Schedule H or X to RMPs, hospitals, dispensaries and nursing homes shall be made only against the signed and written order which should be preserved by the licencee for a period of 2 years.

The prescriptions for Schedule H and X drugs must not be dispensed more than once unless the prescriber has stated thereon that it may be dispensed more than once; however it may be dispensed a stated number of times or at stated intervals of time in accordance with the directions of the prescriber. At the time of dispensing there must be noted on the prescription above the signature of the prescriber, the name and address of the seller and the date of dispensing.

No person dispensing a prescription containing substances specified in Schedule H and X may supply any substitute whether containing the same substance or not in lieu thereof.

Substances specified in Schedule X should be stored under lock and key in cupboard or drawer reserved solely for the storage of these substances; or in a part of the premises separate from the remainder of the premises and to which only responsible persons have access.

Supply of Schedule X drugs should be recorded at the time of supply in a bound and serially numbered register maintained for this purpose and separate pages should be allotted for each drug. The following particulars should be entered in the said register:

1. Date of transaction
2. Quantity received, if any, the name and address of supplier and the licence number of the supplier
3. Name and quantity of the drug supplied
4. Manufacturer's name, batch or lot number
5. Name and address of the patient/purchaser
6. Reference number of the prescription against which supplies were made
7. Bill number and date of receipt of purchase and supply made by him; *and*
8. Signature of the person under whose supervision the drugs have been supplied.

Cancellation and suspension of licences

The LA may, after giving the licencee an opportunity to represent, cancel a licence for the sale and distribution of drugs or suspend it for such period as he thinks fit, either wholly or in respect of some of the substances to which it relates; if the licencee fails to comply with the conditions of the licence or with any provisions of the Act or Rules thereunder.

If, however, such failure or contravention is the consequence of any act or omission on the part of an agent or employee, the licence shall not be cancelled or suspended if the licencee proved to the satisfaction of the LA that:

(a) The act or omission was not instigated or connived at by him or, if the licencee be a firm or company, by a partner of the firm or a director of the company; *or*

(b) that he or his agent or employee had not been guilty of any similar act or omission within twelve months preceding the date on which the act or omission in question took place, or where agent or employee had been guilty of any such act or omission, the licencee had not or could not reasonably have had, knowledge of that previous act or omission, *or*

(c) if the act or omission was a continuing one, he had not or could not reasonably have had knowledge of that previous act or omission; *or*

(d) that he had used due diligence to ensure that the conditions of the licence or the provisions of the Act or the Rules made thereunder were observed.

A licencee whose licence has been cancelled or suspended may prefer an appeal to the State Government, within three months of the order, which shall decide the same.

It was observed by the M.P. High Court in the light of the facts of the case that the Drugs Inspector did not supply to the petitioner a third portion of the sample of the vial in question, which was a mandatory requirement under Sec. 23(4)(iii), read with Sec. 18-A of the Drugs and

Cosmetics Act. Nor did the Collector give notice to the petitioner to show cause why his licence be not cancelled as the drugs supplied by him were found to be spurious. Therefore, the Collector acted in violation of the principles of natural justice which he inflicted the penalty of canceling the licence under the influence of the Government Analyst's report.

Storage of Drugs

Drugs should be stored in a manner as instructions given by the manufacturer on the label.

(a) Storage of Schedule X drugs

Substances specified in Schedule X should be stored under lock and key in cupboard or drawer reserved solely for the storage of these substances or in a part of the premises separate from the remainder of the premises and to which only responsible persons have access.

(b) Storage of veterinary drugs

Veterinary drugs should be stored:

(i)   In a cupboard or drawer reserved for storage of veterinary drugs; *or*

(ii) in a portion of the premises separated from the remainder of the premises to which customers are not permitted to have access.

Maintenance of record Wholesale and Retail drug stores

Proper record should be maintained of sale and purchase of wholesale and retail drug store.

Record of purchase of Drugs

The records should be maintained under the following headings:

(i)   Date of purchase with bill number
(ii)   Name and quantity of the drug its batch number
(iii) Name of the manufacturer of the drug
(iv)   Name and address of the licence drug / good purchased
(v)   Licence number of seller with validity

Records of Sale of Drugs

Sale of drug specified in Schedule X

Schedule X means list of drugs whose import, manufacturing and sale, labeling and packaging are governed by special provisions. For sale and purchase a bound serially numbered register should be maintained and separate page for each drug. In the register particulars are maintained.

1. Date of purchase
2. Name of the drug
3. Quantity of the drug supplied
4. Name and address of the supplier

5. Licence number of the supplier

6. Manufacture's name and batch number

7. Name and address of the purchaser

8. Quantity received

9. Detail of prescription in which the drug used

10. Bill number and date of receipt of purchase

11. Signature with date of the person under whose supervision the drugs have been completed.

Sale of drug other than those specified in Schedule X

The following particulars are required to be entered in a prescribed register maintained for the purchase or credit memo.

1. Serial number of entry

2. Date of supply

3. Name and address of the prescriber

4. Name and address of the patient; if the drug is supplied for veterinary purpose, name and address of the owner should be maintained.

5. Name of drug with quantity should be mentioned in the register

6. Name of manufacturer and its batch number, expiry date are required if Schedule H and C drugs.

7. Signature of the registered pharmacist under whose supervisions the drugs supplied.

Patient Counseling

The pharmaceutical sciences are developing rapidly all over the world. The responsibility of the pharmacist towards through proper utilization of this scientific knowledge in the proper use of modern medicine, is also gradually improving. The pharmacist has to perform dual role:

(a) Counseling and educating the patient

(b) Monitoring of drug levels and also providing relevant information to the physicians.

Patient counseling is defined as providing medication information to the patients or their representatives orally or in written form for proper use of medicament. Following precaution are essential to take while counseling the patient.:

(i) Use language that the patient understands.

(ii) Use appropriate counseling aids such as diagram, photos, pictures, videos, computer etc., to easily understand by the patient.

(iii) Present facts and concepts in simple words and in logical order.

(iv) Use open ended questions.

Patient counseling consists of mainly three stages :

1. Introduction
2. Satisfaction of patient and family person curiosity
3. Technical part and revision.

1. Introduction

   (a) Introduce your self and discuss purpose of counseling
   (b) History taking of the patient – present and past history of patient and family person also if required
   (c) Review the patient's record and familiar with the patient
   (d) Obtain drug related information
   (e) Assess the patients understanding of the reasons for therapy
   (f) Assess any actual and / or potential concerns or problems of importance to the patient.

2. Technical part

   (i)   The medicine's generic and brand name and how it helps the patient.
   (ii)   How to take – with or without milk, before or after meal and breakfast etc.
   (iii) How long it takes to begin working and duration of therapy
   (iv)   How long it will be necessary to take the medicine
   (v)   What to do if you missed to take dose
   (vi)   Restrictions on activities while taking the medicine
   (vii) When to seek help if they are problems
   (viii) How long to wait before reporting no change in symptoms
   (ix)   The cost of the medicine
   (x)   How to have your prescription refilled, if necessary

3. Technical part and revision

   (i)   How to remove the drug from the package
   (ii)   How to administer such as ENT preparations, rectal/vaginal products
   (iii) Importance of medication for his well being.
   (iv)   Side effect medications
   (v)   Drug interactions (Drug-Drug, Drug-Food) and adverse reactions
   (vi)   Storage condition of dosage forms
   (vii) Precaution taken during the treatment
   (viii) Supply medication reminder chart
   (ix)   Necessity to complete the course.

Role of Pharmacist in Health care and Education

Health is a word very known but it carries a lot of complications and troubles. According to the WHO, health is a state of complete physical, mental and social well-being and not merely absence of any illness. Health care system depends upon a health care team. A health care team is the group of community who contribute to a common health goal and common objectives determined by community needs. India with the greatest cultural diversity, health though an important issue is being neglected due to many hindrances. The condition is more worsened due to inappropriate drug use problems. It is in the hands of the pharmacist particularly the community pharmacist, to take up the challenge for providing better health care and better outcomes reasonably. Although community pharmacist is of key importance in providing better health care the patient, in India, Pharmacist has no any recognition in the health care system as compare to other well-established countries. The community pharmacist can take part in health promotion campaigns, locally and nationally, on a wide range of drug related and health related topics. A community pharmacist involvement could play an important role in the following areas of health care.

Pharmacists are dynamic, patient-oriented professionals committed to fulfilling the health care needs of their patients. Pharmacy is a profession that is expanding in new directions to meet the health care needs. There is a movement amongst pharmacists beyond the traditional compounding and dispensing of medication, towards a more professional advisory and primary health care role. Pharmacists can apply their knowledge and skill to become directly involved in the healing and education of patients. Pharmacists form an integral part of the community and serve as an important source of knowledge. A modern-day pharmacist should be trained in providing the knowledge concerning:

- Optimal drug therapy for patients with a focus on drug interactions and potential side effects
- Counseling on various disease conditions
- Education and promotion of the general health of the public
- Information on immunization.

World over pharmacist is one of the important member of the health-team including clinical research. If Indian pharmacist is not fulfilling this role, then he should be appropriately trained and be oriented as a health-care provider to the vast rural population. He can be used intelligently as an alternative manpower towards the sacred goals of :

1. As a communicator
2. As a quality drug supplier
3. As a health promoter
4. As a collaborator
5. As a trainer and Supervisor

The remark of the standing committee that "Pharmacist is the main hurdle in easy accessibility of medicines" is certainly unfounded. With the kind of political, administrative and social structure in our country. The WHO report on "The role of the pharmacist in the health care system" states that the competence of the pharmacist is already proven and evident:

- In the direction and administrative of pharmaceutical services
- In drug regulation and control
- In the formulation and quality control of pharmaceutical products
- In the inspection and assessment of drug manufacturing facilities
- In the assurance of product quality through the distribution chain
- In drug procurement agencies and
- In National and institutional formulary committees.

The main role of community pharmacist is studied under the following category with and without club with health care team.

A. As Pharmacist and health promoter

(a) Immunization

(b) Minor dressing

(c) Preventing tropical diseases

(d) Providing drug-information

(e) Monitoring adverse drug reactions

(f) Monitoring and minimizing adverse drug interactions

(g) Preventing misuse of drugs

(h) Preventing medication errors

B. Health educator

1. Nutrition Counseling
2. Individualization of Drug Therapy
3. Family Planning
4. Alcohols, Drug Abuse and Smoking Cessation
5. Sexually Transmitted Diseases – AIDS
6. Rational Use of Drugs
7. Women Welfare – Pregnancy and Infant Care

1. Nutrition Counseling

Community pharmacist can play significant role in assuring adequate nutrition by advising his patients about basic food needs, keeping to correct improper food habits in children, advising on special requirements, suggesting special diet instructions for diabetic patients and people with food allergy and participating in school lunch programs and schemes like mid-day meals etc., in rural areas. There are certain facts such as women who often eat fish or omega-3-fatty acids are less likely to suffer stroke, symptoms of hyper vitaminosis result in irregular menstrual cycle and excessive intake during pregnancy may cause birth defects, products and their standardization.

2. Women Welfare – Pregnancy and Infant Care

Women health care is the first priority in India. Women are the corner stone for effective public health and investing in women translate into investing in family, community and the Nation. The pharmacist who understands the normal course of pregnancy and infancy is at a distinct advantage as he or she can guide the mother in simple matters of hygiene and management. The community pharmacist can encourage breast feeding and can play a major role by guiding the mother for the protection of the child by following proper immunization schedule. Efforts are definitely underway in this area.

3. Rational Use of Drugs

A community pharmacist can also discuss with administration on the medication, provide information on the storage of the medication and wherever necessary he can counsel the patient. Drug information system should be set up and access to adverse drug reaction system should be made. A community pharmacist should do therapeutic drug monitoring and he should have a sound knowledge of genotype reporting i.e. predictive pharmacology. How many amongst the common people know that drugs such as Action 500, Coldarin can increase blood pressure in patients having hypertension. Even pain shows difference between men and women. Where women respond better to the opiods such as morphine, pentazocine and pethidine men respond better to the non-steroidal anti-inflammatory drug, ibuprofen. In a nut shell there should be rational use of drug i.e., right drug in right patient in right dose at right time. A community pharmacist is one of the inevitable members of the health care team who can help to achieve the goal of rational use of drugs.

4. Sexually Transmitted Diseases – AIDS

India has 3.5 million HIV positive cases, which is about 10% of the global HIV cases and barely second to South Africa. HIV drugs are expensive and beyond the reach of common man. Huge resource of community pharmacist can educate people in the prevention and information of HIV/AIDS. A sensitive issue is the increasing number of women patients suffering from AIDS. The number rose from 7% in 1985 to 18% in 1995. Explaining to what HIV is, its transmission, risk reduction, patient counseling are the components of the counseling that a community pharmacist can provide.

5. Alcohols, Drug Abuse and Smoking Cessation

The pharmacist has a play an important role to help individuals who become dependent upon alcohol. Drug abuse is similar to alcoholism yet different because it has been gaining more acceptances among young people. Annual mortality from tobacco use exceeds that from all other causes combined. Smoking is the greatest single preventable cause of morbidity and mortality in India. The pharmacist can advise on the products available to assist the patient in giving up smoking. Counseling sessions can be made by the community pharmacist to stop smoking.

6. Family Planning

Currently, India's annual population growth rate is 1.74%. India is the second most populous country in the world, contributing about 20% of births worldwide. In 1952, the Indian Government was one of the first in the world to formulate a national family planning programme, which was later expanded to encompass maternal and child health, family welfare, and nutrition. All problems are associated tremendously increasing population in India. The community pharmacist plays a very important role in this case to educate the people and advise various methods available in the market helpful in family planning.

7. Individualization of Drug Therapy

Today the latest concept in medicine is towards individualization of drug therapy. Where judicious patient care is needed individualization of drug therapy becomes a need, and a pharmacist can play a vital role in this. A physician who is preoccupied with patient diagnosis and treatment may not spare time for patient counseling regarding pharmaco-economics, drug information, alternative therapy, moral supporting etc. A pharmacist can set up a separate consultation room and provide counseling to the patient.

Important Terms

Drug includes, all medicines for internal or external use of human beings or animals and all substances intended to be used for, or in the diagnosis, treatment, mitigation or prevention of any disease or disorder in human beings or animals, including preparations applied on human body for the purpose of repelling insects like mosquitoes

Bulk drug means any pharmaceutical, chemical, and biological or plant product including its salts, esters, stereo-isomers and derivatives, conforming to pharmacopoeial or other standards specified in the Second Schedule to the Drugs and Cosmetics Act, 1940, and which is used as such or as an ingredient in any formulation.

Scheduled bulk drug: means a bulk drug specified in the First Schedule.

Non-scheduled bulk drug means a bulk drug not specified in the First Schedule.

Formulation means a medicine processed out of, or containing one or more bulk drug or drugs with or without the use of any pharmaceutical aids, for internal or external use for or in the diagnosis, treatment, mitigation or prevention of disease in human beings or animals.

Scheduled formulation means a formulation containing any bulk drug specified in the First Schedule either individually or in combination with other drugs, including one or more than one drug or drugs not specified in the First Schedule except single ingredient formulation based on bulk drugs specified in the First Schedule and sold under the generic name.

Non-scheduled formulation means a formulation not containing any bulk drug specified in the First Schedule.

Dealer means a person carrying on the business of purchase or sale of drugs, whether as a wholesaler or retailer and whether or not in conjunction with any other business, and includes his agent.

Distributor means a distributor or his agent or a stockist appointed by a manufacturer or an importer for stocking his drugs for sale to a dealer.

Retailer means sale of any goods, includes every person, other than a wholesaler, who sells the goods to any other person; and in respect of the sale of goods by a wholesaler, to any person for any purpose other than re-sale, includes that wholesaler.

Wholesaler means a dealer or his agent or a stockiest appointed by a manufacturer or an importer for the sale of his drugs to a retailer, hospital, dispensary, medical, educational or research institution purchasing bulk quantities of drugs.

Retail price means the retail price of a drug arrived at or fixed in accordance with the provisions and includes a ceiling price.

Ceiling price means a price fixed by the Government for Scheduled formulations in accordance with the provisions.

Manufacture includes any process or part of a process for making, altering, finishing, packing, labeling, packing or otherwise treating or adapting any drug with a view to its sale and distribution, but does not include the compounding or dispensing of any drug or the packing of any drug in the ordinary course of retail business, and "to manufacture" shall be construed accordingly.

Maximum retail price means the retail price arrived at or fixed in accordance with the provisions and includes a ceiling price, at which the drug may be sold to the ultimate consumer and where such price is mentioned on the pack, the words "Maximum or Max. Retail Price Inclusive of all taxes" shall be printed on the pack.

Local taxes means any tax or levy (except excise duty included in retail price) paid and/or payable to the Central Govt. or State Govt. or any local authority under any law, by the manufacturer or his agent or dealer.

Sale turn-over means the product of units of formulations sold by a manufacturer or an importer, as the case may be, in an accounting year multiplied by retail price inclusive of sales tax, if any, paid on direct sales by the manufacturer or importer, but does not include excise duty and local taxes, if any.

Trade means any trade, business, industry, profession or occupation relating to the production, supply, distribution or control of goods and includes the provision of any services.

Goods means goods as defined in the Sale of Goods Act, 1930 and includes:

(i) products manufactured, processed or mined in India,

(ii) shares and stocks including issue of shares before allotment,

Price : in relation to the sale of any goods or to the performance of any services, includes every valuable consideration whether direct or indirect, and includes any consideration which in effect relates to the sale of any goods or to the performance of any services although ostensibly relating to any other matter or thing.

Owner in relation to an undertaking, means an individual, Hindu Undivided Family, body corporate or other association of individuals, whether incorporated or not, or trust (whether public or private or whether religious or charitable) who or which owns or controls, the whole or substantially the whole of such undertaking, and includes any associated person who is a constituent of a group and who has the ultimate control over the affairs of such undertaking.

Registered consumers association means a voluntary association of persons registered under the Companies Act, 1956 or any other law for the time being in force which is formed for the purpose of protecting the interests of consumers generally and is recognized by the Central Government as such association.

CHAPTER 19

Dispensing of Proprietaries

Patent or Proprietary medicine is defined as "a drug which is a remedy or prescription presented in a form ready for internal or external administration of human beings or animals and which is not included in the current edition of the Indian Pharmacopoeia or any other Pharmacopoeia authorized in this behalf by the Central Government after consultation with the Drugs Technical Advisory Board".

Proprietary medicines are now available in ever increasing numbers. Hence traditional compounding of medicines has lost its importance except in hospitals where physician may prescribe compounded prescriptions but to a very limited extent. This means that pharmacists must pay greater attention to dispensing of proprietary medicines. As a matter of fact the number of proprietary medicines available in the market covers a very wide range of therapeutic categories of drugs. Most often proprietary medicines are having similar nomenclature that makes the pharmacist's job much difficult. Pharmacist must clearly understand the wishes of the prescriber and must avoid chances of confusion, error etc., while dispensing proprietary medicines and must make use of computer programs and software in resolving such problems.

Manufacturer's container is defined as container and contents received from the manufacturer with any outer container or covering, literature, if any, and labels removed.

Dispensing label is defined as the label used for dispensing, bearing the name and address of the supplier, the nature of the medicine and any other prescribed directions, the name of patient and the date of dispensing.

Dispensing proprietary medicines may be of two types, (i) dispensing from bulk supplies which may involve transferring the product to a container, and (ii) dispensing of medicines in the original container of the manufacturer.

In the first case all labels of manufacturer must be removed and the pharmacist should apply his own label along with prescriber's direction and name and address of the pharmacy. This amounts to transferring, pouring or counting from the original bulk container. Thus pharmacist assumes the responsibility for the dispensed medicine.

In the second case no labels are removed and pharmacist's label is applied. Thus there is no attempt to conceal the name of the manufacturer.

Many items e.g., aerosols, nasal sprays and ointments are dispensed in the manufacturer's original pack.

Dispensing from Bulk

While dispensing from bulk a container similar to the one in which the bulk has been supplied by manufacturer should be used as far as practicable. However dispensed medicines are not intended for long storage, unlike manufacturers' bulk packs; hence some flexibility is possible, particularly in terms of cost. Special attention should be given to light resistance, the fit of the closure and the size of the mouth.

Dispensing pharmacist must take care not to damage products when repacking. For example, forcing foil packed tablets into a container scarcely large enough to hold them may damage the foil, thus affecting the stability of the contents of chipping or crushing the tablets. The patient can be prevented from accidentally opening more than one compartment of a strip pack if the strips are carefully cut into individually wrapped units before issue.

When more than one type of tablet (or capsule) is prescribed for a patient, risk of confusion can be reduced by packing each in a different kind of container (e.g., glass bottle, plastic vials, etc.). This is particularly helpful if proper name labeling has not been allowed but is unnecessary if the size or number of tablets necessitates containers of different capacities.

Special instruction on the manufacturer's label should also appear on the label used for dispensing. Examples include storage instructions and such warnings as 'inflammable' and 'Avoid driving while under treatment with this medicine.

Dispensing from manufacturer's original pack

When a prescriber orders an original pack (O.P.) the product is dispensed as received from the manufacturer expect that -

(a) Packing leaflets are removed if not intended for the patient. These leaflets are usually designed for doctors and may contain information, such as side effects, that might worry a patient.

(b) A dispensing label is attached without obscuring the manufacturers label if possible. If some overlap is unavoidable, the name and strength of the product, directions for use, and any storage instructions should not be concealed. The dispensing label should give the patient's name and the name and address of the pharmacy.

Proprietary preparations requiring addition of a vehicle during dispensing

Such preparations are to be reconstituted at the time of dispensing or use so as to minimize degradation of a susceptible drug. These include products, such as oral antibiotic suspensions, supplied as a dry powder or granules in a container in which there is space for adding the vehicle at the time of dispensing.

Proprietary preparations in special containers

Such preparations must not be transferred to other containers and must be supplied in manufacturer's original pack. These include products in aerosol cans (e.g., bronchodilators sprays), dropper bottles (e.g., eye and ear drops), collapsible tubes (e.g., creams and ointments) and squeeze bottles (e.g. throat and nasal sprays). Since these have stability and facilitate administration it would be irrational, even if practicable, to transfer them to other containers.

Dispensing of preparations in special containers when an Original Pack has not been ordered - Where the prescriber has not requested an original pack but the item is available only in a specialized container it is difficult to lay down a strict procedure because of the variation in packs and containers. Nervertheless, in general, it is recommended that –

(a) All literature, except any clearly intended for the patient, should be removed.

(b) If possible, the manufacturer's label should be replaced by a dispensing label. Where removal of the original label is impossible it may be necessary to superimpose the dispensing label; this is inelegant but sometimes, as with printed plastics containers, unavoidable. If a label is removed with a solvent, e.g., from a metal container, care must be taken not to contaminate the contents.

Original packs must be dispensed with the same meticulousness as compounded preparations. Labeling, wrapping and other aspects of preparation should clearly indicate to the patient that care and accuracy have been employed in dispensing this medicine.

The literature supplied along with manufacturer's pack need not be removed that is meant to provide essential information directly to the patient, which is his right.

Fundamentally and legally if the manufacturer's bulk container is opened and transferred to pharmacist's container then the manufacturer is no more responsible for the product. While if manufacturer's original container is supplied then manufacturer is responsible for the product. Pharmacist must ensure that the patient has understood the directions for administration; precautions, if any; and storage conditions of prescribed medicines; whether supplied in manufacturer's container or pharmacist's container and his label.

Errors in dispensing of proprietary medicines can be minimized if the pharmacist uses data retrieval system regarding patent and proprietary medicines in the market, their compositions, indications, contraindications etc.

Bioavailability of Proprietary Preparations

There is now significant evidence that chemically-equivalent preparations of the same drug from different manufacturers can be non-equivalent therapeutically. The evidence is particularly strong for products containing chloramphenicol, digoxin, nitrofurantoin, oxytetracyclines, phnindione, phenylbutazone, phenytoin, tetracycline and tolbutamide.

These differences in therapeutic response are divided mainly from differences in bioavailability (i.e., availability of the drug to the body) which, in turn, are caused by differences in the physical nature of the drug, the method of preparation of the dose form, or both.

Physical Form

Use of a different particle size, optical isomer, polymorph or hydrate has, in some instances, been partly, if not entirely, responsible for altered bioavailability.

Preparation of Dosage Form

The factors connected with the preparation of the dosage form that may affect bioavailability include-

(a) Nature and amount of disintegrant in a tablet or diluent in a capsule

(b) Type of base for an ointment or cream

(c) Increase of a surfactant. Small amounts may aid absorption while with large concentrations availability of the drug may be reduced due to entrapment in micelles.

Normally, only the diluent recommended in the official publication or by the manufacturer should be used. If a doctor prescribes another diluent the problems that may arise should be explained to him.

Continuity of Medication

A patient treated in hospital with a drug requiring careful control of dosage should receive the same manufacturer's product when he returns home. Hospital pharmacists should advice the appropriate committee that the proprietary name, or the approved name, followed by manufacturer's name should be stated on the notes sent to the patient's general practitioner. The approved name alone should not be used.

For the guidance of pharmacists' the Pharmaceutical Society of Great Britain states –

'A pharmacist who has accepted a prescription for dispensing will dispense the prescription exactly in accordance with the prescriber's wishes and in particular will not (except with the approval of the prescriber or in an emergency) substitute any other product for a specifically named product even if the pharmacist believes that the therapeutic effect and quality of the other product is identical'.

Nostrums

Nostrums are preparations made by the person who recommends them. They are covered by a provision of the Act exempting products prepared in the course of counter-prescribing i.e., when the pharmacist prepares or dispenses a medicinal product in accordance with this own judgment as to the treatment of the person to whom it is to be administered , who is present in the pharmacy at the time.

For dispensing of nostrums in small-scale manufacturing practice following aspects are maintained.

Quality Control

In the preparation of nostrums full analytical control is not compulsory to follow but a quality control procedure should be confirmed by the pharmacist, of the identity of ingredients and the quality of the final products. In large batches smooth control of quality is recommended and if this is impracticable on the promise, a suitable analytical laboratory should be consult and maintain the proper quality of preparation.

Manufacturing area must be maintain free from source of contamination such as odours and offensive emanations, clean and tidy, well-lit and adequately ventilated and also protected against entry and establishment of birds, insect, rodents and other pests. During the manufacturing, attention should be paid to control of microbial contamination.

Equipment must not contaminate or effect the stability of excipients of preparations. All equipment should be cleaned properly and when the same equipment is used for different products, post process cleaning should be maintain.

Raw Material

Raw material should be bought under warranty from the supplier and when in any suspicion, the pharmacist should assure himself of correct uniqueness or quality of supplied material. Following things are checked and maintain the record.

- Date of receipt
- Full potency and quality
- Storage conditions

If the raw material stocks for long period of time the pharmacist must use his knowledge of drugs to decide when this is necessary to check the quality before use.

Manufacturing Process

Manufacturing must be supervised by a pharmacist and batch made according to a define formula and method of preparation. Contamination of one product by another should be avoided. Clean protective garments should be worn and smoking and eating forbidden during manufacturing. Individuals suffering from a disease in communicable form, carriers of such a disease or persons when open lesions on an exposed part of body should not be allowed to undertake manufacturing processes.

Records should permit identification of the raw materials used for each batch and assist in recalling the product if necessary. A master formula, name and quantity of each ingredient should be kept for each size batch in written. It is also required to maintain manufacturing method, including a specimen label and the number and size of containers in each batch.

At the time of manufacture following details should be recorded-

(a) Method of preparation
(b) Formula of the batch being prepared
(c) Name with quantity of raw materials used in preparations.

(d)   Suppliesr, identification mark and date of receipt of each.

(e)   Name and signature of the pharmacist

(f)   Manufacturing date

(g)   An identification mark that the pharmacist has allocated to the particular batch.

The record of particular batch or preparation must be kept for two years.

Packaging and Labeling

Suitable containers for preparation should be selected and labeled immediately after filling. The labels must have the batch identification mark, date of manufacturing, and quantity. New labels must be printed as specified when any change of composition is made.

***Storage* :** Products must be stored in suitable environment condition to maintain optimum temperature, protection form light and atmospheric moisture.

CHAPTER 20

Drug Interaction

The problem of drug interaction is the one of most serious concern to physicians, pharmacists, nurses and other related professional persons. The complexity of drug treatment and consequently eve greater risk of the patient may be attributed to the introduction of an overwhelmingly large number of potent medicaments particularly in last three decades. The knowledge of drug interactions is most useful to a pharmacist in developing the best medication. In the past, drug interactions were considered as those interactions which occured both in vivo and in vito and could be of physical or chemical nature. Today drug interaction is defined as the phenomenon which occurs when the effect(s) of one drug are modified by prior to simultaneous administration of other drug(s). These interactions may arise either from alteration of the absorption, distribution, metabolism or excretion of one dug by another; or from combination of their actions or effects. The risk of clinical consequences from drug-drug interaction is higher with some drug categories than with others. Drug categories commonly involved in clinically important drug interactions include anticoagulants, cardiac glycosides, oral hypoglycemics, sympahomimetic amines, antihypertensives, anticonvulsants or cytotoxic dugs. Common manifestations are haemorrhage, hypotension, cardiac arrhythmias, severe hypertension, convulsive seizures or hypoglycemia.

Drug interactions are usually considered as undesirable, as detrimental exaggerations or diminutions of the action of the drug upon another on account of the frequency and the clinical importance of adverse drug interactions. Equally important is the fact that the drugs are also used concurrently to enhance or improve their clinical effect. Thus a desirable drug interaction is defined as either a beneficial drug effect that is enhanced or a detrimental drug effect that is mitigated by the concomitant use of another drug.

The term 'incompatibility' should be reserved for those reactions which occur *in vitro*.

It should be remembered that the greatest information available is about those interactions in which the effects of interaction are readily measurable. There may be many more interactions which remain in the practice of clinical medicine and often attributed to patient idiosyncracy or the underlying disease. A glaring example is that of phenylbutazone and coumarin anticoagulants which were given concomitantly to many patients over a period of several years before the adverse interaction was detected.

Classification

Drug interactions may often involve more than one mechanism but a simple classification of drug interaction mechanisms is as follows:

A. **Pharmacokinetic (ADME) interactions** - Where the absorption, distribution, metabolism and excretion of one drug is affected by another drug. Pharmacokinetic interactions are those in which GI absorption of a drug is affected, plasma protein binding is affected, drug metabolism is either stimulated or inhibited; and urinary excretion is either enhanced or inhibited.

B. **Pharmacodynamic (Pharmacologic) interactions** - Where drugs may have additive or synergistic or antagonistic affects and may or may not involve action on the same receptor.

C. **Miscellaneous** - Where the interaction cannot be assigned to any of the above classifications.

Drug interactions may be caused due to (i) interaction(s) with other drugs, (ii) Endogenous physiologic chemical agents, (iii) With components of the diet; and (iv) Chemicals used in diagnostic tests or the results of such tests.

The clinical significance of any drug interaction depends on (i) the patient factor e.g. disease state, renal function, hepatic function, serum protein levels, urinary pH, dietary factors, environmental factors, pharmacogenetic factors, age etc; and (ii) The drug administration factors e.g., order and route of administration, duration of therapy, dose of dug and dosage forms etc.

A discussion of common categories of drug interaction with suitable examples is presented below.

1. *Modification of intestinal absorption :* The drugs being mainly weak acids or bases, ionise depending on the pH of the GI tract and hence their absorption is affected. It should be remembered that the non-ionised forms of drugs are more lipid-soluble and absorbed more rapidly than the ionised ones.

   (a) *Antacid-Aspirin :* Aspirin being weakly acidic, it is expected to be primarily absorbed from the stomach and hence antacids would decrease its absorption. However, since aspirin produces GI side effects it is quite often administered concurrently with antacids. According to some investigators aspirin is less readily absorbed from buffered products and its absorption may, in fact, decrease. Aspirin dissolves faster in alkaline pH though it is in the ionised form. This probably explains the use of aspirin with antacids.

   (b) *Antacid - Penicillin G:* Penicillin G being acid sensitive, its absorption from the stomach will be a function of the pH of the stomach.

   (c) *Antacid-Phenobarbital :* Phenobarbital remains in a non-ionised form in acidic medium and hence its absorption is decreased when antacid is given. Antacid administration will raise the pH of the stomach.

(d)   *Antacid-Pseudoephedrine :* Being a basic drug, the absorption of pseudoephedrine will be enhanced with the simultaneous administration of antacids as the drug remains in a non-ionised form.

(e)   *Antacid - Enteric coated medicines :* If enteric coated medicines are given with antacids, they will disintegrate and cause irritation and vomiting e.g. bisacodyl.

2. Effect on transport system :

(a)   *Food - Antibiotics :* The presence of food slows the process of stomach emptying and affects the dissolution rate. Hence food may influence the absorption of many drugs. Antibiotics like penicillins, tetracyclines, erythromycin and lincomycin are recommended to be given 1 hr before or 2 hr after meal to permit maximum absorption.

(b)   *Griseofulvin -* Phenobarbital : Phenobarbital may increase the secretion of bile and increase peristalsis. This would decrease the transit time in upper portion of the GI tract where griseofulvin is absorbed most efficiently. This phenobarbital reduces the absorption of griseofulvin.

(c)   *Cathartics -* These agents increase the motility of GI tract and influence the passage of other drugs through the tract. The drugs with slow absorption and requiring longer contact may thus be absorbed slowly when given with cathartics.

(d)   *Antimuscarinics -* As these agents decrease the peristalsis, their gastric emptying time is prolonged. The drug may remain in contact with the stomach for a longer time and its absorption may be increased from the stomach or the small intestine. Riboflavine is absorbed from the small intestine. When given with the anticholinergic propantheline, the initial absorption of riboflavine is delayed due to its accumulation in the stomach but subsequently as the drug reaches the small intestine its absorption becomes greater. This may be attributed to inhibitory peristalsis, delayed gastric emptying and longer duration of contact of the drug with the intestine.

(e)   *Antimuscarinics- Levodopa :* The antimuscarinics which are used in Parkinson's disease may have some synergistic effect when administered alongwith levodopa. In such cases the levodopa is poorly absorbed. The greater portion of levodopa is metabolised prior to absorption and hence antimuscarinics should be given in the smallest dose when administered alongwith levododa.

3. Complex formation

Complexation should be considered in a broader perspective and may involve drug-drug, dug-additive or even drug-container interactions. Complexes may be soluble or insoluble and may affect the drug absorption.

(a)   *Tetracycline - Metals :* It is well established that the absorption of tetracyclines is reduced in presence of certain metals like calcium, aluminium, magnesium, bismuth and iron. Antacids containing the slats of these metals would also reduce the absorption of tetracyclines. As milk contains calcium it may also reduce absorption of tetracyclines. However, the absorption of newer tetracyclines like doxycycline and minicycline is not affected by calcium but aluminium may affect. The inhibition of tetracycline salts due to complexation with iron in descending order is as follows ferrous sulphate, ferrous fumarate, ferrous succinate, ferrous gluconate, ferrous tartrate. Thus, inhibition is minimum in a more stable iron complex as sodium edetate.

(b) *Lincomycin - cyclamates* : Food beverages containing sodium or calcium cyclamates reduce the absorption of lincomycin possibly due to formation of a complex. To facilitate the absorption of lincomycin it is recommended that nothing should be given orally except water for a period of 1 to 2 hr before and after oral administration of the drug. The problem has been solved due to introduction of clidamycin which is better tolerated and has the same spectrum of activity.

(c) *Cholestyramine* : Cholestyramine may complex with various agents and drugs e.g., bile salts, thyroid hormone, vitamin K, warfarin etc. Thyroid hormone and cholestyramine should be given at an interval of 4 hours. An interval of 6 hr is necessary for the optimum absorption of warfarin. Prolonged therapy of cholestyramine decreases the absorption of vitamin K.

(d) *Sodium fluoride* : In presence of a large quantity of calcium the absorption of sodium fluoride may be reduced due to complexation. Hence an interval of 1 hr before and 2 hr after the meal is recommended.

(e) *Antidiarrhoeal mixtures* : These mixtures essentially absorb toxic substances causing diarrhoea but then there also exists a possibility of absorption of other medicines. This is evidenced from the finding that the rate and extent of absorption of promazine is decreased by concurrent administration of a mixture of attapulgite and citrus pectin. Lincomycin is reported to be absorbed by kaolin mixture.

4. Displacement of drug from storage tissue components

(a) Drug - Drug : Drugs may be bound to protein and this binding may be competitive or non-competitive. The binding sites being fewer in number there will be a competition for binding and the drug having greater affinity will displace the other having lesser affinity. There will exist an equilibrium between the bound and non-bound drug. Such an interaction is significant when one dug is prone to get bound in a larger quantity and is given with another drug which is able to displace the first one from its site of binding.

(b) *Phenylbutazone - Warfarin* : Because of its greater affinity for binding, phenylbutazone displaces warfarin from the binding site. Thus more free drug is available for the action resulting in haemorrhage. Combination of the two drugs should be avoided. However, the two drugs may be indicated simultaneously as in superficial venous thrombosis.

(c) *Chloral hydrate - Warfarin* : It is reported that prolonged chloral hydrate therapy requires less warfarin during the induction phase of an anticoagulant therapy. But other conflicting reports indicate that chloral hydrate decreases the anticoagulant activity.

(d) *Bilirubin - Sulphonamides :* Bilirubin gets bound with albumin but may be displaced by a number of drugs from the binding sites. Sulphisoxazole and salicylate are reported to have such affect.

(e) *Indomethacin with oral anticoagulants -* The anticoagulant response is increased due to displacement from protein binding sites.

5. Modification of drug action at receptor site

(a) *Physiological antagonism :* This implies that two endogenous substances antagonise the effect of each other by acting at different receptors. Examples are adrenaline and histamine, adrenaline and acetylcholine etc.

(b) *Competitive antagonism :* It involves the competition between agonist and antagonis for the same receptors and the extent to which the antogonist opposes the pharmacological action of the agonist is determined by relative number of receptors occupied by the two receptors.

(c) *Non-competitive antagonism :* Non-competitive antagonism occurs when the agonist and antagonist act on completely different receptors to produce antagonism e.g. acetylcholine and papaverine.

(d) *Interaction at receptor site :* The increased effect of warfarin in the presence of d-thyroxine is attributed to increased affinity of the drug for the receptor site brought about by d-thyroxine. The anabolic steroids like dianabol, norethandrolone and oxymetholone are also reported to increase the affinity of warfarin for the receptor site.

6. Interaction at adrenergic neuron

(a) *MAO inhibitors-Sympathomimetics :* Concurrent administration of MAO inhibitors and sympathomimetics is of potential danger. Hence the patients being treated with MAO inhibitors should be advised to avoid using products containing these sympathomimetic agents. Amphetamine and MAO inhibitors when given simultaneously cause severe headache, hypertension and cardiac arrhythmias.

(b) *MAO inhibitors - Tyramine :* Although this is not considered to be of serious consequences, yet such an interaction cannot be overlooked. When monoamino oxidase is inhibited, large quantities of unmetabolised tyramine can accumulate resulting in release of noradrenaline from adrenergic neurons.

(c) *MAO inhibitors -* Tricyclic antiderpressants : It is recommended that therapy with a MAO inhibitor or a tricyclic antidepressant (amitryptiline, nortryptiline, imipramine etc.) should not be initiated until at least two weeks after the therapy with the other dug has been discontinued.

(d) *Guanethidine -* Tricyclic antidepressants : Tricyclic antidepreseants can inhibit the uptake of guanethidine. A reversal of hypotensive effect of guanethidine following administration of desipramine and protryptiline is also reported.

(e) *Guanethidine - Sympathomimetic agents :* Amphetamine, ephedrine and mehylphenidae antagonise the effect of guanethidine. Amphetamine acts in a way similar to tricyclic antidepressants and in addition it may cause the release of guanethidine from its storage sites in the neuron.

(f)   *Guanethidine   Antipsychotic agents :*   Chlorpromazine, haloperidol and thiothixene can markedly reverse the antihypertensive response of guanethidine by the same mechanism as tricyclic antidepressants.

7. Biotransformation

(a)   *Enzyme inhibition -*   chloramphenicol is reported to inhibit the metabolism of bishydroxycoumarin, tolbutamide and diphenylhydantoin due to inhibition of microsomal enzymes. Disufiram has been used in alcohol addicts due to its inhibitory effect on the enzyme aldehyde dehydrogenase. MAO inhibitors enhance the effect of drugs like babiturates, alcohol, sedatives, hypnotics, tranquillisers and other CNS depressants due to the inhibition of the liver enzyme system. Allopurinol inhibits the enzyme xanthine oxidase and may increase the effect of mercaptopurine azathiopurine etc., as the same enzyme is involved in their metabolism.

(b)   *Enzyme stimulation (induction) :* Barbiturate, chloral hydrate, glutethimide and griseofuvin may cause enzyme induction. Chlordiazepoxide, diazepam and other benzodiazepines donot interfere with the barbiturate action. Decrease in the effect of diphenylhydantoin, steroidal hormones and digitoxin is reported on simultaneous administration due to enzyme induction. Chlorinated hydrocarbons reduce the effect of barbiturates whereas MAO inhibitors increase the effect of barbiturates due to enzyme induction.

It is suggested that pyridoxine accelerates the decarboxylation of levodopa in peripheral tissues and hence less amount of levodopa crosses blood brain barrier and less dopamine is formed in the brain. This ultimately causes a reduction in therapeutic effect.

In alcoholic subjects increased rate of excretion of phenobarbital, meprobamate and increased rate of metabolism of tolbutamide, diphenydantoin and warfarin is reported. This has been attributed to increased activity of liver enzymes.

8. Alteration of urinary excretion : An acidic pH is required for the activity of methenamine but in the same condition there is danger of precipitation of sulphonamides resulting into crystalluria.

In case of drugs such as salicylates there will be large proportion of non-ionised form in acidic urine with increased reabsorption and intensified activity. On the same analogy, for a basic drug e.g., amphetamine, quinidine, pseudoephedrine etc., there will be increased proportion of non-ionised form in basic urine with increased reabsorption and intensified activity.

The antiinfective agents employed for the urinary tract infections are effective in a particular urinary pH. Tetracyclines, nitrofurantoin, methenamine are most active at urinary pH of 5.5 or even less. On the contrary an alkaline pH is required for kanamycin, streptomycin and chloramphenicol.

Antibacterial spectra of many drugs can be modified by appropriate reaction of urine. Thus, erythromycin is active against gram positive bacteria but its spectrum can be expanded to include gram negative organisms by making the urine alkaline. Novobiocin can be made active against gram negative organisms if urine is name acidic.

The acidification of urine enhances the excretion of methadone but its metabolite is less affected by urinary changes. In a number of drugs reabsorption and excretion are influenced by the urinary pH.

9. **Direct effect on kidney :** Probenecid, phenylbutazone, sulphapyrazone, aspirin, indomethacin etc., are reported to increase the half-life of penicillin by blocking its tubular excretion. Probenecid apart from penicillin also increases the half-life of aminosalicylic acid, sulphonamides and dapsone. It also increases the half life of acetoheximide and causes hypoglycemia. This is attributed to the interference in the renal excretion of hydroxyhexamine, the active metabolite of acetohexamide.

It has been suggested that high doses of salicylates should be given cautiously when administered alongwith frusemide as there is a competition between these drugs for renal excretory sites and patients may experience salicylate toxicity at lower dose.

Sodium depletion enhances lithium toxicity. It is suggested that lithium carbonate should not be given to the patient on diuretic therapy.

10. **Increase or decrease of synthetics**

Antibiotics like chloramphenicol, neomycin, tetracyclines and sulphonamides enhance the anticoagulant effect due to the interference with the synthesis of vitamin K by microorganisms in GI tract. Similarly, quinidine enhances anticoagulant effect by suppressing prothrombin formation.

CHAPTER 21

Future of Dispensing Pharmacy

In view of the highly specialised and responsible nature of the job, a pharmacist throughout the world has been entrusted with the handling of drugs and most countries have enacted laws to give protection to the society. In India Pharmacy Act 1948 and the Drugs and Cosmetics Act 1940 and Rules, 1945 regulate the profession of pharmacy and dispensing of medication.

With changing times, compounding of drugs is being gradually replaced by manufactured drugs on the following grounds :

1. Advances in pharmaceutical technology of dosage forms have rendered compounded medication almost obsolete both for scientific reasons and convenience.

2. Increase in the number of in-patients and ambulant patients have forced the pharmacist to over-the-counter (OTC) dispensing.

3. Patient psychology has undergone changes with time. Previously a patient felt convinced that a `coloured' mixture or liquid preparation was the answer to his ailment but today unless he is given a costly prescription embodying an injection etc, he underrates the prescriber and the medication.

4. There is an acute shortage of qualified pharmacists all over the world and in course of time supply of manufactured drugs has evolved as the substitutes of traditional dispensing.

   Increasing population and awareness of health matters have contributed to an increase in the number of prescriptions thus making the task of a pharmacist more difficult if he sticks to compounding individual prescriptions.

5. Solid dosage forms like tablets and capsules which are difficult to prepare at the dispensing counter are preferred by the patient and the physician over liquid dosage forms for obvious reasons.

6. A pharmacist's role in the health care team is better recognised today. It has been accepted that he is the expert on drugs. This means a departure from the conventional role of a compounder/dispenser. Today he advises the physician on dosage forms, dosage regiment, side effects, bioavailability and drug interaction.

7. A compounded dosage form can not be subjected to quality control whereas manufactured products are subjected to such a testing and therefore considered more reliable.

The paradigm shift from compounded to manufactured products will be more prominent in course of time and greater emphasis is likely to be placed on unit-dose dispensing systems, which appear to be an answer to manifold problems. The following are some advantages attributed to unit-dose dispensing system.

1. Patients receive improved pharmaceutical service 24 hours a day and are charged for only those doses which are administered to them.

2. All doses of medication required at the nursing station are prepared by the pharmacy thus allowing the nurse more time for direct patient care.

3. Allows the pharmacists to interpret or check a copy of the physician's original order thus reducing medication errors.

4. Eliminates excessive duplication of orders and paper work at the nursing station and pharmacy.

5. Eliminates credits.

6. Transfers intravenous preparation and drug reconstitution procedures to the pharmacy.

7. Promotes more efficient utilization of professional and non-professional personnel.

8. Reduces revenue losses.

9. Conserves space in nursing units by eliminating bulky floor stock.

10. Eliminates pilferage and drug wastage.

11. Extends pharmacy coverage and control throughout the hospital from the time the physician writes the order to the time the patient receives the unit-dose.

12. Communication of medication orders and delivery systems are improved.

13. The pharmacists can get out of the wards where they can perform their intended function as drug consultants and help provide the team effort that is needed for better patient care.

The removal or withdrawal of a single dose from a drug container and its administration to a patient on the order of a physician or dentist is purely a nursing function and this has to be viewed quite distinctly from the act of dispensing which is the exclusive domain of a pharmacist.

Till the unit-dose dispensing becomes universal it may be advisable to adopt pre-packaging in hospitals. Thus pharmacist will be performing the compounding function to the least extent and dispensing function will be in the form of pour and count and handover.

In course of time a pharmacist will be required to dispense radiopharmaceuticals and the pharmacists must prepare themselves to discharge this function.

To keep pace with the modern developments and in order to facilitate the dispensing function, it will be a common practice to make use of electronic data processing machines and computers etc. Use of appropriate software and websites would eliminate chances of prescription errors, would facilitate information on drug-drug, drug-food and drug-excipient interactions; as well as irrational combinations, banned drugs and drug combinations.

However, the pestle and mortar on traditional basis may retain its importance as the symbol of both dispensing and the dispenser.

Appendix A

List of Life Saving Drugs

1. 32 P Sodium Phosphate
2. Flucytosin
3. 5-Fluorouracil
4. 6-Isoguanine
5. Aclarubicin
6. Dactinomycin
7. Agglutinating Sera
8. Allopurinol
9. Ambenonium Chloride
10. Amikacin
11. Amino-glutothemide
12. Amiodarone
13. Amiphenazole
14. Amphotericin-B
15. Amrinone
16. Amsacrine
17. Amylobarbitone Sodium
18. Anti-Diphtheria Normal Human Immunoglobulin
19. Anti-Haeomophilic Factor concentrate (VIII and IX)
20. Anti-human lymophocyte immuniglobulin IV
21. Anti-human thymocyte-immunoglobulin IV
22. Anti-Pseudomonas Normal Human Immunoglobulin
23. Anti-Plague serum
24. Anti-Pseudomonas Normal Human Immunoglobulin
25. Anti-Rabies Normal Human Immunoglobulin
26. Aprotinin
27. Atracurium besylate
28. Baclofen
29. Beclamide
30. Bemergide
31. Bleomycin
32. Blood group sera
33. Burn therapy dressing soaked in gel
34. Bovine Thrombin for in vitro test for diagnosis in Haemorrhagic disorders
35. Bovine Albumin
36. Broxuridine
37. Bretyleum Tossylate
38. Busulphan
39. Calcium Disodium Edetate

40. Carbidopa with Levodopa
41. Carmustine
42. Cefoperazone
43. Ceftizoxime
44. Cesium Tubes
45. Chenodeoxycholic Acid
46. Chlorambucil
47. Chlormerdrin 197 Hg.
48. Chloestyramine
49. Christmas Factor Concentrate (Coagulation factor IX prothrombin complex concentrate)
50. Chorionic Gonadotrophin
51. Cobalt-60
52. Clindamycin
53. Colistin
54. Carboquone
55. Corticotrophin
56. Cyclocytidine
57. Cyclophosphamide
58. Cyanamide
59. Dacarbazine
60. Daunomycin
61. Daunorubicin
62. Desmopressin
63. Desferrioxmine
64. Diagnostic Agent for Detection of Hepatitis B Antigen
65. Diagnostic kits for detection of HIV antibodies
66. Diphtheria Antitoxin Sera
67. Dimercaprol
68. Diazoxide
69. Dobutamine
70. Dispyramide Phospate
71. Edrophonium
72. Dopamine
73. Enzyme Linked Immunoabsorbent Assay Kits (ELISA KITS)
74. Epirubicin
75. Fibrinogen
76. Floxuridine
77. Follicle Stimulating Hormone (FSH)
78. Fospestorol
79. Gallium Citrate
80. Gasgangrene Anti-Toxin Serum
81. Glucagon
82. Heptamine
83. Hepatitis B Immunoglobulin
84. Hexamethymelamine
85. Histoglobulin
86. Hydralazine
87. Hydroxyurea
88. Idraubicine
89. Idoxuridine
90. Ifosfamide
91. Isoprenaline
92. Immunoassay kit for blood Fibrinogen degradation product for direct estimation of diagnostic test in D.I.C.
93. Inactivated rabies vaccine (Human diploid cell)
94. Inactivated rabies vaccine (Vero-cell)
95. (a) Indium (III) in bleomycin (b) Indium 113 Sterile generator and elution accessories (c) Indium 113 in brain scanning kit (d) Indium 113 in liver scanning kit.
96. Interferon alpha -2b/interferon alpha -2a/Inteferon NL/Inteferon alpha NL (LNS)
97. Intravenous amino acids

98. Intravenous Fat Emulsion
99. Iopamidol
100. Iohexol
101. Ketamine
102. Isoflurane
103. Selenium-75
104. Asparaginase
105. Calcium folinate
106. Lactulose
107. Levodopa with benserazine
108. Levodopa (L-Dopa)
109. Mannitol Busulphan preparations
110. Lomustine
111. Meningococcoal A and C combined vaccine with diluant solvent
112. Melphalan
113. Mercaptopurine
114. Mesna
115. Methisazone
116. Methicillin
117. Methoxy isobutyl Isonitrile
118. Methotrexate
119. Methyl prednisolone
120. Methoxyflurane
121. Metrizamide Inj with diluant
122. Metraminol
123. Mithramycin
124. Nimustine
125. Mitotane
126. Mitomycin
127. MMR (Measles, mumps and rubella) vaccine
128. Latamoxef
129. Monocomponent insulins
130. Nalorphine
131. Mustin Hydrochloride
132. Netilmicin
133. Naloxone
134. Nitroglycerine
135. Normal Human plama
136. Normal Human immunoglobulin
137. Nuclear magnetic resonance contrast agent
138. Normal Human serum Albumin
139. Penicillamine
140. Pancuronium Bromide
141. Pentamidine
142. Penicillinase
143. Peplomycin
144. Pilocarpine
145. Podohyllotoxin
146. Piperacillin
147. Poliomvelitis vaccine (inactivated and live)
148. Laureth 9
149. Poly myxin B
150. Polyestradiol
151. Potassium Aminobenzoate
152. Porcine Insulin Zinc Suspension
153. Praziquantel
154. Pralidoxime
155. Prednimustine
156. Prazosin
157. Porcine and Bovine insulin
158. Procarbazine
159. Purified Chick Embryo Cell Rabies Vaccine
160. Protamine
161. Pyridostigmine
162. Pyridinol Carbamate

163. Radio-immunoassay kit for hormones (T3, T4, TSH Insulin, Glycogen, Growth Hormone, Cortisol, L. H., FSH and Digoxin)
164. Quinidine
165. Radioisotope T1 201
166. Tribavarin
167. Septopal beads and chains
168. Sodium Arsenate
169. Sodium Cromoglycate spincaps and cartridges
170. Sodium Hyalauronate sterile1% and 1.4% solution
171. Solution containing Human Follicle Stimulating and Luteinising hormones
172. Solution of Nucleotides and Nucliosides
173. Somatostatin
174. Somatropin
175. Specific Desensitizing Vaccine
176. Sterile Absorbable Haemostat for control of surgical vessel bleeding
177. Streplokinase and Streptodomase preparations
178. Strontium Chloride (85 Sr.)
179. StrontiumSR-89 Chloride
180. Suxamethonium Chloride
181. Testolactone
182. Technitium-99M
183. Thioguanine
184. Thallium 201
185. Ticarcillin
186. Tobramycin
187. Tissue Plasminogen Activator
188. Tranexamic Acid
189. Tocainide
190. Tri-iodothyronine
191. Triethylene Tetramine
192. Triethylene Thiophosphoramide
193. Trofosfamide
194. Tubocurarine
195. Urokinase
196. Ursodeoxycholic Acid
197. Vancomycin
198. Vasopressin
199. Vecuronium Bromide
200. Vindesin Sulphate
201. X-ray diagnostic agents, the following :- (i) Propylidone (ii) Ethyl iodopheny-lun decylate (iii) lodipammide methyl glucamine (iv) Lipidoll utra fluid (v) Patent blue
202. Anti -D Immunoglobulin
203. Aurothiomalate Sodium
204. Botulinum Toxin Type 'A'
205. Triptorelin
206. D.K.line 100% purified perflurodicalin liquid
207. Fligrastim/Molgramostim (G-CSF/GM-CSF)
208. Flecainide
209. Foetal Bovine Serum (FBS)
210. GadoliniumDTPA Dimeglumine
211. HTLV - 1 Western Blot Kits
212. Tetanus Immunoglobin
213. BCG vaccine, Iopromide, lotrolan
214. Legionella Pnuemophilis IF kits
215. Muromonab-CD3
216. Octreotide
217. Typhoid Vaccines : (i) VI Antigen of Salmonella Typhi, and (ii) Ty 21a cells and attenuated non-pathogenic strains of S.Typhi

218. (a) Rabbit brains thromboplastin for PT test; (b) Reagent for PT tests; (c) Human Thrombin for TT tests
219. Pnuemocystis carinij IF Kits
220. Puenoxytelzamins
221. Rabies immunoglobulin of equine origin
222. Thrombokinase
223. Teniposide
224. Vidarabine
225. Iscador, CLIA Diagnostic kits
226. Lamivudine
227. Zalcitabine
228. Saquinavir
229. Zidovudine
230. Ritonavir
231. Amifostine
232. Gemcitabine
233. Goserlin Acetate
234. Teicoplanin
235. Recuronium Bromide
236. Abeciximab
237. Disodium Pamidronate
238. Savoflurane
239. Ticarcillin Disodium and Potassium Clavulante combination
240. Trans 1-Diamino cyclohexane Oxalatoplatinum
241. Letrozole
242. Irinotecan
243. Leuprolide Acetate
244. Fludarabine Phosphate
245. Lenograstim
246. Tretinoin
247. Enoxaparin
248. Eptifibatide
249. Mycophenolate Mofetil
250. Prostaglandin E1 (PGE1)
251. Natural Micronised Progesterone
252. Latanoprost
253. Riluzole
254. Cefpirom

Appendix B

Most of these combinations are not approved by the Drugs Controller General, India and hence illegal or not recommended.

1. Alprazolam + Sertraline
2. Alprazolam + Imipramine
3. Alprazolam + Fluoexetine
4. Alprazolam + Melatonin
5. Imipramine + Diazepam
6. Risperidone + Trihexyphenidyl
7. Norfloxacin + Tinidazole
8. Norfloxacin + Tinidazole + Dicyclomine
9. Norfloxacin + Tinidazole + Loperamide
10. Norfloxacin + Metronidazole
11. Norfloxacin + Ornidazole
12. Ciprofloxacin + Tinidazole
13. Ciprofloxacin + Metronidazole
14. Ofloxacin + Tinidazole
15. Ofloxacin + Metronidazole
16. Ofloxacin + Ornidazole
17. Fluconazole + Tinidazole
18. Doxycycline + Tinidazole
19. Tetracycline + Metronidazole
20. Mefenamic Acid + Drotaverine
21. Nimesulide + Paracetamol
22. Nimesulide + Diclofenac
23. Nimesulide + Dicyclomine
24. Nimesulide + Chlorzoxazone
25. Nimesulide + Methocarbamol
26. Nimesulide + Camylofin
27. Nimesulide + Serratiopeptidase
28. Nimesulide + Tizanidine
29. Nimesulide + Paracetamol + Chlorzoxazone
30. Nimesulide + Tizanidine + Paracetamol
31. Rofecoxib + Tizanidine
32. Ibuprofen + Tizanidine
33. Diclofenac + Tizanidine
34. Diclofenac + Famotidine
35. Diclofenac + Paracetamol + Tizanidine
36. Diclofenac + Serratiopeptidase

37. Diclofenac + Paracetamol + Serratiopeptidase
38. Ibuprofen + Paracetamol + Magnesium Trisilicate
39. Ranitidine + Dicyclomine
40. Sucralfate + Oxethazine
41. Cisapride + Simethicone
42. Cisapride + Omeprazole
43. Mosapride + Methylpolysiloxane
44. Magaldrate + Simethicone + Oxethazine + Dicyclomine
45. Diazepam + Dried Alum. Hydrox. Gel + Alum. Glycinate + Oxyphenonium
46. Diazepam + Dried Alum. Hydrox. Gel + Mag. Trisilicate + Dimethylpolysiloxane
47. Diazepam + Magaldrate + Oxyphenonium
48. Diazepam + Propantheline + Dihydroxy. Alum.
49. Amoxycillin + Serratiopeptidase
50. Pipenzolate + Phenobarbitone
51. Amoxycillin + Probenecid + Tinidazole
52. Cefuroxime + Serratiopeptidase
53. Roxithromycin + Ambroxol
54. Ciprofloxacin + Ambroxol
55. Cefoperazone + Sulbactum
56. Ramipril + Losartan
57. Amlodipine + Lisinopril
58. Amlodipine + Enalapril
59. Amlodipine + Ramipril
60. Amlodipine + Losartan
61. Atenolol + Alprazolam
62. Propranolol + Alprazolam
63. Propranolol + Diazepam
64. Cinnarizine + Domperidone
65. Domperidone + Ranitidine
66. Domperidone + Omeprazole
67. Domperidone + Famotidine
68. Mebendazole + Pyrantel
69. Mebendazole + Levamisole
70. Simvastatin + Nicotinic Acid
71. Cetirizine + Paracetamol + Phenylpropanolamin

Fixed Dose Combinations and Rational Drug Therapy

The list of combination drugs recommended by the WHO

S.No.	Combination	Concentration	Dosage Form
1.	Neomycin + Bacitracin	5 mg + 500 IU	Ointment
2.	Amoxicillin + Clavulanic acid	500 mg + 125 mg	Tablet
3.	Imipenem + Cilastatin	250 mg + 250 mg	Injection
4.	Sulfamethoxazole + Trimethoprim	100 mg + 20 mg 400 mg + 80 mg	Tablet

Contd...

S.No.	Combination	Concentration	Dosage Form
5.	Sulfamethoxazole + Trimethoprim	80 mg + 16 mg/ml (in 5 ml ampule)	Injection
6.	Isoniazid + Ethambutol	150 mg + 400 mg	Tablet
7.	Rifampicin + Isoniazid	150 mg + 75 mg 300 mg + 150 mg	Tablet
8.	Rifampicin + Isoniazid + Pyrazinamide	150 mg + 75 mg + 400 mg	Tablet
9.	Thiacetazone + Isoniazid	50-150 mg + 100-300 mg	Tablet
10.	Benzoic acid + Salicylic acid	6% + 3% (w/w)	Ointment
11.	Ethinylestradiol + Levonorgestrel	30 µg + 150 µg	Tablet
12.	Ethinylestradiol + Levonorgestrel	50 µg + 250 µg (Pack of four)	Tablet
13.	Ethinylestradiol + Norethisterone	35 µg + 1 mg	Tablet
14.	Levodopa + Carbidopa	100 mg + 10 mg 250 mg + 25 mg	Tablet
15.	Ferrous salt + Folic acid	60 mg + 400 µg	Tablet
16.	Sulfadoxine + Pyrimethamine	500 mg + 25 mg	Tablet
17.	Lidocaine + Epinephrine	1 or 2% + 1:200,000	Injection
18.	Oral Rehydration Salts Sodium chloride Trisodium citrate dihydrate Potassium chloride Glucose	 3.5 g/L 2.9 g/L 1.5 g/L 20.0 g/L	Powder

Appendix C

Important Websites

Important Search Engines

Web Address	Engine Name
www.altavista.com	Alta vista
www.lycos.com	Lycos
www.yahoo.com	Yahoo
www.excite.com	Excite
www.google.com	Google
www.infoseekguide.com	Infoseekguide
www.msn.com	Microsoft

Pharmaceutical Associations

Web Address	Particulars
www.pharmweb.net	Pharmacy Institutions
www.nim.nih.gov	National Library of Medicine
www.who.ch	World Health Organization
www.acs.org	American Chemical Society
www.pharmainfo.com	Pharmaceutical Info-net works
www.pharmabiz.com	Pharmaceutical Industry Information
www.kar.nic.in	Rajeev Gandhi University of Health Sciences
	International Pharmaceutical Federation (FIP)
www.pharmaweb.net	Pharmaceutical Companies
www.nppainindia.com	National Pharmaceutical Prizing Authority India
www.cpv.uoknsc.edu	Virtual Pharmacy Libraries
www.rpsgv.org	Royal Pharmaceutical Societies

Web Address	Particulars
www.npa.co.uk	National Pharmaceutical Association (NPA)
www.ama.org	American Medical Association
www.fda.gov	Food and Drug Administration USA
www.eudra.org	European Medicines Evaluation Agencies
www.mcc.ac.uk	International Federation of Pharmaceutical Manufacturers
www.pitt.edu	American College of Clinical Pharmacy
www.niper.nic.in	National Institute of Pharmaceutical Education and Research (NIPER)
www.bath.ac.uk	Pharmacy Consortium for computer added learning
www.mcc.ac.uk	Pharmaceutical Meetings
www.abpi.org.uk	Association of British Pharmaceutical Industries
www.pharma.onweb.com	Indian Formulation Units

Journals

Important Organizations of Pharmacy

Web address	Site	Particulars
ww.aaps.org	AAPS	Detail information of American Association of Pharmaceutical Sciences
www.who.int	Action Programme on essential drugs	Information world health organization program supporting and co-ordinating comprehensive national policies
www.accp.org	American college of clinical pharmacy	Information of clinical pharmacy and research in American colleges
www.aacp.org	American association of colleges of pharmacy	Detail of American bodies, pharmaceutical information and a software library
www.ualberta.ca	CSPS	Canadian Society for pharmaceutical Sciences, provides research, journals and also some useful links of pharmaceutical sciences
www.cdnpharm.ca	Canadian Pharmaceutical Association	Canadian Professional Organisation site, providing publication, news and benefits to pharmacist.
www.compassnet.com	Compounding Pharmacists	International academy of compounding pharmacist
www.crsadmhadq.org	Controlled Release Society	Provide advancement of sciences and technology of drug delivery systems

Contd…..

Web address	Site	Particulars
www.fda.gov	Food and Drug Administration	Links with other sites, news, publications and research report
www.netlink.co.uk	Guild of Hospital Pharmacists	Information of part of manufacturing science and finance union
www.npa.co.uk	National Pharmaceutical Association	Organisation of Britain's Community and retail Pharmacist.
www.psa.org.au	Pharmaceutical Society of Australia	Organisation detail and activities in the field of pharmacy in India
www.earnet.in	All India Council for technical Education	All Technical course detail and different types of scholarships and grants
www.pci.org	Pharmacy Council of India	Pharmacy Council of India, list of PCI approved college, Standard Inspection form and schedule and detail of council
www.escp.nl	European Society of clinical Pharmacy	
www.ismp.org	Institute of safe Medication Practices	Information regarding medication errors and safety issues
www.rpsgb.org.uk	Royal Pharmaceutical Society of Great Britain	
www.aadmc.org	Allergy and Asthma Disease Management Centre	It provides detail of allergy and management of asthma
www.allergy.org.au	Australian Society of Clinical Immunology and Allergy	Information regarding allergy and web address of different sites
www.njc.org	National Jewish Medical and Research Centre	Provide information to pharmacist and doctors
www.menopause.org	North American Menopause Society	Comprehensive site that includes information aimed at consumers and health professionals
www.healthwomen.org	National Women's Health Resource Centre	Main aim of this site to provide knowledge to public

Appendix D

Schedule N

List of minimum equipment for the efficient running of a Pharmacy : -

(i)   **Entrance :** The front of a pharmacy shall bear an inscription "Pharmacy" in front.

(ii)   **Premises :** The premises of a pharmacy shall be separated from rooms for private use. The premises shall be well built, dry, well lit and ventilated and of sufficient dimension. To allow the good in stock specially medicament and poisons to be kept in a clearly visible and appropriate manner. The area of the section to be used as dispensing department shall be not less than 6 square meters for one pharmacist working there in with additional to square meters for each additional pharmacist. The height of the premises shall be atleast 2.5 meters.

The floor of the pharmacy shall be smooth and washable. The walls shall be plastered or tiled or oil painted so as to maintain smooth, durable and washable surface devoid of holes and cracks and crevices.

A pharmacy shall be provided with ample supply of good quality water.

The dispensing department shall be separated by a barrier to prevent the admission of the public.

(iii)   **Furniture and apparatus :** The furniture and apparatus of a pharmacy shall be adapted to the uses for which they are intended and correspond to the size and requirements of the establishment.

Drugs, chemicals and medicaments shall be kept in a room appropriate to their properties and in such special containers as will prevent any deterioration of the contents of contents of containers kept near them. Drawers, glasses and other containers used for keeping medicaments shall be of suitable size and capable of being closed tightly to prevent the entry of dust.

Every containers shall bear a label of appropriate size, easily readable with names of medicaments as given in the pharmacopoeias.

A pharmacy shall be provided with a dispensing bench, the top of which shall be covered with washable and impervious material like stainless steel, laminated or plastic, etc. A pharmacy shall be provided with a cupboard with lock and key for the storage of poisons and shall be clearly marked with the worked 'poison' in red letters on a white background.

Containers of all concentrated solutions shall bear special label or marked with the works "To be diluted"

A Pharmacy shall be provided with the following minimum apparatus and books necessary for making of official preparations and prescriptions :-

Apparatus

- Balance, dispensing, sensitivity 30 mg
- Balance, counter, capacity 3 Kg, sensitivity 1 gm.
- Beakers, lipped, assorted sizes
- Bottles, prescription, undergraduated, assorted sizes
- Cork assorted sizes and tapers.
- Cork, extractor
- Evaporating dishes, porcelain
- Filter paper
- Funnels and glass
- Litmus paper blue and red
- Measure glasses cylindrical 10 ml, 25 ml, 100 ml and 500 ml
- Mortars and pestles, glass
- Mortars and pestles, Wedgwood
- Ointment pots with bakelite or suitable caps
- Ointment slab, porcelain
- Pipettes, graduated, 2 ml, 5 ml and 10 ml
- Ring, stand(retort) iron, complete with rings
- Rubbers stamps and pad
- Scissors
- Spatulas, rubber or vulcanite
- Spatulas, stainless steel
- Spirit lamp
- Glass stirring rods
- Thermometers $0°$ to $200\ °C$
- Tripod stand
- Watch glasses
- Water Bath
- Water distillation still in case eye drops and eye lotions are prepared
- Weights, Metric, 1 mg to 100 gm

- Wire guaze
- *Pill finisher, boxwood
- *Pill machine
- *Pill Boxes
- *Suppositories mould

Books

- The Indian Pharmacopoeia (Current edition)
- National Formulary of India
- The drug and cosmetics Act 1940
- The drugs and Cosmetics Rules, 1945 The Pharmacy Act, 1948
- The Dangerous Drugs Act, 1930

General Provisions : A pharmacy shall be conducted under the continuous personal supervision of a registered pharmacist whose name shall be displayed conspicuously in the premises.

The shall always put on clean white overalls.

The premises and fittings of the pharmacy shall be properly kept and everything shall be in good order and clean.

All records and registers shall be maintained in accordance with the laws in force. Any containers taking from the poison cupboard shall be replaced their in immediately after use and the cupboard locked. The keys of the poison cupboard shall be kept in the personal custody of the responsible person.

Medicament when supplied shall have labels conforming to the provisions of laws in force.

Note : The above requirements are subject to modifications at the discretion of the licensing authority, if he is of opinion that having regard to the nature of the drugs dispensed, compounded or prepared by the licensee. It is necessary to relax the above requirements or to impose additional requirement in the circumstances of a particular e case. The decision of the licensing authority in that regard shall be final.

* These items are to be provided only by those who intend to dispense pills or suppositories, as the case may be.

Index

A

Absorption and adsorption 28

Absorption bases 222

Academics 6

Addition 73, 168, 284, 293

Adjustment of ph, stabilization and preservation 253

Adjustment of tonicity and specific gravity 271

Adverse drug reaction 120, 289

Aerosols 132, 293

Aim of packaging and labelling 32

Air distribution 257

Air-conditioned atmosphere 256

Alligation 58, 59

Aluminium 36, 188

Ampoule 29, 266

Analysis and testing 7

Antagonism 73, 302

Antimicrobial agents 214, 270

Antioxidants 270

Apothecaries' weights and measures 42

Applications 9, 36

Asbestos 26

Aseptic 254, 256, 266, 272, 274

Aseptic technique 274

Avoirdupois weights and measures 42

B

Bacteriostatic water for injection (bwfi) 269

Bastedo's formula 76

Binders and adhesive 146

Bioavailability of Proprietary Preparations 319

Bolus 141

Bottle method 213

Bougies 242

Bubble wrap 33, 36

Buccal and sublingual tablets 150

Bulk powders for external use 132

C

Cachets 9, 135

Calculation in powder dispensing 128

Calculation of dose 74

Capsules 9, 160-164

Career scope for pharmacy professionals 5

Chemical incompatibility 286

Chewable tablets 150

Clark's formula 77
Classification of dosage form 8
Classification of douches 184
Classification of powders 131
Classification of suppositories bases 243
Classification of suspensions 197
Classification of tablets 145
Clean 248, 257, 266
Cleaning and sterilization of rubber closures 277
Cleaning and sterilization of vials 277
Cleaning of air 257
Closures 36, 38, 271
Coating and polishing 153
Cobalt chloride test 216
Cognitive component 14
Colation 27
Cold 31, 209, 245
Cold compression 243, 245
Collodions 183
Coloring agent 147, 176
Common Design of Drug Stores 296
Common polymers and their typical uses 35
Community pharmacy 5, 292
Comparison of flocculated and
    deflocculated suspension 197
Compounding, labelling and packaging 109, 111
Compressed tablets 147
Compression coating 157
Compression mould suppositories 245
Conductivity test 216
Consultancy 7
Contraindicated drugs 290
Cool 31, 180, 277
Copolymers 35

Cotton filters 26
Cowling's formula 76
Cracking or coalescence 216
Creaming 217
Creams 9, 223, 234, 235

D

Dental powders 133
Depot 197
Design of an aseptic laboratory 256
Determination of capsule fill weight 161
Dilling's formula 75
Diluents 146
Dilution of creams 234
Dilution of linctuses 176
Dilution of lotions 177
Dilution test 215
Direct compression 148
Disadvantages of powder 125
Disintegrants 146, 150
Disintegration 141, 151, 160, 163
Dispensing of proprietaries 292
Dispensing of suspensions 198
Dispensing procedures 14
Dissolution 21, 152, 163
Douche powders 132
Douches 184
Draughts 9
Drugs and Cosmetics Act 292
Drug inspector 6
Drug interaction 298
Dry granulation 148
Dry gum method 213
Dry heat sterilization 274
Dusting powders 132, 141

Dye solubility test 216

E

Ear drops 188, 189
Effervescent granules 131, 134
Effervescent tablets 149
Efflorescent substances 137, 139
Elixirs 9, 170, 171
Emulsifying agents 210, 211, 270
Emulsifying cream 235
Emulsion 9, 205, 206-210, 214, 216, 223
Emulsion bases 223
Emulsion types 206
Enemas 9, 185, 210
Enteric coating 157
Equipment in small scale 23
Essential Commodities Act 292
Evaluation of capsules 163
Evaluation of emulsions 214
Excessive heat 31
External 10, 124, 132, 166, 178, 184, 192, 209
External emulsions 209
External liquid preparations 166, 177, 184, 192
Eye drops 259
Eye lotions 261
Eye ointments 261

F

Factors affecting selection of
    packaing materials 32
Factors affecting the dose and
    action of drugs 72
Film coating 155
Film defects 156
Filter paper 25
Filtering media 25

Filtration 25, 26
Filtration equipment 26
Filtration through bacteria proof filters 274
Flavoring agent 147, 176
Fluorescence test 216
Formulation of solution 174
Freezing point method 62
Friability 151
Fried's formula 76
Fusion 228, 246
Future of dispensing pharmacy 305

G

Gargles 9, 192
Gels 9
Glass wool 126
Glidants 146
Granules 9

H

Hand homogenizer 25
Hand mould suppositories 245
Hard gelatin capsules 160
Hardness 151
Health care team 292
Hermetically sealed container 30
Higher education 6
Homogenization 24
Hompolymers 34
Hospital pharmacy 5
Household measures 43
How to use ear drops 187
How to use eye drops 260
Hygroscopic and deliquescent substances 137
Hypodermic tablets 151

I

Ideal ointment base 221

Ideal suppository base 242

Ideal suspension 195

Idiosyncracy 74

Imperial system 42

Important Terms 314

Implants 13

Incompatibility 282, 286

Infusion 56, 266

Inhalations 10, 191

Injection 12, 276, 281

Instability of emulsion 216

Insufflation 132

Insufflations 10, 133

Internal 72, 133

Internal liquid preparations 16

Internet 19

Intrauterine devices 13

Ion exchange resin systems 13

Irrigations 10

Isotonic solution v-values 63

Isotonic solutions 62, 253

J

Jellies 10, 237

Journalism 7

Journals 17

L

Labelling 32, 111, 112, 178, 180, 228

Large scale equipment 23

Large volume parenteral (lvp) 26

Latin terms commonly used in prescription 104

Legal provisions 115

Legal Requirements for Establishment of Drug Stores 298

Levigation 23, 128

Light-resistant container 30

Liniments 10, 179

Liposomes 11

Liquid dosage forms 16

Lotions 10, 177, 161

Lozenge tablets 149

Lozenges 143

Lubricants 146

M

Maintenance of record Wholesale and Retail drug stores 308

Marketing 7, 32

Measures of capacity 41, 42

Measures of length 41

Measures of mass 40, 42

Measuring 20

Medicated elixirs 170

Medication errors 119, 122

Membrane filters 26

Metals 36, 38

Method based on body surface : 77

Method based on weight of the child 77

Methods for calculating isotonicity 62

Metric system 40

Metrology 39

Microcapsules 121

Mixing 24, 126

Mixtures 286, 288

Moist heat sterilization 274

Molecular weight method 65

Monoclonal antibodies 12

Mortar and pestle 227

Mould lubricant 248

Mouth washes 10

Multiple dose container 31

Multiple emulsions 207

Multiple unit container 31

Multiple-dose vial 26

N

Nanoparticles 12

Nasal bougies 242

Nasal drops 10, 190

Nasal drug delivery systems 13

Nasal sprays 190

Negative mixtures 24

Neutral mixtures 24

New drug delivery systems 11

Non-medicated elixir 170

Nosocomial 26

Nostrums 295

Novel drug delivery system 7

O

Official books 16

Oil-in-water (o/w) emulsion 206

Ointment bases 221

Ointment jars 228

Ointment mill 227

Ointment slab 227

Ointment tubes 228

Ointments 10, 220, 227

Operational aspects 19

Ophthalmic 23, 36, 229, 258

Ophthalmic ointments 220, 229

Ophthalmic preparations 252

Ophthalmic products 252

Oral emulsions 208

Organoleptic properties 151, 214

Organisation and structure of retail and wholesale drug store 293

Osmotic pumps 12

Over proof 50

P

Packaging 29, 32, 33, 228

Paints 11, 181

Paper 26, 33, 129

Parenterals 266, 275

Pastes 10, 237

Pastilles 142

Patient Counseling 308

Percentage of solid in liquid 47

Percentage solution 47

Pessaries 10, 242

Pharmaceutical calculation 39

Pharmaceutical profession and ethics 1

Phase inversion 217

Physical incompatibility 28

Pills 10, 140

Plasters 239

Plastic /polymer 33

Polymer characterization 34

Positive mixtures 24

Posology 72

Poultices 239

Powder parenterals 275

Powder rapping in papers 131

Powders 10, 124, 131

Precautions for aseptic work 317

Preparation of ointments 227

Preparation of suppositories 245

Prescription 3, 15, 101, 104

Prescription processing 15

Preservatives for ophthalmic preparations 255

Primary packaging component 29

Principle of size reduction 23

Production 6

Proof spirit 50

Properties of ointment bases 226

Protection from heat 122, 128

Pulverization by intervention 153

Purpose of coating 153

Purpose of emulsion 206

Purpose of suspension 196

Pyrogen 26

R

Reading and checking the prescription 109, 110

Receiving the prescription 109, 110

Rectal emulsions 210

Rectal ointments 230

Rectal suppositories 242

Reducing and enlarging recipes 52

Reference books 16

Regulatory affairs 7

Role of Pharmacist in Health care and
     Education 311

Renewal of Licence 300

Resealed erythrocytes 12

Research 7

Retail Sale of Drugs 302

Room temperature 31

Routes of administration 73, 197

Rubber 35

S

Safety cover 38

Scope abroad 7

Scope for diploma students 5

Scope for pharmacy graduates 5

Secondary packaging component 29

Sedimentation and decantation 27

Semisolid preparations 29

Sifting 127

Silverson mixer-homogenizer 25

Site Selection 294

Single dose container 31, 260

Single unit container 30

Sintered glass filters 26

Siphoning 27

Size reduction 23

Size separation 24

Small volume parenteral (svp) 26

Snuffs 132

Soap method 214

Sodium chloride equivalent method 66

Sodium chloride equivalents 66

Soft gelatin capsules 164

Solid dosage forms 11, 108

Solubilization 21

Soluble tablets 149

Solution 11, 47

Solutions 26, 62

Sources of information 16

Spatulation 127

Special powders 136

Spirits 176
Sprays 11, 190
Sterilization 254, 259, 273, 274
Storage of Drugs 308
Storage under non-specific conditions 31
Subscription 102
Sugar coating 154
Superscription 102
Supply of Schedule C and C_1 Drugs 306
Supply of Schedule H and X Drugs 306
Suppositories 11, 24, 243, 245
Surfactants 211
Suspending agents 199, 286
Suspension 195
Suspensions 197, 198, 201
Suspensions containing diffusible solids 198
Suspensions containing indiffusible solids 198
Synergism 73
Synergistic or antagonistic drugs 290
Syrups 11, 16

T

Tablet defects 152
Tablet triturate 8, 146
Tablets 11, 144, 145, 147
Tamper-evident container 31
Temperature 28, 31, 217
Tests for identification of emulsion type 215
The aseptic room 256
Therapeutic incompatibility 289
Throat paints 181
Tightly-closed container 30
Tolerance 73
Tonicity contributors 270

Transcription or signatura 102
Transdermal drug delivery systems 13
Trituration 22, 126
Tumbling 127
Types of mixtures 24
Types of Drug Store and Design 294

U

Under proof 50
Unit dose container 31
Urethral suppositories 242
Use of equivalents 43
Using aseptic techniques 274

V

Vaginal suppositories 242
Vaginal tablets 149, 150
Viscosity of the eye medication 254
Volatile substances 137
Volume of injection 276

W

Warm 31
Water for injection (wfi) 277
Water in oil (w/o) emulsions 201
Water-soluble bases 224
Weighing 10
Weight variations 151, 163
Well-closed container 30
Wet granulation 147
Wet gum method 213
Wrapping 128, 129

Y

Young's formula 75

www.ingramcontent.com/pod-product-compliance
Lightning Source LLC
LaVergne TN
LVHW081722210726
843527LV00005B/281